The Health Professional's Guide to
Food Allergies and Intolerances

Janice Vickerstaff Joneja, PhD, RD

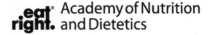
eat right. Academy of Nutrition and Dietetics

Diana Faulhaber, Publisher
Laura Pelehach, Acquisitions and Development Manager
Elizabeth Nishiura, Production Manager

10 9 8 7 6 5 4 3

ISBN 978-0-88091-453-6

Contents

Also Available from the Academy of Nutrition and Dietetics

Visit the Academy's online store (www.eatright.org/shop) to purchase a related package of downloadable client education materials, *Food Allergies and Intolerances: Client Education Tools for Dietary Management,* also by Janice Vickerstaff Joneja (available in 2013).

Acknowledgments

A book such as this depends on the painstaking work of many dedicated researchers and their meticulously scrutinized reports in peer-reviewed publications. By citing their work in the extensive bibliographies in each chapter, I gratefully acknowledge their expertise and contribution to the growing body of knowledge on adverse reactions to foods.

I am also grateful to all my colleagues in various branches of science and dietetics, to my many students, and to the clients and patients I have known during my more than 35 years of conducting research, teaching, and clinical practice. Each one has provided valuable information, insight, perspective, support, and stimulus to enable me to further my knowledge and proficiency. In return, I hope this book will help them in their own work in this field.

I especially wish to thank Laura Pelehach, acquisitions and development manager, Academy of Nutrition and Dietetics, who urged me to write this book. She has acted as my editor, critic, and supporter throughout the process of its development. I am convinced that without her continued encouragement and editorial expertise, this book would not have been completed.

Thank you as well to the reviewers of the manuscript: Wendy Busse, MSc, RD; Louise Goldberg, RD, CSP, CNSC; Kathy S. Kendall, MS, RD; Emily McCloud, MS, RD; Monique Ryan, MS, RD, CSSD, HFS; Mary K. Sharrett, MS, RD, CNSD; and Diana Sugiuchi, RD, CNSD, ACSM-HFS.

This book is dedicated to Katelyn Eve and Michael Edward Joneja.

—Janice Joneja

Preface

In 1990, when my first book on the immunology of allergy was published,[1] I was unable to find a dietitian to help me with a chapter on food allergy. I felt quite competent and comfortable with the science of allergy, having studied the subject since my postgraduate years in science. However, the science of food allergy, in contrast to the immunological processes involved in respiratory allergy, was still in its infancy. In fact, there was outright denial by many practitioners that food allergy even existed.

Having realized the tremendous need for information on all aspects of food allergy, I returned to the university where I had earlier held a faculty position as an assistant professor in medical microbiology. There, I took all the courses and the subsequent internship that qualified me to become a registered dietitian (RD). I wanted an opportunity to apply the science of allergy to the practical management of adverse reactions to foods. In my years of practice and research in food allergy since then, I have witnessed an amazing change both in the approach to food allergy and in the quality of science in the field. Whereas previously the field tended to be avoided by "traditional" clinicians and scientists because of the lack of good evidence-based research, as an increasing number of highly reputable practitioners entered the field, the science and practice of food allergy moved into the mainstream. Now, more than 20 years later, all new editions of every journal on allergy and clinical immunology from countries around the world seem to carry reports of innovative research on some aspect of food allergy.

Even the definition of allergy has changed over the same period of time. Previously, the definition of food allergy was reserved for IgE-mediated reactions (referred to as *type 1 hypersensitivity*); now the designation encompasses any immunologically mediated reaction to food that results in an adverse effect.

While the consequence of all this research activity is a greatly expanded and enhanced basis for the practice of food allergy, there is unfortunately the inevitable downside that results from any new field of interest in science and medicine: For every article reporting a positive outcome, there are two that report conflicting results. This is unsurprising, because parameters of practice in the application of science in food allergy have not yet been standardized. Furthermore, there is a great deal that we still need to discover regarding the precise immunological, biochemical, and physiological mechanisms responsible for the adverse reactions to foods that are being observed in clinical practice.

The greatest challenge that we face in food allergy management is the lack of any definitive laboratory tests that would identify the specific food responsible for the clinical signs and symptoms that result from its ingestion. This is not surprising because science shows us that there are many different ways in which foods can trigger an immunological or biochemical response in the body, so to expect that a single test would reveal the causative agent when we do not even understand the mechanisms responsible for the adverse reaction is completely unrealistic. Hopefully, this dilemma will be resolved as more evidence-based research and well-controlled large-scale clinical trials provide the information to fill the enormous gaps with which we are still striving to cope as we apply science to practice.

This book is designed as a practice-ready manual for dietitians and other health care professionals in the field of food sensitivity management. In 1995, the first of its kind (now out of print) was published.[2] The current manual is greatly expanded and updated from that early publication and incorporates the latest research and practice in the field, which has increased rapidly in the intervening years and continues to evolve. Because this is designed as a practical tool, the science and reports of clinical trials have been carefully chosen to provide the information required for the practitioner to understand the basics of each subject. Relevant references are provided in each chapter for readers who require further information. The Academy of Nutrition and Dietetics is also the publisher of the companion product *Food Allergies and Intolerances: Client Education Tools for Dietary Management* (available in 2013), which includes handouts for the practitioner to give to their patients and clients who must manage adverse reactions to foods.

References

1. Joneja JMV, Bielory L. *Understanding Allergy, Sensitivity and Immunity: A Comprehensive Guide*. New Brunswick, NJ: Rutgers University Press; 1990.
2. Joneja JMV. *Managing Food Allergy and Intolerance: A Practical Guide*. Vancouver, BC: McQuaid Consulting Group; 1995.

Introduction

Adverse reactions to food are arguably some of the most confusing and misunderstood conditions in medical practice. Physicians, registered dietitians, other health care professionals, and patients alike are often unsure about what symptoms are caused by food allergy, food intolerance, and other adverse reactions to foods, as well as the diverse methods of diagnosis and the best way to manage them.

There is a heightened interest in food allergies, but no clear consensus exists regarding their prevalence or the most effective diagnostic and management approaches to them. IgE-mediated food allergy is estimated to affect more than 1% to 2% but less than 10% of the population. Although the perception is that the incidence of food allergy is increasing, it is unclear whether this is a real increase or if it is due to a greater awareness of the condition and an escalation in the number and range of tests available for diagnosis.

The evidence for the prevalence and management of food allergy is significantly limited by a lack of uniformity for criteria for making a diagnosis.[1] Food allergy does not fit into the medical paradigm of "one cause, one disease," and the definitive tests required to confirm a diagnosis are not available. Consequently, constant questions and controversy surround definitions of each of the different ways in which the body responds to diverse components of foods.[2] Consensus documents and professional guidelines are published regularly as new evidence-based data dictate changes in clinical practice.[3] Furthermore, the definition of the most severe reaction to food, anaphylaxis, is also open to frequent debate.[4]

The greatest obstacle in understanding the problems involved in food sensitivity diagnosis, prevention, and management is the misconception that "food allergy" is a distinct disease. In medicine, the typical scenario is the appearance of specific symptoms, which are diagnosed as a disease by well-authenticated tests. Based on the diagnosis, the cause is understood and a specific treatment plan is put in place, which usually controls the disease. Unlike a specific medical disease, the food that causes food allergy in one person may not trigger the same symptoms in others who eat it; in fact, most people eating the food will have no adverse response at all.

Food does not cause allergy. The symptoms are caused by the allergic person's unique response to the food, not by the food itself. Furthermore, to complicate the situation, many adverse reactions to foods are not caused by an allergic reaction, but by *food intolerances*. Food intolerance reactions are quite different from food allergy both in the way the body responds to the food and the management of the condition. The term *food sensitivity* describes when eating a food results in distressing symptoms. This term covers both food allergy and food intolerances. Both of these topics will be covered more fully in the first section of this book.

Food Allergy

The term *food allergy* is reserved for an immune system response that is triggered when a food is eaten by a person who has been sensitized to it. The key event in food allergy is recognition of the food by components of the immune system, which cause the release of chemicals (inflammatory mediators) that act on body tissues and result in a specific set of symptoms. In the 1960s, Professors Philip Gell and Robin Coombs[5] used the term *hypersensitivity reactions* for all immune system reactions that are not involved in protection against diseases caused by viruses, bacteria, and other threats to the body. They classified these reactions into four distinct types: type I, II, III, and IV. Such reactions include allergy. Therefore, another term for an allergic reaction is a *hypersensitivity reaction*, which often is used in medical texts in place of *allergy*.

However, with the broadening of the definition of allergy to encompass any immunological reaction to a component of food that results in symptoms, several diseases not previously considered as "allergies" are now included in this term. Previously, only reactions that resulted from production of IgE in response to consuming the food that elicited the initial reaction were defined as "allergies." Now many conditions that cause immunologically mediated reactions to foods but that do not involve IgE are included under the umbrella of "allergy." Consequently, tests designed to diagnose IgE-mediated reactions are of no value in these situations.

Under the current definitions, for convenience we may classify the different types of immunologically mediated reactions into the following broad categories:

- Reactions resulting from ingestion of food that elicits production of food-specific IgE. Anaphylactic reactions typify this type of response, but symptoms can occur in every organ system as a result of the release of inflammatory mediators from granulocytes, principally mast cells. Tests for food-specific IgE may determine the foods responsible in up to 50% of cases.
- Reactions that result from release of inflammatory mediators in response to IgE produced against nonfood material such as inhaled pollens or inhaled latex. In sensitive individuals, food antigens that are structurally identical to those of the pollen or latex respectively will result in symptoms. These are termed *oral allergy syndrome* (OAS) and *latex-food syndrome*, respectively. Tests for allergen-specific IgE will identify the pollen or latex, but usually not the food responsible for the reaction.
- Reactions that result from inflammatory mediators released from granulocytes such as eosinophils in the digestive tract, without any evidence that

antigen-specific antibody is involved. In these cases, foods are clearly involved in the reaction, but because the mechanism responsible for the infiltration of the areas by eosinophils is unknown, there are no tests that will reveal the identity of the foods involved.

■ Food protein enteropathies, such as milk protein enteropathy or soy protein enteropathy, where the mechanism of response has not been determined.

■ Food-associated diseases such a gluten-sensitive enteropathy (celiac disease) in which food is implicated as the trigger, but the IgA antibodies are produced against body tissues, not the food. Celiac disease is not usually considered to be an allergy; it is more correctly designated an autoimmune disease. However, because it involves an immunological response to a food component, it is often included under the umbrella of allergy for convenience.

Food Intolerances

In addition to the increasing list of immunologically mediated adverse reactions to foods, we have the diverse conditions loosely classified as food intolerances, which are considered to encompass any adverse reaction to a food or food additive that is not caused by an immune system response. This term covers a large number of different biochemical and physiological processes, many of which are poorly understood; therefore, very few definitive tests are available to effect a diagnosis. The subject of food intolerances is discussed in more detail in Chapter 3.

Sensitization and Tolerance in Food Allergy

One of the significant advances in the approach to food allergy prevention and management in recent years has resulted from the increased understanding about the mechanisms involved in the immunological response in food allergy. Our immune systems are designed to prevent disease from external agents such as viruses, bacteria, and toxins and from internal agents such as cancer cells by recognizing the "invader" as foreign to the body and mounting a powerful defense against it. All food is foreign to the body. It is derived from plants, fungi, fish, poultry, and animals unrelated to humans, yet in most cases such foreign material is absorbed and incorporated into the human body without difficulty.

In order for this to happen, a complex series of events takes place that suppresses the natural immunological rejection and results in a state we call *tolerance*. Immunological tolerance is achieved after an initial active response orchestrated by T helper cells, followed by suppression of the response by activation of suppressor cells (sometimes called *T regulatory cells* [T_{reg}]) and production of suppressive cytokines. In order for tolerance to food to occur, the immune cells must encounter food molecules in an environment that will promote the process of recognition, activation, and suppression.

This all takes place in the gut-associated lymphoid tissue (GALT) of the digestive tract; the process is called *oral tolerance*. In most cases we first encounter food early in life, often from our mother's breastmilk, which contains molecules of food from her diet. We then develop tolerance during the process of low-dose, continuous exposure that is optimal for the development of immunological tolerance. As we continue to encounter an increasing number of foods, develop early tolerance, and continue to eat the foods throughout life, such tolerance is maintained and allows us to eat all foods with impunity.

Food allergy presents a different immunological profile. Instead of developing immunological tolerance, the immune system in individuals with allergies mounts a nonprotective resistance, resulting in disease. This process is called *immunological* (or allergic) *sensitization*. Following sensitization, whenever the same food molecules are encountered, the immune system mounts an allergic defense and symptoms develop. This is designated *atopy* and the individual as *atopic*. (Details of this process are provided in Chapter 1.)

Previously it was thought that sensitization and the allergic response to food developed early in life as a result of exposure to foods during the period in which an infant's immune system was immature—predominantly the first year of life. It was argued that if the infant could be protected from encountering the highly allergenic foods during this early period, the more mature immune system of the 2-year-old or even 3-year-old would be better equipped to deal with the food components and thus avoid sensitization. However, after several years of parents being given strict directives to avoid exposing their children to highly allergenic foods such as peanuts, tree nuts, fish, shellfish, and other "high allergenicity" foods in the early months and even years, the enormous increase in allergic children in the population suggested that the approach was somehow not working.

Recent research now indicates that oral tolerance develops early in life and that there may be specific "windows of opportunity" in which exposure to allergenic foods leads to tolerance rather than sensitization. If these opportunities are bypassed as a result of avoiding the food, allergy may result. Exactly what the process of oral tolerance entails, the optimal circumstances in which it takes place, and the best time for exposing the infant to highly allergenic foods still remain to be determined. Nevertheless, current research indicates that early exposure in a "safe environment" rather than complete avoidance of the food is likely to promote tolerance and that, in fact, early avoidance may lead to later sensitization—a complete reversal of the teaching from learned societies just a few years ago (this topic is discussed in detail in Chapter 44).

In addition to early exposure of the potentially allergic infant to food as a measure to prevent food allergy, inducing tolerance by exposure to allergenic foods later in life is being increasingly explored in the management of established food allergy. Previously, anyone, especially a child, who was allergic to a food was instructed to strictly avoid the food as a measure to prevent symptoms, and, as a result of avoidance, to develop tolerance over time as their immune system became more mature. However, research studies are now indicating that exposure to the allergenic food in a "safe environment" using the "low-dose continuous exposure" criterion can result in tolerance. This is important research, as it may lead to greater safety for those individuals at risk of a life-threatening anaphylactic reaction to a food, and preclude a lifetime of fear and stress associated with eating. The topic of specific oral tolerance induction (SOTI) is discussed in Chapter 44.

Allergy, Microorganisms, and Probiotics

Another focus of recent research that may promote tolerance to foods is based on the concept that the microorganisms residing in the large intestine can strongly influence the immunological processes taking place in the area. Interactions of the resident microflora with the cells of the surrounding GALT, interactions of the members of the microflora with each other, and the results of the activity of the microorganisms on the materials available in the colon (such as undigested food materials) seem to impact the immunological responses involved in allergy. This topic is discussed in Chapter 47. This is a rapidly evolving field and promises interesting developments in food allergy prevention and management in the future.

Foods That Cause Food Sensitivity Reactions

Any food is capable of triggering allergy in a person sensitized to it. All foods contain molecules that can elicit a response of the immune system. However, for many reasons that include both the structure of the food molecules and peoples' immunological responses, the foods that cause the majority of allergic reactions tend to be few in number.

Food intolerances, which result from the body's inability to digest, absorb, or efficiently metabolize a food or a component of food, add another layer of complexity to the problems associated with adverse reactions to foods. In most cases of food intolerances, there are no tests available for their identification because the mechanisms responsible for the development of symptoms are incompletely understood.

Many attempts have been made to classify adverse reactions to foods, but because of the paucity of information regarding mechanisms in many cases, none are entirely satisfactory. A generalization of the types of reactions involved is represented in Figure 1.

Dietary Management of Adverse Reactions to Foods

Adverse reactions to foods and beverages can appear in many forms and can result in a confusing array of symptoms. Sometimes, the realization that a person's ill health is caused by their diet is reached only when all other causes have been ruled out, often after many and varied diagnostic tests. At other times, the culprit food is

FIGURE 1

Classification of Adverse Reactions to Foods According to the Pathogenic Mechanisms

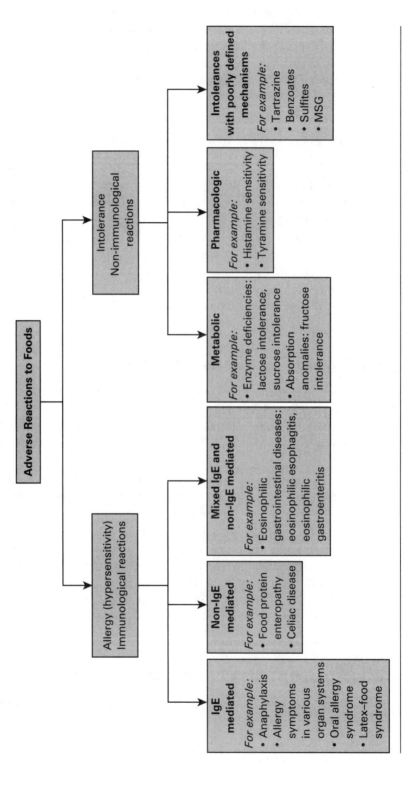

instantly recognized, especially when the result is an immediate, frightening, severe anaphylactic reaction.

The ultimate aim in managing and living with food sensitivity is detecting and eliminating the specific antagonistic foods and formulating a nutritionally sound diet to ensure optimum health. This is often a tedious, time-consuming process and requires a tremendous amount of knowledge, skill, commitment, and dedication on the part of both the food-sensitive individual and the clinician who is supervising his or her treatment.

However, when a person has been feeling chronically sick and then suddenly feels well for the first time in many years, as so often happens, the reward more than justifies the time and effort that have gone into the endeavor. The successful management of food sensitivity has four distinct phases:

- Accurate identification of the foods responsible for the symptoms, which ultimately will involve elimination of the suspect foods and challenge (reintroduction of the foods) to identify those that elicit symptoms on ingestion
- Provision of a diet that excludes all the offending foods and supplies complete balanced nutrition from alternative sources
- Recognition of the development of tolerance to the foods that have previously caused adverse reactions
- Regular consumption of the foods to ensure the maintenance of tolerance

Although people often look for the ideal "hypoallergenic diet," such a thing does not exist. What is "hypoallergenic" for one person could be life-threatening for another. Each person's inherited tendencies, previous medical history, lifestyle, and response to both food and nonfood factors (such as airborne and environmental allergens) will contribute to the way in which his or her body reacts to the "foreign" foods and chemicals that enter it.

This book is designed to provide the information and tools that are required to identify the specific foods, food additives, and other ingested materials that are responsible for a person's adverse reactions and to devise nutritionally adequate diets to ensure the best possible health of the food-sensitive individual.

The first part of the book explains exactly what "food allergy" and "food intolerance" mean in terms of how the food-sensitive person's body responds and copes with food, and what actually causes a person to react in a certain way. The subsequent sections provide detailed instructions for the application of this information in practice.

References

1. Chafen JJ, Newberry SJ, Riedl MA, et al. Diagnosing and managing common food allergies: a systematic review. *JAMA*. 2010;303(18):1848-1856.
2. Johansson SGO, Hourihane JOB, Bousquet J, et al. A revised nomenclature for allergy. An EAACI position statement from the EAACI nomenclature task force. *Allergy*. 2001;56: 813-824.

3. Boyce JA, Assa'ad A, Burks AW, et al. Guidelines for the diagnosis and management of food allergy in the United States: report of the NIAID-sponsored expert panel. *J Allergy Clin Immunol.* 2010;126(6):S1-S58.

4. Sampson HA, Munoz-Furlong A, Campbell RL, et al. Second Symposium on the Definition and Management of Anaphylaxis: Summary Report—Second National Institute of Allergy and Infectious Disease/Food Allergy and Anaphylaxis Network Symposium. *Ann Emerg Med.* 2006;47:373-380.

5. Gell PGH, Coombs RRA, eds. *Clinical Aspects of Immunology.* Oxford, UK: Blackwell; 1963:317-337.

PART I

Food Allergies and Intolerances: Scientific Background

CHAPTER 1

Food Allergy: The Science

Food allergy does not readily fit into the medical paradigm of "one cause, one disease," and it lacks the definitive tests required to confirm a cause. Consequently, the appropriate treatment or management strategy is often difficult to determine. Many components of foods are capable of triggering an immunological response, and the reactions and their results (symptoms) vary among individuals. Therefore, constant questions and controversy surround definitions of food allergy and the various immunological responses to food components that result in symptoms.[1,2] Furthermore, the definition of the most severe reaction to food, anaphylaxis, is also open to frequent debate.[3] This chapter will detail the processes involved in the immunological response to foods that result in the adverse reactions we loosely term *allergy*.

The Simple Explanation of Food Allergy

Food allergy is an inappropriate response of the immune system that results in symptoms. Our immune systems fight disease by recognizing a "foreign invader" when it enters the body and releasing a battery of defensive chemicals (called *inflammatory mediators*) into local tissues and into circulation to defend us from the threat. All the food we eat comes from foreign sources—plants, animals, birds, fish, and fungi—that we consume as nourishment. Normally, our immune systems see this material as "foreign but safe" due to a complex process of tolerance that occurs when food is processed through the digestive system. When something goes wrong in this processing, a person becomes "sensitized" to the food and thereafter the immune system perceives it as foreign and a threat. Whenever the food enters the body again, the immune system treats it as if it could cause disease. The symptoms that we experience from this defensive action are called *allergy* or *atopy*.

The Simple Explanation of Food Intolerance

Unlike allergy, food intolerance does not involve an immune system response. Most intolerance reactions that we understand (and there are many that we do not) involve a defect in the processing of the food, either during digestion or later, after the food constituents have been absorbed into the body. The symptoms are often caused by an excess of a component that has not been digested completely (eg, lactose intolerance) or cannot be processed efficiently after it has entered the body.

Whatever process is involved in an adverse reaction to food, a critical factor in effectively managing the condition is understanding the physiological mechanisms contributing to the development of symptoms. Such understanding will lead to the development of interventions that can relieve the person's distress. This chapter deals with the immunological processes involved in food allergy. Later chapters deal with the mechanisms implicated in other adverse reactions to foods.

The Science of Allergy

The symptoms of an allergic reaction are caused by biologically active chemicals that the immune system produces in its attempt to protect the body from a foreign invader. Usually this invader is a microorganism, such as a virus, bacterium, or other pathogen, or perhaps cancer cells that arise within the body. However, the immune system of an allergic (atopic) person attempts to protect the body not only from potential pathogens, but also from harmless substances such as pollens, animal dander, dust mites, mold spores, and food. The question that has always puzzled clinicians and scientists is, "What causes the immune system of one individual to fight a harmless substance, while another's system recognizes the same materials as innocuous?" Although we do not know the entire answer to that question, research is starting to reveal parts of the puzzle. The difference lies at the beginning of the process of recognizing what is safe and what may harm the body.

Unless it is overtly poisonous or contains toxins from external agents such as microorganisms, food itself is incapable of causing disease in the way that viruses, bacteria, and cancer cells can. It is the body's response to components of the food that results in the symptoms we call *food allergy*, *food intolerance*, *food sensitivity*, or *adverse reactions to foods*. The reason that one person's body develops distressing symptoms and another's body uses the same food for comfort and nurture is due to several factors, including:

- Inherited genetic predisposition
- The circumstances under which the food was first encountered
- The microorganisms that colonize the digestive tract
- The medications that have been taken by mouth
- Other factors that we are only just beginning to understand

Moreover, food sensitivity is unlike any other disease entity in that it has many different causes, because *any* food is capable of triggering allergy in a person who has been sensitized to it or who lacks the systems required to process it adequately when it enters the body. The same food may be absolutely safe for others.

Furthermore, food allergy can result in many different symptoms in diverse organ systems. For example, people can develop symptoms in the skin, such as eczema or hives; in the digestive tract, such as stomachache, diarrhea, nausea, or vomiting; in the lungs, such as asthma; in the upper respiratory tract, such as a stuffy, runny nose or earache; or in all body systems at the same time (anaphylaxis), which sometimes results in death. All this may occur as a result of eating the *same* food. Each person with allergies differs in the way his or her immune system responds to certain foods.

The usual medical model of disease that a physician traditionally follows (the medical paradigm) has several distinct steps that lead from symptoms to therapy:

■ The symptoms ("presentation") suggest several possibilities as to their cause.
■ Tests that will lead to a diagnosis are carried out.
■ The diagnosis arrived at, as a result of the tests, determines the treatment.
■ Treatment typically consists of medications, or perhaps surgical intervention.
■ As a result of treatment (therapy), the symptoms are alleviated.

This protocol works well for conditions that are caused by a single entity such as a bacterium, virus, cancer, injury, or other agent that harms the body. It does not work well for food allergy where there are many different agents responsible for triggering an immune system response, which results in a diverse array of symptoms that differ from person to person, and even within the same person from time to time.

Because several different processes can occur when body systems deal with the diverse chemicals that make up a food, it would be unrealistic to expect that the food responsible for triggering the body's adverse reaction could be identified by any single laboratory test. Consequently, even a clear definition of the term *food allergy* using symptoms, causative factors, physiological processes, or diagnostic tests (which are the usual ways we define a disease) has always eluded clinicians and scientists.

In the popular literature, it has become convenient for all adverse reactions that result from eating to be labeled "food allergy," but in medical and scientific fields, there are several defined conditions within this broad category that indicate the probable mechanism of the reaction that is taking place within the body. This helps determine the possible cause of the symptoms, predicts the probable severity and duration of the reaction, and suggests the most appropriate treatment.

Definition of Food Allergy Terms

One of the most comprehensive attempts at defining adverse reactions to foods was made in 2001 by the European Academy of Allergy and Clinical Immunology[1] and includes the following:

- ▪ *Allergy* is a hypersensitivity reaction initiated by immunological mechanisms.
- ▪ An adverse reaction to food should be called *food hypersensitivity*.
  - • When immunological mechanisms have been demonstrated, the appropriate term is *food allergy*.
  - • If the role of immunoglobulin E (IgE) is highlighted, the correct term is *IgE-mediated food allergy* (we shall discuss IgE and other antibodies later in this chapter).
  - • All other reactions, previously sometimes referred to as *food intolerance*, should be referred to as *nonallergic food hypersensitivity*.
- ▪ *Anaphylaxis* is a severe, life-threatening, generalized, or systemic hypersensitivity reaction.
- ▪ *Atopy* is a personal or familial tendency to produce IgE antibodies in response to low doses of allergens, usually proteins, and to develop typical symptoms such as asthma, rhinoconjunctivitis (hay fever), or eczema/atopic dermatitis.

Previously, the American Academy of Allergy and Clinical Immunology and the National Institute of Allergy and Infectious Disease (NIAID) of the National Institutes of Health (NIH)[4] defined the diverse terms in use as follows:

- ▪ An *adverse food reaction* is a generic term referring to any untoward reaction after the ingestion of a food.
- ▪ An adverse food reaction can be either a food allergy or a food intolerance. A *food allergy* is the result of an abnormal immunological response after ingestion of a food. A *food intolerance* is the result of nonimmunological mechanisms.

In spite of (or, more likely, because of) these seemingly precise but sometimes conflicting academic definitions, authors of research papers and articles on food allergy now frequently define their own use of the terms in any published work so that the reader is clear about their meaning in that specific context.[5] In accordance with this sensible practice, I will do likewise. See Box 1.1.

The Science of Food Sensitivities

From the time the food enters the mouth until symptoms occur, processes involved in an adverse reaction to a food component are complex. The most important of these processes will be discussed in some detail. This chapter covers food allergy. Later chapters will deal with food intolerances.

The Immunological Process in an Allergic Reaction

The events involved in an allergic reaction involve activation of the immune system in response to a foreign antigen and the consequent production and release of diverse reactive chemicals that act on body tissues to produce the symptoms of allergy. These events are summarized in the following sections.[6]

BOX 1.1 Definition of Terms as Used in This Book

- *Adverse food reaction* and *food sensitivity* are generic terms referring to any troublesome reaction after the ingestion of a food.
- Adverse food reactions can be (a) food allergy or (b) food intolerance.
- A *food allergy* is the result of an abnormal immunological response after ingestion of a food.
- A *food intolerance* is the result of nonimmunological mechanisms.
- *Anaphylaxis* is a severe, life-threatening, generalized (systemic) allergy or hypersensitivity reaction.
- *Atopy* is a term used to indicate IgE-mediated allergy resulting in the development of symptoms.
- When it is unclear whether the reaction is immunologically mediated or due to a biochemical or physiological defect, the generic term *food sensitivity* will be used. Examples include sulfite sensitivity and nickel sensitivity.

Antigen Enters the Body

The immune system responds when a foreign antigen enters the body. An *antigen* is defined as anything that will elicit an immune system response. All antigens contain proteins. Some antigenic proteins are linked to carbohydrates; they are referred to a *glycoproteins*. Recent research[7] suggests that the carbohydrate linked to protein in a food antigen is important in influencing the immune response that leads to allergy (see later in this chapter for details about this process). When the antigen elicits a hypersensitivity reaction of the immune system (allergy), the antigen is called an *allergen*. All allergens are antigens; however, not all antigens are allergens. For example, bacteria, viruses, and other disease-causing entities contain antigens, but they are not allergens. They elicit a protective response of the immune system; they do not induce allergy.

A complex series of events is set in motion when an allergen enters the body of a person at risk for allergy. The process finally results in the release of chemicals (called *inflammatory mediators*) that act on body tissues to cause allergy symptoms. All immunological processes involve the various white blood cells (leukocytes) and the different types of chemicals they produce.

T-Cell Lymphocytes Detect a Foreign Invader

Whenever a foreign antigen enters the body, a group of specific white blood cells called *lymphocytes* are activated. Lymphocytes are the sentinels of the immune system. They are the first cells that recognize and respond to anything foreign entering the body. Two different types of lymphocytes are in blood: T cells and B cells. T-cell lymphocytes are the ultimate "gatekeepers" and controllers of the immune system. B cells are primarily involved in producing antibodies and are discussed later in this chapter.

Certain types of T cells, *helper T-cells* (Th cells), are responsible for identifying foreign materials that enter the body through any route from the exterior environment. They initiate and direct the subsequent activities of the immune system if the foreign material is deemed a threat to the body's health.

T cells exert their control of the whole immune response by means of several different types of "messenger chemicals" called *cytokines*. The responses of Th cells of allergic and nonallergic individuals are different. The two types of responses have been designated Th2 response and Th1 response, respectively. Different cytokines are released in each response and control the way in which the body reacts to the foreign material.

Cytokines Direct the Immune Response

When a pathogen (disease-causing microorganism) enters the body, the immune system activates a Th1 response. Cytokines such as interleukin 1 (IL-1), interleukin 2 (IL-2), interferon-gamma (INF-γ), and others are produced. They stimulate the formation of immunoglobulin G (IgG) antibodies,[5] which eventually destroy the invading microorganism by means of a complex series of events known as the *complement cascade*.[a] Symptoms such as fever, aching muscles, fatigue, and general malaise that are typical of an infection such as the flu are the result of the body's response to cytokines and other inflammatory mediators produced during this battle between the immune system and the foreign invader.

In an allergic reaction, a similar series of events is engaged, but this time it is between the immune system and a nonthreatening invader such as a food. In this case, the Th2 cytokines control the immune response. Instead of the IL-2, INF-γ, and similar cytokines of the Th1 response, an entirely different set of cytokines are produced. Interleukins 4, 5, 6, and 13 (IL-4, IL-5, IL-6, and IL-13) are typical of the Th2 response and result in production of IgE antibodies. (The different types of antibodies and their functions will be discussed later in this chapter.) Unlike IgG, IgE antibodies do not trigger the complement cascade. Instead, they initiate a series of reactions that result in the release of inflammatory mediators such as histamine and other reactive chemicals from specialized cells called *mast cells*. The inflammatory mediators act on body tissues and produce the itching, swelling, reddening (flushing), and smooth muscle contraction (eg, the bronchospasm of asthma) that are typical of allergy.[5]

Simply stated:

■ The Th1 response protects the body from disease, and IgG antibodies are responsible for destroying the invader.
■ The Th2 response results in allergy, and IgE antibodies are responsible for the release of inflammatory mediators that cause the symptoms of allergy.

---

[a] *Complement* is a group of more than 20 enzymatic proteins in the blood that act together, in response to antigen and antibody, to destroy foreign cells by splitting them apart (lysis). This process is known as the *complement cascade*, which releases various chemical by-products that act as opsonins, chemotaxins, and anaphylatoxins to help destroy a threat to the body and results in inflammation in various tissues.

To understand the process that may lead to either of these reaction pathways in an allergic reaction to food, we need to look at how the immune system of the digestive tract functions.

The Immune System of the Digestive Tract

The immune system of the digestive tract is different from that in other parts of the body. It is composed of specialized cells that make up the gut-associated lymphoid tissue (GALT). Processing of food through this system allows the uptake of nutrients through the walls of the digestive tract (the intestinal epithelium) without triggering the protective response that would otherwise form a barrier to the foreign materials in food. At the same time, any potentially disease-causing microorganisms taken in through the same route are effectively excluded by the GALT. So we have a system that can recognize foreign material that is safe (food) and foreign material that is a threat (microorganisms, toxins, and other noxious agents) at the same time and in the same place.

In addition to distinguishing between food and potential pathogens, the GALT must also distinguish between invading microorganisms and others that are permanent residents of the large intestine—called the *gut microflora* or *microbiota*. It is estimated that there are about 10^{12} to 10^{14} fairly innocuous microorganisms per mL in the gastrointestinal tract of the healthy human, mostly in the large bowel. They break down undigested food that moves into the bowel from the small intestine (where most of the digestion of food and absorption of nutrients takes place). Micronutrients such as vitamin K, biotin, thiamin, vitamin B-12, and folate are produced as a result of their metabolic activities. These vitamins are absorbed and form an essential part of a body's nutritional resources.

In addition, microorganisms in the large bowel defend the bowel from invasion by nonessential, or harmful, microorganisms by competing with them for space and nutrients. Microorganisms in the large bowel also perform a vital role in keeping the surrounding tissues healthy by stimulating the GALT in a positive manner. These resident microorganisms will be discussed in the chapter on probiotics (Chapter 47).

In summary, the GALT is responsible for:

- Allowing innocuous food materials to pass through into circulation
- Preventing potential pathogens from entering the body
- Allowing members of the resident microflora to flourish in the large intestine

So what goes wrong in food allergy? To answer this, we need to examine the mechanisms that determine how the immune system responds to food.

The process that enables us to eat food without any adverse effects, which is the experience of most people to most foods, is called *tolerance*. In immunological tolerance, the immune system recognizes that the food is foreign to the body, but any defensive action is suppressed by means of a series of specific responses.

The Process of Immunological Tolerance to Food in the Digestive Tract

As in all immunological responses, T cells and their messenger cytokines are involved in the process of oral tolerance. As far as we know at present, in the normal, healthy (nonallergic) human, T cells that first encounter the "foreign food" when it enters the body for the very first time (perhaps in mother's breast milk or as a solid food after weaning) are of the Th1 type.[b] They are picked up by special cells (usually dendritic cells) in the infant's digestive tract and transported in the lymphatic system to the thymus gland. Here the regulatory T cells (sometimes written as T_{reg} cells) stop any further action on the part of the Th1 cells when it is discovered that the foreign molecules pose no threat to the body. This process of inhibiting T-cell action is carried out by cytokines, especially TGF-β (transforming growth factor–beta) and possibly IL-10 (interleukin-10) and IL-13 (interleukin-13).

The "educated" T cells are then transported in the blood circulatory system, back into the digestive tract GALT, as "memory cells." Whenever the same food is eaten again, the memory T cells remember that this substance is safe and remain quiescent, without any further attempt to protect the body from this particular foreign material. As far as we know, this process occurs every time a food enters the body for the first time.[8]

The process of oral tolerance allows the healthy (nonallergic) human to eat any food, absorb its essential nutrients, and excrete the residue that is unnecessary to the body in the form of feces, while maintaining healthy tissue along the whole length of the digestive tract. However, not all food is tolerated by all people. The immune system of individuals who have food allergies rejects the foreign proteins in food. But the process is not the same as when the immune system fights the foreign protein in a virus or bacterium, even though both the food and the invading microorganism enter the body through the same route—the mouth and digestive tract.

In food allergy, the process of oral tolerance is diverted; instead of the Th1 response leading to oral tolerance via immunological suppression, the Th2 pathway is activated. The allergen in the food is recognized by the immune system of the potentially allergic person, and a series of reactions ensues that result in the release of the inflammatory chemicals that act on body tissues to produce the symptoms of allergy. This process of recognition, activation, and finally the production of antibodies specific to the food allergen is called *sensitization*.

Figure 1.1 is a diagrammatic representation of the pathways involved in the processes of oral tolerance and allergic sensitization. Readers who wish more detailed information about the immunological response in allergy and immunological tolerance are directed to publications on the subject.[6,9]

The B-cell lymphocytes are the link between the response of the Th cells and the release of the inflammatory mediators that cause allergy. These cells produce the extremely important *antibodies*.

---

[b] Sometimes these cells are called *Th3 cells* to distinguish them from the Th1 response that results in immunological protection.

FIGURE 1.1

Any foreign protein (antigen) entering the body is assessed by the immune system. The protein is broken down by an antigen-presenting cell and presented to an appropriate T cell coupled to a surface receptor, together with a "self-antigen" (MHC class II) for comparison. The first T cell encountered is designated Th0 and produces a range of cytokines (IL-2, IL-3, IL-4, etc; only the significant cytokines are listed in this illustration. T cells produce several others). If the foreign protein is part of a pathogenic microorganism, such as a virus or bacterium, T cells of the Th1 class respond with their own cytokines. The immune system is triggered to provide protection against the invader with the production of specific IgG antibodies. This destroys the invader by way of a complex series of immunological events involving the complement proteins in what is known as the *complement cascade*. If the foreign protein is a food allergen, T cells of the Th2 class are activated. Specific cytokines are produced that result in the production of IgE against the foreign invader. This results in release of inflammatory mediators from mast cells that produce the symptoms typical of allergy. The normal response to food is tolerance, which involves several regulatory T cells (Th3, T_{reg} cells, T suppressor cells [CD8]) and their cytokines. Oral tolerance can develop following food allergy by activating regulatory T cells (T_{reg}) and their associated cytokines. Arrows indicate the direction of reactions. A double-sided arrow indicates the reaction pathway can proceed in either direction depending on the conditions of response.

Lymphocytes

Th1: Type I T helper cell; Th2: Type 2 T helper cell; Th3: Occasional designation of T cells involved in tolerance that produces regulatory cytokines; Th0: "Naïve" T helper cell prior to differentiation for a specific function; T_{reg}: T cells involved in regulatory functions leading to tolerance; Tr1: A type of T regulatory cell that produces cytokines involved in tolerance; CD: indicates the type of lymphocyte antigen (marker) on the cell: T helper cells express CD4 antigen; T suppressor cells or T regulatory cells usually express CD8 antigen; other T cells are identified with numbers (eg, CD25) that indicate their structure and function; all T cells express CD3 antigen.

Cytokines

IL: Interleukin—each interleukin is identified by a numeral (IL-1, IL-2, etc); INF: Interferon—interferons are usually identified with Greek letters (INF-α, INF-γ, etc); GM-CSF: granulocyte macrophage colony-stimulating factor; TGF-β: Transforming growth factor beta; MHC: major histocompatibility complex—the antigen expressed by the cell identifying it as "self." The Roman numeral (I, II) indicates the histocompatibility type.

Immunological Pathways to Protection, Allergy, or Oral Tolerance:

T helper (CD4+) cells respond

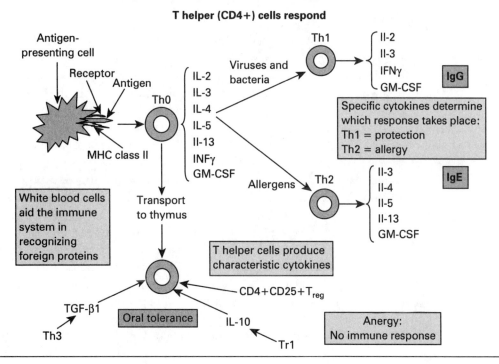

Antibodies and the Immune Response

B Cells

The main function of B cells is to produce antibodies. Antibodies are complex molecules produced by the immune system in response to antigens. As we have already seen, antigens are foreign proteins, or glycoproteins, that trigger the immune response. Every living cell produces several different proteins, unique to its own cell type and species. The antibody produced against the antigen is entirely specific to that antigen and fits with it like a lock and key, forming an antigen-antibody complex. When the body is invaded by a microorganism, such as a bacterium or virus, B cells will make an antibody precisely designed to couple with molecules of that specific microorganism. The molecules of the microorganism that trigger that response are antigens. Similarly, if a pollen or a food causes B cells to make antibody in the allergic response, the molecules of the pollen or food causing the antibody production are antigens. As mentioned earlier, antigens are called *allergens* in the case of allergies.

In the process of making antibodies, B cells first convert into plasma cells. The antibody is generated from plasma cells.

The antibodies produced by B cells are five different types of immunoglobulin: IgA, IgG, IgM, IgE, and IgD. Each antibody molecule is made up of a special protein called a *globulin*. Because the globulin is associated with the immune system, the prefix *immuno-* is attached to it. Each of the five antibodies has a specific role in immune protection and in the reactions that are responsible for adverse reactions to foods.[6]

IgM

IgM, the largest of the antibodies, is found circulating in blood. It acts by seeking out antigens and attaching them at one end of one or more of its five "arms." It has ten attachment sites (two per arm) and can mop up many antigens at a time. IgM is the first line of defense against a foreign molecule when it reaches the bloodstream. It is the first *protective* antibody the fetus produces in utero, and a rise in the level of fetal IgM often accompanies an in utero viral infection.

IgA

IgA is found mainly in mucous secretions (secretions from surfaces exposed to the outside world through orifices such as the mouth, respiratory tract, vagina, etc), where it is called *secretory IgA* (sIgA) to distinguish it from the IgA found in blood (usually called *serum IgA*). sIgA acts as the first line of defense against foreign molecules entering through external orifices, before they can enter the bloodstream. It is important in defending the digestive tract of the neonate against anything entering through its mouth. However, as we shall discuss in Chapter 42, the neonate has no sIgA of its own, and its early digestive tract protection comes entirely from its mother's colostrum (the first fluid that passes through the breast before mature milk is produced), which contains an abundant supply of sIgA.

IgG

IgG is the most important antibody in the immune system's defense against invading disease-causing microorganisms. It is found in the bloodstream after the first-line IgM has started to mop up the invader. B cells first produce IgM and then switch over to IgG once the invader is established to be a real threat to the body. IgG remains long after the disease has been successfully suppressed; this ensures that the same microorganism is "neutralized" when it enters the body on a subsequent occasion and therefore will not cause the same infection again. This same process occurs when one receives an immunization shot containing killed or live attenuated microorganisms (microorganisms with reduced disease-causing potential) and defends the body against the real live virus or bacterium if it does get in later.

There are four different subtypes of IgG antibodies, which function in different situations: IgG1, IgG2, IgG3, and IgG4. In general, IgG4 antibodies are important in certain types of immunological (or hypersensitivity) reactions against foods. IgG1, IgG2, and IgG3 are important in the defense against invading pathogens and other agents that can cause disease in the body.

IgE

IgE is the most important antibody in the majority of allergies—the classic allergy of hay fever, asthma, hives, angioedema (tissue swelling), and the potentially life-threatening anaphylactic reactions. Apart from the allergic reaction, the only other currently known role for IgE is in fighting parasites and intestinal worms (helminths and nematodes).

IgD

The role of IgD is less well defined and is usually associated with aiding other immune functions, such as switching from one antibody type to another. It is mentioned here simply for completeness. Its role in allergy is probably minimal.

IgE-Mediated Hypersensitivity (Allergy)

After the Th2 reaction produces IgE in response to an allergenic food, a series of events takes place that finally results in the symptoms of allergy. Biologically active chemicals, called *inflammatory mediators*, are released from mast cells. Mast cells are specialized white blood cells that are present in all tissues but are particularly abundant in the digestive tract, lungs, respiratory tract, and skin. These cells produce and store the inflammatory mediators that are then ready to defend cells and tissues whenever an event that threatens the body's health takes place. In the case of food allergy, this event is eating the allergenic food that has triggered the Th2 response and thus sensitized the individual to the allergen.

The reaction can be considered as occurring in two phases, the early and the late response:

■ The early phase results in the release of inflammatory mediators from mast cells in tissues.

■   The late phase results in the recruitment of additional granulocytes,[c] which are drawn to the reaction site by chemotactic factors (agents that move cells by a process of chemical attraction) released in the early phase. The newly recruited granulocytes are stimulated to release their own inflammatory mediators, which augment the allergic reaction by increasing the levels of those already present.

Early Phase: Release of Inflammatory Mediators

As soon as IgE antibodies are produced by the activated B-cell lymphocytes, they migrate to the surface of specific white blood cells that have receptors on their surface with which to couple with the antibody. These receptors are designated Fcε R1 receptors, indicating that they are compatible with the IgE antibody. Mast cells in tissues possess these IgE-compatible receptors. The mast cell is the essential granulocyte in the IgE-mediated allergic response. It has been estimated that there may be as many as 500,000 receptors for antibody molecules on the surface of each mast cell.

The process of degranulation is initiated when an allergen cross-links two IgE molecules on adjacent receptors on the surface of a mast cell, forming a bridge between them.[6] The allergen needs to be a certain size (estimated at 10 to 70 kilodaltons[d]) to effect this bridging. At the same time, it is necessary that there be a sufficient number of IgE molecules on the cell's surface to ensure that two would be close enough for the allergen to bridge them.

Often the first exposure to an allergen does not result in a sufficient number of IgE molecules to allow the allergen-antibody bridges to form, so a single exposure to an allergen rarely results in the release of inflammatory mediators and is usually symptom free. The process in which a person is exposed to an allergen but does not exhibit symptoms is generally referred to as the *sensitizing event*. On subsequent exposure, when sufficient IgE molecules are present on the surface of the mast cells, degranulation will occur and overt symptoms may be experienced. Each of the inflammatory mediators released during degranulation has a specific effect on the body, resulting in the symptoms typical of allergy (see later discussion for details).

Late Phase: Amplification of the Allergic Response

During the late phase of the allergic response, neutrophils, eosinophils, monocytes, and basophils are attracted to the reaction site by the chemotaxins produced in the early phase. A measurable increase in eosinophils may indicate that the symptoms are due to a hypersensitivity reaction. When the granulocytes release their intracellular inflammatory mediators, the allergic reaction is powerfully augmented. This can be experienced in the late-phase reaction of asthma or anaphylaxis when an initial reaction seems to be resolving but suddenly becomes extremely acute, putting

---

[c] A *granulocyte* is a white blood cell with a lobed nucleus, characterized by numerous granules within its cytoplasm. The granules contain *inflammatory mediators,* a variety of biologically active chemicals that are important in immunological protection. Mast cells, basophils, neutrophils, and eosinophils are examples of granulocytes.

[d] Daltons and kilodaltons are the units used to measure the size of molecules.

the person in serious danger. The second phase of an anaphylactic reaction may be fatal, especially if the patient is discharged from care too soon. The second phase may occur several hours after the initial response but usually is exhibited within a maximum of 4 to 6 hours after the first phase.

The process of mediator release from basophils, eosinophils, and other granulocytes differs from that of the IgE-mediated response. Not all the mast-cell mediators listed are produced from all of these auxiliary cells (eg, mast cells release tryptase but basophils do not), but those that are have a similar effect on body systems.

Mediators Released from Mast Cells and their Effects

Histamine   Histamine is a potent inflammatory mediator that controls several different tissue responses, the most important of which include:

- Vasodilation (widening of small blood vessels)
- Increase in the permeability of the membrane around the blood vessels, allowing fluids and protein to leak out
- Bronchoconstriction (contraction of smooth muscle surrounding the lungs)
- Stimulation of nerves, resulting in itching
- Increased secretion of mucus

Chemotactic Chemicals (Chemotaxins)   Chemotaxins are chemicals that can facilitate the movement of cells by means of a concentration gradient (the cells move from an area with a high concentration of the chemical to one where the chemical is less concentrated). Chemoattractants from mast cells are mainly involved in the movement of granulocytes such as neutrophils and eosinophils to the reaction site. These granulocytes contain their own inflammatory mediators, which are released in the late phase of the allergic response.

Enzymes   Enzymes such as tryptase, kininogenase, and phospholipases result in further activation of inflammatory processes and can cause tissue damage. Sometimes the level of enzymes, especially tryptase, is measured as an indicator to confirm mast cell degranulation.[10] Basophils do not release tryptase, so this is one method of differentiating between mediators released from mast cells and those from other granulocytes,[11] which may prove useful in determining anaphylaxis due to mast cell degranulation.

Phospholipase A2 is the key enzyme that leads to the production of several different types of powerful inflammatory mediators in a series of enzymatic reactions:

- The omega-6 lipid, arachidonic acid, is released from its position in the membrane of the cell.
- Arachidonic acid is then metabolized by two pathways to form the *secondary mediators of inflammation* (known as eicosanoids) of two very important groups: (a) prostaglandins and (b) leukotrienes.
- The enzyme systems responsible for their production are (a) the cyclo-oxygenase pathway and (b) the lipoxygenase pathway.

The *cyclooxygenase system* results in the production of prostanoids of the "2 series" (contain two double bonds in their structure), written as PG_2. They include the prostaglandins prostacyclin and thromboxane, which have important functions in many body systems. In allergy, their most important functions include:

▪ Mediation of atopic symptoms; for example, PGD_2, like histamine, causes vasodilation, bronchoconstriction, nerve stimulation, and mucus secretion.
▪ Regulation; for example, $PGF_{2\alpha}$ stimulates mast cell degranulation, whereas PGE_1 and PGE_2 tend to inhibit mast cell degranulation.

The *lipoxygenase system* produces the leukotrienes of the "4 series" (four double bonds in their structure), written as LT_4. Some of the leukotrienes are powerful inflammatory chemicals. For example:

▪ LTB_4 is a vigorous chemoattractant for granulocytes and thus is responsible for augmenting the allergic response when the newly recruited granulocytes release their own battery of inflammatory chemicals.
▪ LTC_4, LTD_4, and LTE_4 cause smooth muscle contraction and are key factors in the bronchospasm of asthma. They also mediate mucus secretion and mucosal edema, which are frequent symptoms of allergy.

Figure 1.2 shows this system of development of secondary mediators of inflammation.

Clinical Expression of Allergy (Atopy)

Even when the potential to produce antigen-specific IgE has been inherited, further genetic elements seem to be required for atopic disease to be expressed clinically and for symptoms to occur. For example, the ability of granulocytes such as basophils to release inflammatory mediators seems to be determined by genetic factors, but exposure to the allergens that trigger the response is dependent on lifestyle events.

Other Antibodies in Food Sensitivity

It is common to find anti-food IgG antibodies circulating in blood, even in people who have no signs or history of adverse reactions to foods. In fact, an increase in anti-food IgG might be indicative of successful resolution of an IgE-mediated allergy.[12] The subject of IgG-mediated food allergy is complicated because of the nature of the antibody and the immunological reactions associated with it. Present knowledge about food allergy–associated IgG may be summarized as follows:

▪ Four distinct subclasses of IgG have been identified: IgG1, IgG2, IgG3, and IgG4.
▪ IgG4 has a high affinity for food antigens.
▪ IgG4 represents a very small proportion of total IgG in normal sera; reports of the level of IgG4 differ from laboratory to laboratory, the range being 0.7% to 4.9% of total IgG.[13]

FIGURE 1.2

Phospholipase A2 acts on cell membranes and releases arachidonic acid. Arachidonic acid is metabolized by two pathways: (a) the cyclooxygenase pathway or (b) the lipoxygenase pathway. The cyclooxygenase pathway produces the prostanoids, which include (a) prostaglandins (PG_2); (b) prostacyclin (PGI_2); (c) thromboxane (TX). The lipoxygenase pathway produces leukotrienes (LT_4), which include several different leukotrienes in a sequence (A, B, C, D), as shown by the arrows. Each of these mediators (prostanoids and leukotrienes) has different effects on body systems as discussed in the text.

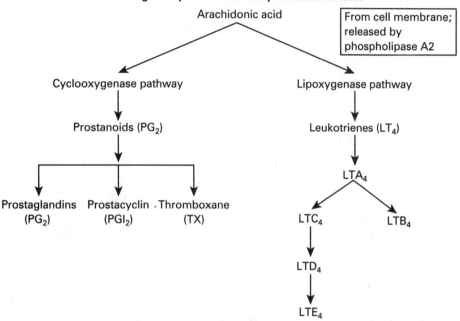

- In the newborn baby, levels of IgG1 and IgG3 rise rapidly, and IgG1 may reach concentrations close to the adult level at 8 months. In contrast, IgG4 is still only a fraction of the adult level at 2 years of age and may not reach adult levels until the age of 12 years.
- Anti-food IgG4 may be associated with allergy, in particular to the milk protein β-lactoglobulin in atopic dermatitis (eczema) in children.[14]
- There is some evidence that *total* anti-food IgG (all classes of IgG measured together) might represent some protection from IgE-mediated food allergy. In one study, symptom-free children had higher levels of IgG antibodies to milk and egg proteins than those who developed allergic symptoms, and a high IgG-to-IgE ratio in cord blood was suggested to be a sign of a decreased risk for food allergy.[15]

▪   Food allergy in infants is frequently associated with an increase in gut permeability ("leaky gut"). It is likely that antigenic food molecules passing into circulation trigger production of anti-food IgG. Thus, in cases of IgE-mediated food allergy that results in inflammatory reactions within the gastrointestinal tract, causing a nonintact digestive epithelium, it is logical to expect to find higher than normal levels of anti-food IgG. Some authorities think that these anti-food IgG antibodies represent a protective mechanism, rather than a source of allergic pathology.[16]

It remains for future research to determine the role of IgG, and especially IgG4 anti-food antibodies in allergy. Later we will discuss the role of IgG in allergic sensitization and tolerance in the fetus and newborn (Chapter 44). In Chapter 4, we shall look at the consequences of all this immunological activity in our discussion of the symptoms of allergy.

Incidence of Allergy

Estimates of the incidence of IgE-mediated food allergy range from 0.1% to 7% of the overall population, with a male to female ratio of approximately 2:1.[17] However, these statistics are based on numerous reports that use different diagnostic criteria (skin tests, intradermal tests, radioallergosorbent test [RAST], enzyme-linked immunosorbent assay [ELISA], fluorescent allergosorbent test [FAST], and double-blind placebo-controlled food challenge [DBPCFC]; refer to Chapter 5 for details of these tests) as well as self-reported questionnaires, so it is very difficult to provide reliable statistics for the prevalence of food allergy in any population.

Based on reports in the current medical literature, the prevalence of "adverse food reactions" was recently estimated to be approximately 2% to 8% in infants and 1% in adulthood.[18] Reports of cow's milk protein allergy in infants range from 0.5% to 2.5% of children younger than 5 years. Many studies have suggested a rise in prevalence of food allergy during the past 10 to 20 years.[19]

The public tends to believe that the incidence of food allergy is much higher than these figures suggest. In studies from various countries, up to 50% of the population believe that they or their children have some degree of sensitivity to foods or food additives. A meta-analysis of data from 51 publications[20] indicated a self-reported incidence of food allergy in children and adults to five foods (milk, egg, peanut, fish, and crustacean shellfish) that was notably higher than the rates determined on the basis of evidence of IgE-mediated sensitization and DBPCFC. The incidence of allergy to specific foods varies widely among populations and countries and depends on methods of diagnosis and reporting that can be diverse and variable.[21]

The present consensus guidelines state that babies who have a first-degree relative (ie, parent or sibling) with a diagnosed food allergy are at high risk for allergy.[22] There is no definition of "moderate" or "no risk," because even with an absence of any family history of allergy, there is a 15% chance that a baby will develop allergy.

Why One Person Experiences an Immunological Reaction and Another Does Not

As discussed earlier, immunological responses to foods vary from individual to individual. What determines why one person experiences a Th2 response, while another does not? The answer could be one of several reasons.

Allergy as an Inherited Characteristic

The potential to develop allergy is an inherited characteristic. It is probable that the characteristic that is inherited is the potential to experience a Th2 response when harmless foreign materials, such as food, pollens, animal dander, and other allergens enter the body. There is no evidence that allergy to a specific allergen, such as peanut, shellfish, grass pollen, animal dander, and so on, is inherited. Hopefully, in the future, indicators for the inherited potential, such as specific gene sequences will identify which babies are likely to develop allergy prior to, or at birth, so that appropriate precautions can be taken to avoid early allergic sensitization.

The Circumstances Under Which the Allergen Is Encountered

Early infancy is a time when the baby might be at maximum risk of being sensitized to allergens. At birth, the baby's immunological response tends to be the Th2 reaction. It is theorized that this is because the fetus exists within a Th2 milieu in utero to preclude a maternal Th1 response from rejecting the developing fetus. After birth, the immunological response switches to the protective Th1 (this is discussed in more detail in Chapter 42). If this switch does not occur, the tendency will be for the baby to respond to food and other foreign but safe materials with an allergic rather than protective reaction.

From birth to about 2 years of age, the baby's immune system is relatively immature. During this period, a baby with an inherited potential to develop allergy is likely to respond to a foreign protein with the Th2 response that results in allergy unless the allergen has been introduced in such a way that tolerance develops. As the immune system matures, the chance of a Th2 response is substantially reduced. In addition, the lining of the digestive tract changes and becomes less permeable to food molecules of the size required for an allergic reaction to occur. From the age of 2 years onward, most children start to outgrow their early food allergies.

In the past, many experts believed that if a baby can be protected from allergic sensitization during the period in which the immune system and the digestive tract are in the most vulnerable state for allergy to develop, the incidence of lifelong food allergy and potentially life-threatening anaphylactic reactions to foods will be reduced and hopefully prevented. However, this thinking is changing in light of new evidence-based findings.

Recent research suggests that pregnancy, lactation, and early feeding are critical stages during which tolerance to foods occurs. Immunological tolerance is a fairly new concept in food allergy, but it is the most important event in digestive tract immunology. See the earlier discussion in this chapter and Chapter 44 for details.

The Microorganisms That Colonize the Digestive Tract

The microorganisms that colonize the large intestine, and in some cases the lower part of the small intestine, may play an important role in determining the way in which an individual responds to foods and may influence whether the immune system develops a Th1 or Th2 response. The influence of the resident microflora on allergy is discussed in more detail in Chapter 47.

References

1. Johansson SGO, Hourihane JOB, Bousquet J, et al. A revised nomenclature for allergy: an EAACI position statement from the EAACI nomenclature task force. *Allergy.* 2001;56:813-824.
2. Boyce JA, Assa'ad A, Burks AW, et al. Guidelines for the diagnosis and management of food allergy in the United States: report of the NIAID-sponsored expert panel. *J Allergy Clin Immunol.* 2010;126(6):S1-S58 (section 2.1.1).
3. Sampson HA, Munoz-Furlong A, Campbell RL, et al. Second Symposium on the Definition and Management of Anaphylaxis: Summary Report—Second National Institute of Allergy and Infectious Disease/Food Allergy and Anaphylaxis Network Symposium. *Ann Emerg Med.* 2006;47(4):373-380.
4. American Academy of Allergy and Clinical Immunology/NIAID. *Adverse Reactions to Foods.* Bethesda, MD: National Institutes of Health; 1984. NIH Publication 84-2442:1-6.
5. Boyce JA, Assa'ad A, Burks AW, et al. Guidelines for the diagnosis and management of food allergy in the United States: report of the NIAID-sponsored expert panel. *J Allergy Clin Immunol.* 2010;126(6):S1-S58 (2.1)
6. Joneja JMV, Bielory L. *Understanding Allergy, Sensitivity and Immunity: A Comprehensive Guide.* New Brunswick, NJ: Rutgers University Press; 1990.
7. Vickery BP, Chin S, Burks AW. Pathophysiology of food allergy. *Pediatr Clin North Am.* 2011;58(2):363-376.
8. Strobel S, Mowat A. Oral tolerance and allergic responses to food proteins. *Curr Opin Allergy Clin Immunol.* 2006;6(3):207-213.
9. Holgate ST, Church MK, Broide DH, Martinez FD. *Allergy.* 4th ed. Expert Consult Online and Print. Philadelphia, PA: Elsevier, Mosby, Saunders; 2012.
10. Schwartz LB, Metcalfe DD, Miller JS, Earl H. Sullivan tryptase levels as an indicator of mast-cell activation in systemic anaphylaxis and mastocytosis. *N Engl J Med.* 1987;316:1622-1626.
11. Sanz ML, Gamboa PM, García-Figueroa BE, Ferrer M. In vitro diagnosis of anaphylaxis. *Chem Immunol Allergy.* 2010;95:125-140.
12. Stapel SO, Asero R, Ballmer-Weber BK, et al. Testing for IgG4 against foods is not recommended as a diagnostic tool: EAACI Task Force Report. *Allergy.* 2008;63(7):793-796.
13. Aalberse RC, van Milligen F, Tan KY, Stapel SO. Allergen-specific IgG4 in atopic disease. *Allergy.* 2003;48(8):559-569.

14. Jenmalm MC, Bjorksten B. Exposure to cow's milk during the first 3 months of life is associated with increased levels of IgG subclass antibodies to beta-lactoglobulin to 8 years. *J Allergy Clin Immunol.* 1998;102(4 pt 1):671-678.

15. Dannaeus A, Inganas M. A follow-up study of children with food allergy. Clinical course in relation to serum IgE- and IgG-antibody levels to milk, egg and fish. *Clin Allergy.* 1981;11:533-539.

16. Sampson HA. Food allergy. Part 1: Immunopathogenesis and clinical disorders. Current reviews of allergy and clinical immunology. *J Allergy Clin Immunol.* 1999;103(5 pt 1):717-728.

17. Osterballe M, Hansen TK, Mortz CG, Host A, Bindslav-Jensen C. The prevalence of food hypersensitivity in an unselected population of children and adults. *Pediatr Allergy Immunol.* 2005;16(7):567-573.

18. Chafen JJ, Newberry SJ, Riedl MA, et al. Diagnosing and managing common food allergies: a systematic review. *JAMA.* 2010;303(18):1848-1856.

19. Branum AM, Lukacs SL. Food allergy among children in the United States. *Pediatrics.* 2009;124(6):1549-1555.

20. Rona RJ, Keil T, Summers C, Gislason D, Zuidmeer L, Sodergren E. The prevalence of food allergy: a meta-analysis. *J Allergy Clin Immunol.* 2007;120(3):638-646.

21. Boyce JA, Assa'ad A, Burks AW, et al. Guidelines for the diagnosis and management of food allergy in the United States: report of the NIAID-sponsored expert panel. *J Allergy Clin Immunol.* 2010;126(6):S1-S58. (2.2.2)

22. Greer FR, Sicherer SH, Burks AW, American Academy of Pediatrics Committee on Nutrition, American Academy of Pediatrics Section on Allergy and Immunology. Effects of early nutritional interventions on the development of atopic disease in infants and children: the role of maternal dietary restriction, breastfeeding, timing of introduction of complementary foods, and hydrolyzed formulas. *Pediatrics.* 2008;121(1):183-191.

CHAPTER 2

The Allergenic Potential of Foods

To what extent should a known allergen be avoided? For example, if an individual is allergic to soy, should all forms of soy be strictly eliminated from the diet, including hydrolyzed soy protein, lecithin made from soy, fermented soy (soy sauce), tofu, and so on? Few practitioners can answer this question with certainty, and so for safety, the allergic person is usually advised to avoid all forms of the food, even when this may lead to a great deal of work, social and economic stress, annoyance, and fear when food ingredients are inadequately or ambiguously labeled. It can also possibly lead to nutritional deficiency.

The degree to which an allergic individual will react to a food allergen depends on several factors, especially that person's atopic (allergic) potential and the food's allergenic potency. A small number of foods are considered most likely to cause a severe, sometimes anaphylactic reaction in the hypersensitive individual. For babies and young children in the United States, eggs, cow's milk, soy, peanuts, tree nuts, fish, crustacean shellfish, and wheat proteins tend to be the most problematic;[1] for adults, peanuts, tree nuts, shellfish, finfish, and sulfites are the most frequently reported allergens. All sources of these should be strictly avoided if the allergic person has shown signs of an anaphylactic reaction to them.

However, the question remains, "What about foods that may not have triggered an anaphylactic reaction but are known to cause symptoms of allergy, albeit mild ones, in an individual?" Authorities in the field agree that if a person is mildly allergic to a food, less stringent precautions need to be taken in detecting the food as a "hidden ingredient" than if the food is likely to precipitate a life-threatening anaphylactic reaction. But how do we determine the degree of vigilance required in avoiding the food, and how do we assess its potential to trigger a life-threatening reaction in the future? To begin answering this question, we first discuss what exactly a food allergen is.

What Is a Food Allergen?

Many scientists have tried to answer this question, but currently our best definition of food allergen is "an antigen present in a food that causes an allergic reaction."

The major difficulty with this statement is that a precise definition of food allergy is still lacking. Several controversial aspects of food allergy make reaching consensus on a precise definition difficult. For example, there is a lack of agreement about the symptoms triggered by foods and their frequency and severity. This is related to several factors:

■ The target organ for many food allergies varies from person to person. The same food can induce a reaction in entirely different organ systems in different individuals; for example, cow's milk protein may induce digestive tract symptoms in one child, skin reactions in another, and a life-threatening anaphylactic reaction in a third.

■ Some foods more frequently provoke an allergic reaction than others that are very similar; for example, peanuts have a greater allergic potential than lentils, although both are legumes.

■ There are multiple opinions regarding the importance of immunological processes other than IgE-mediated hypersensitivity reactions in triggering allergy to food. Some clinicians restrict their definition of allergy to those reactions that they can prove are triggered by IgE; others include all reactions to foods that involve any activation of the immune system.[2,3] The definition of food allergy proposed in 2010 by the NIAID-Sponsored Expert Panel in the United States is "an adverse health effect arising from a specific immune response that occurs reproducibly on exposure to a given food."[4]

■ The persistence of food allergy differs. Some food-induced reactions persist for years, whereas others do not. The majority of children outgrow most of their early food allergies by the age of 5 years.

Most research on allergens has been carried out on the foods that trigger an IgE-mediated reaction; these foods have a component that induces the production of, and reacts with, IgE antibodies to cause mediator release from mast cells and other granulocytes, resulting in an immediate hypersensitivity reaction (see Chapter 1). These characteristics allow the food component to be identified, separated, and studied. Once the antigenic/allergenic component has been isolated, its structure and molecular characteristics can be determined.[5]

Scientists are beginning to determine the structure of some specific molecules that cause the immune system to produce IgE antibodies to them. This is certainly increasing our understanding of what an allergenic food component looks like. However, the reason why one particular molecule will trigger an allergic reaction, and why one person will respond to the molecule while another does not, are great topics for debate, but unfortunately we have very little scientific data to answer the questions.[6]

Chemical Structure of Allergens

Most food allergens are either proteins or glycoproteins. *Glycoproteins* are proteins to which a carbohydrate chain is attached to the protein or peptide structure. Although huge numbers of different proteins and glycoproteins are consumed in the diet, only a few are capable of causing an allergic reaction. In addition, only sensitized individuals will exhibit symptoms of allergy when they eat a potentially allergenic food.

Some nonprotein molecules, called *haptens*, can cause an allergic response. Haptens are small molecules that are unable to trigger an allergic response on their own. Many are inorganic compounds or elements such as nickel or sulfur. Haptens become allergens when they attach to a protein. The "carrier protein" with its attached molecule forms a new antigen, called a *neoantigen*. The carrier protein may be part of the food in which the hapten exists, or it may be a protein from the body to which the hapten attaches after it is consumed. The neoantigen is then capable of triggering a hypersensitivity response, leading to allergy. The IgE antibodies are specific to the hapten part of the new antigen; therefore, if the hapten is nickel or sulfite, the IgE is produced against the nickel or sulfite, not the protein to which it is attached. Penicillin allergy is typical of an allergic reaction in which the reactive molecule (penicillanic acid) is not allergenic on its own, but when bound to a body protein becomes a powerful allergen.

Characteristics of Food Allergens

The characteristics that are required for a molecule to initiate an allergic response include:

- Solubility: It must be soluble in water.
- Size: It must be the appropriate *size* to effect bridging of two adjacent IgE molecules on the mast cell surface. This has been estimated to be a molecular weight of between 10,000 and 70,000 daltons.[a] However, much smaller molecules may be allergenic when they act as haptens. The neoantigen formed when the hapten combines with a carrier protein is the correct size to bridge the two IgE molecules.
- Attachment sites: It must have two or more antigenic sites along its length that are available for coupling with two adjacent IgE molecules. This may depend on the *shape* of the allergenic molecule.
- Intestinal permeability: The molecule must pass the barrier of the intestinal mucosa to contact cells of the immune system. Proteins in excess of 70,000 daltons in molecular weight are unlikely to pass through a healthy mucosa. However, the increased mucosal permeability resulting from certain conditions (eg, intestinal inflammation, immaturity in young infants, concomitant ingestion of alcohol) may allow access to much larger molecules.
- Stability: It must retain its allergenicity through various food-processing treatments. Most food allergens are heat and acid stable.

---

[a] Molecular weight is measured in daltons. A kilodalton (kDa) is 1,000 daltons. Refer to Glossary for details.

▪ Resistance to digestion: It must survive the digestive process and reach the intestinal mucosa in an immunogenic form. This means that it must be resistant to the effects of proteolytic enzymes and must be stable in the acidic environment of the stomach.

Structure and Function of Allergenic Molecules in Natural Food

Many laboratories are studying the molecule structure and characteristics of food allergens after they have been separated from the whole food. A variety of analytical methods are used to determine the size (measured in kilodaltons [kDa]) and the activity of the antigenic fraction of the food. Based on these data, the possible function of the molecule in the natural food may be assumed or suggested. Several important allergens such as those in peanut, apple, peach, and codfish have been separated and studied in this way. The database of the Food Allergy Research Resource Program (FARRP) under the auspices of the University of Nebraska contains numerous proteins of known sequence that are classified as food allergens.[7]

This type of research is increasing in importance as a growing number of novel, genetically engineered foods are being produced all over the world. The potential to incorporate allergens into or to develop new allergenic molecules within the novel species necessitates the availability of methods to detect them using defined characteristics. Most research into the function of allergenic molecules has been carried out on plants.

As discussed earlier, the allergenic component of food always contains a protein. Proteins comprise amino acids linked together to form the specific protein coded in the plant's or animal's DNA. Up to 22 different amino acids combine in numerous different sequences to form all of the proteins in nature. Based on the amino acid structure of the allergenic molecules, current research indicates that a surprisingly small number of amino acid sequences within the enormous range of proteins in plant foods are capable of initiating a hypersensitivity response of the immune system. Furthermore, the function of these proteins within the plant seems to be restricted to a small number of categories. These include:

▪ Storage proteins, especially in nuts, seeds, and cereal grains
▪ Inhibitors of enzymes that may be destructive to storage factors (eg, inhibitors of alpha amylases that might break down starches and trypsin that might destroy proteins in cereal grains)
▪ Structural proteins
▪ Regulatory proteins, such as profilins, that are important in plant fertilization (eg, in pollens)
▪ Pathogenesis-related proteins[8] (proteins involved in the defense-related activities of the plant). Hevamines are examples; they are lysozyme-like enzymes that break down fungal cell walls and defend the plant against fungal attack.
▪ Lipid transfer proteins (LTP) that are essential in the functioning of a cell

Allergenic Storage Proteins

Albumin is an example of an allergenic storage protein that can be found in a wide range of foods. Albumins are produced by animals, fish, and plants. Eggs from all species contain ovalbumin, milk from all species contains lactalbumin, fish contains parvalbumin, and plants contain seed storage albumins. Because a great deal of plant foods are seeds (grains, flours, peas, beans, lentils, nuts, edible seeds), most people consume many plant albumins daily. Albumins from different species tend to be distinct, so allergy to one does not always predict allergy to another, even within the same genus. One of the predominant characteristics of the albumins seems to be their resistance to a variety of adverse conditions. For example, they tend to be resistant to enzymes that degrade proteins, such as trypsin, chymotrypsin, and pepsin, which are released in the alimentary tract to digest food proteins. They also tend to be highly resistant to heat and survive cooking temperatures as high as 88°C (190.4°F).

Class 1 and Class 2 Allergy

In 1987, Amlot and his colleagues[9] reported a unique type of food allergy that differed from the usual presentation in which sensitization to the food takes place within the digestive tract (see Chapter 1 for details). In the new syndrome, initial (primary) sensitization was discovered to be due to an inhaled pollen. The food allergy component developed as a local reaction within the oral cavity in response to consumption of certain raw foods. This was labeled oral allergy syndrome (OAS).

Research revealed that the primary sensitizing allergens were inhaled pollens from a variety of plants, which induced pollen-specific IgE that triggered respiratory symptoms such as hay fever. IgE antibodies from the pollen then attached to mast cells localized in the upper respiratory tract tissues that released inflammatory mediators when the allergens entered the body. Because oral tissues are located in areas adjacent to the upper respiratory tract, IgE-primed mast cells also infiltrate the oral tissues. The unique aspect of OAS is that molecules of certain raw food plants have structures so similar to the pollen allergen that they can couple with the pollen-specific IgE attached to the mast cell surface. The bridging of two IgE molecules by the food allergen then starts the process of degranulating the mast cell that releases inflammatory mediators. The inflammatory mediators act on local tissues, causing the symptoms of OAS (see Chapter 33).

Subsequent research revealed that the characteristics of food allergy resulting from primary sensitization to the food in the digestive tract differs significantly from when reaction to the food is secondary to an inhalant allergy. Research also found that the allergens involved in the two processes are different. The two types of response have been designated class 1 and class 2 allergy, respectively.[10]

Characteristics of Class 1 Allergens

Class 1 food allergens:

▪ Encounter the immune system through the digestive tract
▪ Induce allergic sensitization directly via the intestine
▪ Are resistant to digestive enzymes
▪ Are stable in response to gastric acid
▪ Are heat-stable and are not deactivated by cooking

Characteristics of Class 2 Allergens

Class 2 food allergens:

▪ Do not induce allergic sensitization
▪ Rapidly dissolve in the oral cavity
▪ Are readily broken down by digestive enzymes
▪ Are susceptible to acid in gastric secretions
▪ Are heat-labile and are generally deactivated by cooking

Table 2.1[11] summarizes the characteristics of the two classes of allergens.

TABLE 2.1
Characteristics of Class 1 and Class 2 Food Allergies

Characteristic	Class 1 Allergy	Class 2 Allergy
Route of sensitization to allergens	Digestive tract	Respiratory tract
Typical age of onset	Infancy and early childhood	Adolescence and adulthood; usually after some years of respiratory allergy
Symptoms	May affect any organ system, especially skin and mucous membranes, digestive tract, respiratory tract, systemic (anaphylaxis)	Typically confined to the oral cavity and adjacent areas (eg, throat): itching; tingling, swelling of the lips, palate, tongue or oropharynx; occasional sensation of tightness in the throat.
Foods implicated	Any, but most frequently: peanuts, tree nuts, soy, fish, shellfish, egg, milk, wheat, sesame seeds, additives such as sulfites	Raw fruits, raw vegetables, raw nuts
Response to heat, acid, digestive enzymes	Stable	Labile

Source: Data are from Yasuto K, Atsuo U. Oral allergy syndrome. *Allergol Int.* 2009;58:485-491.

Foods Frequently Associated with Allergy

Although any food protein can be potentially allergenic, relatively few are known to cause most allergic reactions. In addition, an allergenic protein can only induce an allergic reaction in an atopic person who has been sensitized to it. As previously mentioned, most of the severe allergic reactions to foods occur in response to a surprisingly small number of foods.

■   The foods most commonly associated with allergic reactions in children are milk, egg, wheat, soy, peanut, tree nuts, and sometimes fish and shellfish.

■   Allergies to milk, egg, wheat, and soy are often outgrown in early childhood.

■   Adults tend to experience allergic reactions to the foods that persist as allergens beyond infancy, predominantly peanuts, tree nuts, shellfish, and certain species of fish.

■   Oral allergy syndrome is more common in adults than in children. The foods that most frequently elicit symptoms depend on the inhalant allergen to which the person is sensitized (for details of these foods, see Chapter 33).

■   In people allergic to latex, foods with allergens that are structurally homologous with latex allergens are those most frequently associated with allergy (see Chapter 34).

Allergens Eliciting Allergy via the Digestive Tract

Lists of the most allergenic foods in which the primary route of sensitization and response is via the digestive tract vary according to the source of the data and differ between countries, probably indicating a cultural bias.

In general, the top eight allergenic foods include:

■   Peanut and peanut products
■   Soy and soy products
■   Egg and egg products
■   Milk and milk products
■   Tree nuts and tree nut products: the most allergenic of these are almond, Brazil nut, cashew, filbert (hazelnut), macadamia, pecan, pine nut, pistachio, and walnut.
■   Fish and fish products (not all species of fish have the same allergenicity)
■   Shellfish: crustaceans (shrimp, prawn, lobster, crab, crayfish) and mollusks (clams, mussels, oysters, scallops)
■   Wheat and wheat products

However, the severity of reactions associated with these foods varies. For example:

■   Peanuts, tree nuts, shellfish, fish, milk, and egg account for most reported cases of anaphylactic reactions in children and adults in Western countries.

▪ Soy is less frequently reported as a highly allergenic food, although it is often associated with severe cases of allergy and atopic dermatitis in childhood.

▪ Wheat allergy (quite distinct from gluten-sensitive enteropathy or celiac disease, which is not usually considered to be an allergic condition) is usually mild. However, wheat tends to be the food most frequently associated with food-associated exercise-induced anaphylaxis (see Chapter 4).

Other allergenic foods, present on some lists, absent on others include:

▪ Sesame seed and products containing sesame seed
▪ Mustard seed
▪ Lupine
▪ Celery
▪ Corn

Food additives rarely cause IgE-mediated hypersensitivity reactions and therefore do not appear on allergen lists. The exception is sulfite, which is included on many food allergen lists.

Relatedness of Allergens

Cross-reactivity among foods in the same botanic or zoological family is uncommon. For example, cross-reactivity among members of the legume family (peanuts, soy, peas, beans, lentils, etc) is uncommon, and allergic individuals usually demonstrate hypersensitivity to only one or two of this group. Dietary restriction of all members of a botanic family when a person is allergic to one is unjustified and may lead to nutritional deficiencies; for instance, if a person is allergic to peanuts, it is not necessary to exclude all legumes from his or her diet. Each food needs to be tested separately.

Shellfish tends to be an exception to this generalization. Crustaceans such as crab, lobster, prawns, shrimp, and similar shellfish do seem to exhibit a high degree of antigenic cross-reactivity. In addition, there is evidence that people who are sensitive to crustaceans are typically more likely than the general population to be allergic to mollusks, which include mussels, clams, scallops, winkles, squid, edible snails, and so on. Individuals who are allergic to these types of shellfish are advised to avoid *all* shellfish.

The same restrictions usually do not always apply to finfish (free-swimming species, such as salmon, trout, white fish, etc), which do not exhibit the same degree of cross-reactivity: hypersensitivity to each bony fish seems to be species-specific, unless the allergy is to a parvalbumin, which occurs in all fish species in differing amounts. Parvalbumin serves the same function in all types of fish and is localized in their fast-contracting muscles, brain, and some endocrine tissues. If a person is sensitized to parvalbumin, it is likely that he or she will need to avoid all types of fish.[12]

Polysensitization (multiple sensitization) to various fish species is linked to reactivity to their parvalbumins. The degree of allergy (reactivity) to different species is likely due to the level of the parvalbumin; for example, amounts of parvalbumins from cod were recorded as 20 times and from whiff 30 times higher than from swordfish, which may explain the higher allergenicity of cod compared to other species of fish, such as swordfish.[13]

Panallergens

The panallergen concept encompasses families of related proteins, which are involved in general vital processes and are thus widely distributed throughout nature. Plant panallergens share molecules with the same structure and function. They are responsible for many IgE cross-reactions even between unrelated pollen and plant food allergen sources. Although panallergens are usually considered minor allergens, sensitization to them might be problematic, as there is the risk of developing multiple sensitizations.[14]

Known panallergens presently comprise only a few protein families, including profilins, polcalcins, and nonspecific lipid transfer proteins (nsLTP). Multiple allergies to both pollen and food allergen sources seem to be determined by sensitization to such allergens.[15] This is discussed in more detail in Chapter 33.

The list of panallergens and foods with related allergenic molecules will likely expand as research uncovers more details about the molecular structure of allergens and the immunological response to them. In the meantime, a few attempts have been made to predict the likelihood of a person who is allergic to one type of food to be reactive to others with similar structures. A 2001 publication[16] provides a list of the degree of risk for several foods. If a person is allergic to:

- A legume such as peanut, there is a 5% risk that he or she would be allergic to other legumes
- A tree nut such as walnut, there is a 37% risk that he or she would be allergic to other tree nuts
- Fish such as salmon, there is a 50% risk that he or she would be allergic to other fish
- Shellfish such as shrimp, there is a 75% risk that he or she would be allergic to other shellfish
- A grain such as wheat, there is a 20% risk that he or she would be allergic to other grains
- Cow's milk, there is a 92% risk that he or she would be allergic to goat's milk, but only a 4% risk of allergy to mare's milk
- Pollen from birch or ragweed, there is a 55% risk that he or she would be allergic to certain fruits and vegetables
- A peach, there is a 55% risk that he or she would be allergic to other fruits in the rose (*Rosaceae*) family

■ Melon, there is a 92% risk that he or she would be allergic to fruits such as banana, watermelon, and avocado

■ Latex, there is a 35% risk that he or she would be allergic to fruits such as kiwi, banana, and avocado

■ Fruits such as kiwi, banana, and avocado, there is an 11% risk that he or she would be allergic to latex

Quantity of Food Required to Cause an Allergic Reaction

The amount of food that needs to be ingested in order to cause an allergic reaction depends on the potency of the allergen and the individual's response to it. The notion of threshold doses is common in the field of toxicology, where animal experimentation and epidemiological studies allow determination of the level at which no adverse effect is observed—the no observed adverse effect level (NOAEL). There is no measure of nonreactivity to an allergen (NOAEL), so the majority of studies report the lowest dosage required to elicit symptoms in the smallest number of subjects in a sample population (LOAEL—lowest observed adverse effect level).

In the case of food allergy, neither animal models nor epidemiological studies help to determine the range of reactive doses in humans.[17] No studies have determined a "safe dose" for any food allergen. Therefore, minimal reactive doses are measured based on the LOAEL. LOAELs are expressed in quantity of allergen causing a reaction in the smallest measured percentage of a sensitive population. In addition, the LOAEL varies significantly among atopic individuals, so it is not possible to specify a minimal dosage of an allergenic food that will elicit symptoms in a population.

An example of this measurement system is reported thus:[9] Data from 125 positive oral challenges to egg, peanut, milk, and sesame seeds indicated the LOAEL for each food to be less than:

■ 2 mg egg
■ 5 mg peanut
■ 0.1 mL milk
■ 30 mg sesame seed

In manufactured foods, the detection limits for each allergen was determined to be:[18]

■ 10 ppm egg to ensure the safety of 99% of people allergic to egg
■ 24 ppm peanut to ensure the safety of 96% of people allergic to peanut
■ 30 ppm milk to ensure the safety of 98% of people allergic to milk

The Food and Drug Administration (FDA) Ad Hoc Committee on Hypersensitivity to Food Constituents attempted to define "allergenic levels" of foods in their 1986 report:[19]

- The usual amount of food that produces an allergic reaction in a sensitized adult is 20 g.
- Shrimp allergy will be provoked with 1 to 2 g of shrimp.
- Peanut allergy can be precipitated by as little as 25 mg of peanut.

A few studies[20] have attempted to define a specific threshold level for a variety of food allergens; for example:

- An open food challenge of ovalbumin determined that 10 mg was required to elicit symptoms in egg-allergic children.
- Challenge testing with increasing quantities of allergenic food has demonstrated that 6 mg of cod was required to elicit symptoms.
- The amount of peanut required to elicit an allergic reaction in another test was reported to be 0.1 to 0.2 mg.

However, there are reports that inhalation of food components (such as being in a room where fish is being cooked) or merely handling the food can precipitate a reaction in highly sensitive individuals.[21] As more sophisticated analytical tools become available, more data on this subject likely will be collected. In the meantime, the directive is that all sources of the most highly allergenic foods, especially those that have been demonstrated to cause a severe or anaphylactic reaction in an individual, should be completely avoided. To achieve this, a sensitive individual must be aware of:

- All types of natural foods that contain the allergen
- All terms in a food ingredient list that indicate the presence of the allergen or its derivatives (refer to individual chapters on food allergens for complete details)
- Foods and nonfood products that are likely to contain the culprit allergen

Additives Derived from Potentially Allergenic Foods

In a number of cases, ingredients in processed and manufactured foods are derived from natural food sources, but information about their origins is sometimes difficult to access. Table 2.2 provides examples of some common ingredients and their food origins.[22] This list is by no means exhaustive. Highly sensitive individuals are encouraged to obtain information from food manufacturers concerning hidden sources of their particular allergens and to become familiar with terms on food ingredient labels that would indicate the presence of their allergens.

TABLE 2.2
Sources of Additives in Common Foods: Presence of Potential Allergens

Name of Additive	Sources (Potential Allergens)	Foods Likely to Contain Additive	Function in Foods
Lecithin	• Egg • Egg yolk • Soy beans • Corn	• Ready-to-eat break-fast cereals • Candy • Chocolates • Bread • Rolls • Buns • Margarines	Antioxidant and emollient Composed of choline, phosphoric acid, fatty acids, glycerin
Starch	• Wheat • Potatoes • Rice • Corn • Beans • Other plants The plant source may not be identified on an ingredient label	"Thickened" or "creamed" products	Thickening agent in a number of manufac-tured foods Usually used in its "modified" form
Modified starch	• Derived from plants (above) and modified with acid to make the starch more digestible	• Baby foods • Nonfood products such as dusting and face powders, baby powders, and bath salts	Present in foods as bleached starch; acetylated distarch adipate; distarch phosphate; others with "distarch" in the name
Carotene (provitamin A; beta-carotene)	Carrots	• Margarines • Butter • Shortening • Fat-free milk • Buttermilk • Cottage cheese • Beet juice • A number of red-colored foods	Coloring agent A source of vitamin A in "enriched" foods
Annato (bixin; norbixin)	Extract from the seed of a tropical tree, *Bixa orellana*	• Dairy products (cheese, butter) • Breakfast cereals • Baked goods • Margarines • Meat-product cas-ings (eg, bologna, frankfurters) • Beverages • Ice cream	Coloring agent (yellow to pink) Spice flavoring

Continues

TABLE 2.2

Sources of Additives in Common Foods: Presence of Potential Allergens (*Continued*)

Name of Additive	Sources (Potential Allergens)	Foods Likely to Contain Additive	Function in Foods
Hydrolyzed vegetable protein (HVP) Hydrolyzed plant protein (HPP)	• Soy beans (soy; the most frequently used source) • Peanuts • Wheat • Corn	• Soups • Meat-based entrées • Stews • Flavoring and seasoning mixes	Flavor enhancer Plant protein is hydrolyzed (broken down) by enzymes or acids High glutamate and salt content (high MSG)
Carrageenan	Algae (seaweed) "Irish moss"	• Milk products • Pressure-dispensed "whipped cream" • Cheese spreads • Ice cream • Custards • Sherbets • Salad dressings • Sauces • Chocolates and chocolate products • Artificially sweetened jams and jellies	Emulsifier (blender) and stabilizer, prevents separation of ingredients Thickening agent; gelling agent
Malt extract	Germinated barley	• Beers • Meat and poultry products • Ice cream • Flavored milks • Sour cream • Chocolate syrup • Candy • Cough drops • Condiments • Salad dressings • Breakfast cereals	Flavoring agent
Xanthan gum	Product of the fermentation of dextrose (derived from corn syrup) by the microorganism *Xanthomonas campestris*	• Dairy products • Salad dressings • May replace starch, sugar, and oil in low-calorie products • Xanthan gum is not digested by the body and passes out mostly unchanged	Thickener, stabilizer, emulsifier, suspending agent Prevents ingredients from separating
Locust bean gum	Carob seed	• Ice creams • Sauces • Salad dressings • Sausages (acts as a binder)	Thickening and stabilizing agent Used to blend ingredients and prevent separation Binding agent Texture modifier

References

1. Burks AW, Jones SM, Boyce JA, et al. NIAID-sponsored 2010 guidelines for managing food allergy: applications in the pediatric population. *Pediatrics.* 2011 Nov;128(5):955-965.

2. Sampson HA. Food allergy. Part 1: Immunopathogenesis and clinical disorders. Current reviews of allergy and clinical immunology. *J Allergy Clin Immunol.* 1999;103(5 pt 1):717-728.

3. Johansson SGO, Hourihane JOB, Bousquet J, et al. A revised nomenclature for allergy. An EAACI position statement from the EAACI nomenclature task force. *Allergy.* 2001;56:813-824.

4. Boyce JA, Assa'ad A, Burks AW, et al. Guidelines for the diagnosis and management of food allergy in the United States: report of the NIAID-sponsored expert panel. *J Allergy Clin Immunol.* 2010;126(6):S1-S58 (section 2.1.1).

5. Sicherer SH, Sampson HA. Food allergy. *J Allergy Clin Immunol.* 2010;125(2 suppl 2):S116-S125.

6. Traidl-Hoffmann C, Jakob T, Behrendt H. Determinants of allergenicity. *J Allergy Clin Immunol.* 2009;123(3):558-566.

7. Food Allergy Research Resource Program (FARRP) database. Department of Food Science and Technology at the University of Nebraska in Lincoln. http://www.allergenonline .com.

8. Van Loon LC, Van Strien EA. The families of pathogenesis-related proteins, their activities, and comparative analysis of PR-1 type proteins. *Physiol Molec Plant Pathol.* 1999;55:85-97.

9. Amlot PL, Kemeny DM, Zachary C, Parkes P, Lessof MH. Oral allergy syndrome (OAS): symptoms of IgE-mediated hypersensitivity to foods. *Clin Allergy.* 1987;17:33-42.

10. Sampson HA. Food allergy. Part 1: Immunopathogenesis and clinical disorders. Current reviews of allergy and clinical immunology. *J Allergy Clin Immunol.* 1999;103(5 pt 1):717-728.

11. Yasuto K, Atsuo U. Oral allergy syndrome. *Allergol Int.* 2009;58:485-491.

12. Griesmeier U, Vázquez-Cortés S, Bublin M, et al. Expression levels of parvalbumins determine allergenicity of fish species. *Allergy.* 2010;65(2):191-198.

13. Griesmeier U, Vázquez-Cortés S, Bublin M, et al. Expression levels of parvalbumins determine allergenicity of fish species. *Allergy.* 2010;65(2):191-198.

14. Hauser M, Roulias A, Ferreira F, Egger M. Panallergens and their impact on the allergic patient. *Allergy Asthma Clin Immunol.* 2010;6(1):1.

15. Mari A. Multiple pollen sensitization: a molecular approach to the diagnosis. *Int Arch Allergy Immunol.* 2001;125:57-65.

16. Sicherer SH. Clinical implications of cross-reactive food allergens. *J Allergy Clin Immunol.* 2001;108(6):881-890.

17. Moneret-Vautrin DA, Kanny G. Update on threshold doses of food allergens: implications for patients and the food industry. *Curr Opin Allergy Clin Immunol.* 2004;4(3):215-219.

18. Morisset M, Moneret-Vautrin DA, Kanny G, et al. Thresholds of clinical reactivity to milk, egg, peanut and sesame in immunoglobulin E-dependent allergies: evaluation by double-blind or single-blind placebo-controlled oral challenges. *Clin Exp Allergy.* 2003; 33(8):1046-1051.

19. Food and Drug Administration Ad Hoc Committee on Hypersensitivity to Food Constituents. *Report*. Washington, DC: Food and Drug Administration; 1986.

20. Crevel RW, Ballmer-Weber BK, Holzhauser T, et al. Thresholds for food allergens and their value to different stakeholders. *Allergy*. 2008;63(5):597-609.

21. Roberts G, Golder N, Leack G. Bronchial challenges with aerosolized food in asthmatic, food-allergic children. *Allergy*. 2002;57:713-717.

22. Winter R. *A Consumer's Dictionary of Food Additives*. 7th ed. New York, NY: Three Rivers Press; 2009.

CHAPTER 3

Food Intolerances

An adverse reaction to food that results in clinical symptoms but is not caused by an immune system reaction is classified as *food intolerance*. In contrast to food allergy, which is the immune system's response to antigenic proteins, food intolerance is usually triggered by small-molecular-weight chemical substances and biologically active components of foods. The physiological mechanisms that are responsible for these reactions can be diverse and complex, and many are presently poorly understood.

Classification of Nonimmunologically Mediated Adverse Reactions to Foods

Nonimmunologically mediated adverse reactions to foods may, for convenience, be classified into three main categories:

- Metabolic dysfunction (eg, enzyme dysfunction such as lactase deficiency causing lactose intolerance)
- Pharmacological responses (eg, a reaction to a pharmacologically active agent such as histamine or tyramine in food)
- Reactions with incompletely understood mechanisms (eg, sensitivity to food additives such as sulfites, benzoates, tartrazine and other azo dyes, monosodium glutamate [MSG])

Some classification schemes[1] include toxic reactions, such as food poisoning due to microbial toxins, and food aversions. However, in this discussion, food intolerances are limited to those that result from an idiosyncratic response that is experienced as a result of individual deficiencies in metabolism, absorption, or other anomalies in the body's handling of food.

Although convenient for classification purposes, the categories defined earlier are not easily separated in practice. Often, a reaction that may be classified in one category because of the symptoms (effect) may have its cause in another. For example, a response to a pharmacologically active agent such as tyramine or histamine may be caused by a reduced ability of an enzyme to break down the chemical—in the case of tyramine, a reduction in monoamine oxidase, or in the case of histamine, a reduction in diamine oxidase. In other words, the cause is an enzyme deficiency; the effect is a pharmacological response.

Food Intolerances as Dose-Related

Food intolerances are dose-related, meaning that the higher the dose of the intolerance trigger, the more severe the symptoms. In practice, most—if not all—intolerance reactions would occur in any individual if the level of the inciting dietary factor were sufficiently high. However, everyone has their own unique limit of tolerance, often dependent upon the amount of enzyme produced to maintain the metabolite within the normal range. When a person develops symptoms at a much lower level than in the majority of the population, he or she is intolerant to the food or food ingredient.

An example of this distinction is scombroid fish poisoning or toxicity. When fish such as mahimahi, tuna, mackerel, sardines, or anchovies are not properly processed or stored, they may start to decay, and high levels of histamine can develop within the fish. Bacteria in the gut of the fish (typically *Morganella morganii*) convert histidine in the fish protein to histamine by means of the enzyme histidine decarboxylase. When the level of histamine is extremely high, anyone eating the fish will become ill; typical symptoms include skin flushing, throbbing headache, oral burning, abdominal pain, nausea, diarrhea, drop in blood pressure, palpitations, a sense of unease, and occasionally collapse or loss of vision. The symptoms of poisoning can show anywhere from within minutes up to 2 hours following consumption of the fish, and usually last for approximately 4 to 6 hours and rarely exceed 1 to 2 days. However, histamine intolerance, or more accurately, sensitivity, occurs in sensitive people after consuming foods that have a much lower level of histamine, to which the majority of the population will not react adversely. They develop the symptoms listed earlier after the level of histamine in the body exceeds their limit of tolerance.

Many food intolerance reactions can be explained on the basis of metabolic dysfunction or pharmacological ("druglike") responses to components of foods that may be naturally occurring, added to foods, or arise during their manufacture. In many cases, the mechanism responsible for the adverse response is not clearly defined. The reactions discussed in this chapter provide an overview of the research findings and current understanding of a few of the more common causes of food intolerance. Refer to Table 3.1 for examples of the factors frequently implicated in food intolerance reactions; these are discussed in individual chapters in Parts III and IV.

TABLE 3.1

Factors Most Frequently Implicated in Food Intolerance Reactions

Intolerance Factors	Site of Action	Symptoms Associated with Intolerance	Type of Foods Represented	Discussion and Management
Carbohydrates: disaccharides (lactose, sucrose, maltose) and monosaccharide (fructose)	Digestive tract	• Excessive gas • Abdominal bloating • Abdominal pain • Diarrhea, loose stool • Occasional nausea • Occasional vomiting	• Sugars • Starches • Polysaccharides	Disaccharide Intolerance (Chapter 23) Lactose Intolerance (Chapter 11) Fructose Intolerance (Chapter 24)
Biogenic amines: histamine, tyramine	Systemic, but with localized foci	• Skin (hives, angioedema, itching, reddening) • Mucous membranes (itching, swelling, reddening) • Headaches • Digestive tract disturbances • Migraine headache • Hives • Itching	• Fermented foods • Alcoholic beverages • Some vegetables and fruits • Some spices • Some artificial colors • Some preservatives • Fermented foods • Alcoholic beverages (eg, red wine) • Vinegars • Yeast extract • Some vegetables and fruits • Chicken liver	Histamine Sensitivity (Chapter 31) Tyramine Sensitivity (Chapter 32)
Salicylates	Systemic: Inhibition of cyclooxygenase pathway and imbalance in inflammatory mediators	• Hives • Angioedema • Asthma in people with asthma • People sensitive to aspirin at particular risk for developing symptoms of intolerance	• Mostly naturally occurring in a variety of foods, including many fruits and vegetables, some spices	Salicylate Intolerance (Chapter 26)
Artificial colors: tartrazine and other azo dyes	Systemic: • Inhibition of cyclooxygenase pathway and imbalance in inflammatory mediators • Release of histamine	• Asthma in people with asthma, especially aspirin-sensitive people with asthma • Hives • Nausea • Headaches • Rashes • Hyperactivity in a few sensitive individuals	• Manufactured foods • Do not occur naturally	Intolerance of Tartrazine and Other Food Colors (Chapter 27)
Benzoates	Unknown. Suggested to be due to inhibition of the cyclooxygenase pathway, release of histamine, and imbalance in inflammatory mediators	• Asthma in people with asthma • Hives • Angioedema • Nasal congestion • Headache • Skin irritation (contact dermatitis) • Digestive tract disturbances	• Manufactured foods as antimicrobial preservatives; color preservatives; bleaching agent • Naturally occurring in foods such as berries, cinnamon and a few other spices, tea, prunes	Benzoate Intolerance (Chapter 25)

Continues

TABLE 3.1
Factors Most Frequently Implicated in Food Intolerance Reactions (*Continued*)

Intolerance Factors	Site of Action	Symptoms Associated with Intolerance	Type of Foods Represented	Discussion and Management
Butylated hydroxyanisole (BHA); butylated hydroxytoluene (BHT)	Unknown	Usually skin reactions, such as hives	• Manufactured foods as antioxidants for delaying rancidity in fats, oils, and fat-containing foods • Often used in treatment of food packaging materials (eg, cereal packaging)	Intolerance of BHA and BHT (Chapter 28)
Sulfites	Systemic and local: lungs	• Asthma in people with asthma • Reactions in skin and mucous membranes • Anaphylaxis in people with asthma	• Manufactured foods as antimicrobial preservative, especially on grapes where mold occurs naturally; as color preservative, to control browning, especially in dried fruits, cut potatoes, apples, coconut; as bleaching agent in maraschino cherries, glacé fruits, and citron peel; and as texturizer, especially for frozen, uncooked dough • Used in fermentation control in wine and other alcoholic beverage manufacture	Sulfite Sensitivity (Chapter 21)
Monosodium glutamate (MSG)	Systemic	• Suggest involvement of the central nervous system, such as flushing, facial numbness, tingling and numbness in hands and feet, tightening of the chest, dizziness, balance problems, blurring of vision, visual disturbances, "psychological" reactions • Asthma in people with asthma • Digestive tract disturbances	• Manufactured foods with "added flavor"; added as a flavor enhancer to cooked natural foods • Glutamates occur naturally in some foods, such as cheeses, mushrooms, and tomatoes	MSG Sensitivity (Chapter 30)

Reference

1. Boyce JA, Assa'ad A, Burks AW, et al. Guidelines for the diagnosis and management of food allergy in the United States: report of the NIAID-sponsored expert panel. *J Allergy Clin Immunol.* 2010;126(6):S1-S58.

PART II

Determining the Offending Foods: Diagnosis

CHAPTER **4**

Symptoms of Food Allergy

Because there are currently no reliable laboratory tests that can unequivocally iden-tify the precise food responsible for a person's allergy or intolerance symptoms, controversy exists among medical practitioners as to which symptoms are caused by food allergy or by intolerance of foods or food additives and which are not.

The medical community universally acknowledges that conditions such as hay fever, asthma, and atopic conjunctivitis are often triggered by airborne allergens; that hives, mouth and facial swelling, throat tightening, and itching can result from food allergies; and that rashes can result from direct contact with allergens such as nickel, latex, and poison ivy. Anaphylactic reactions to injected allergens such as x-ray dyes, local anesthetics, and wasp and bee stings are well recognized. Anaphy-lactic reactions to foods, although rare, are always headline news.

However, the popular literature will often report on an array of symptoms that are purported to be due to "food allergy." In fact, it is difficult to cite a symptom that has not been ascribed to this cause. Often, traditional medical practitioners discount many so called subjective symptoms, which depend on anecdotal reports from the per-son with the symptoms. When symptoms cannot be validated by standard laboratory tests, they are sometimes written off as psychological in nature, resulting in frustration and resentment on the part of both patient and doctor. (Note: Details of symptoms specifically associated with pediatric food allergy are discussed in Chapter 42.)

Site of Symptoms of Adverse Reactions

Traditionally, the lungs and respiratory tract, the digestive tract, and the skin and mucous membranes have been targeted as sites of reactivity to antigens in the atopic response. However, as knowledge has progressed, it is increasingly apparent that ad-verse reactions to foreign antigens and "reactive chemicals" can occur in any organ system.[1] Box 4.1 summarizes the types of reactions presently accepted as possibly due to adverse reactions to allergens, when all other causes for the pathology have been ruled out.[1]

BOX 4.1   Examples of Allergic Conditions and Symptoms

Respiratory tract
Allergic or perennial rhinitis (stuffy nose, hay fever)
Rhinorrhea (runny nose)
Allergic conjunctivitis (itchy, watery, reddened eyes)
Serous otitis media (earache with effusion)
Asthma, bronchospasm
Laryngeal edema (throat tightening due to swelling of tissues)

Skin and mucous membranes
Atopic dermatitis (eczema)
Urticaria (hives)
Angioedema (swelling of deeper tissues, especially the mouth and face)
Pruritus (itching of skin, eyes, ears, mouth)
Contact dermatitis
Oral allergy syndrome (OAS)

Digestive tract
Diarrhea
Constipation
Nausea and vomiting
Abdominal bloating and distention
Abdominal pain
Indigestion
Belching

Nervous system
Migraine
Other headaches
Spots before the eyes
Listlessness
Hyperactivity
Lack of concentration
Tension-fatigue syndrome
Irritability
Chilliness
Dizziness

Other
Frequent urination
Bed-wetting
Excessive sweating
Pallor
Hoarseness
Dark circles around the eyes
Muscle aches
Low-grade fever

Anaphylactic Reactions to Foods

An anaphylactic reaction can be defined as a severe reaction of rapid onset, involving most organ systems and resulting in circulatory collapse and a drop in blood pressure.[2] In the most extreme cases, the reaction progresses to anaphylactic shock with cardiovascular collapse, resulting in death. Because of the risks associated with such a reaction, anyone at risk of severe food allergy and their caregivers should be aware of the signs suggesting the potential for anaphylaxis and the dietary measures necessary for its prevention.[3]

Incidence of Anaphylaxis

The true incidence of anaphylaxis is unknown. Some clinicians reserve the term for the full-blown syndrome (see details of symptoms of anaphylaxis later), whereas others use it to describe milder cases.[4] Anaphylactic reactions to foods are reported less frequently than anaphylactic reactions to nonfood triggers such as medications; radiocontrast dyes used in diagnostic procedures; injected anesthetics; and wasp, bee, and insect stings. A 2001 report[5] estimated that 1% to 15% of the global population is at risk of experiencing an anaphylactic reaction to all triggers of anaphylaxis. The estimated rate of actual anaphylaxis to food was reported as 0.0004%, 0.7% to 10% to penicillin, 0.22% to 1% to radiocontrast media (RCM), and 0.5% to 5% to insect stings.

However, statistics from the United States present a different picture. A population-based study from Rochester, Minnesota,[6] found that ingestion of a specific food was responsible for 33%, insect stings were responsible for 18.5%, and medications were responsible for 13.7% of reported cases of anaphylaxis. In a study of patients referred to an allergy-immunology practice in Memphis, Tennessee,[7] food was the cause of anaphylaxis in 34% of patients, medications in 20%, and exercise (exercise-induced anaphylaxis [EIA]; see discussion beginning on page 46 for details) in 7%.

Symptoms of an Anaphylactic Reaction to Food[8,9]

The first symptoms may be in the mouth, with burning, itching, or irritation of the lips, mouth, and throat. This may be followed by nausea, vomiting, abdominal pain, and diarrhea as the food enters the digestive system. Digestive tract symptoms are reported in 40% of cases. As the food antigen enters the general circulation, a feeling of being unwell, anxious, warm, itchy, or faint develop, and sometimes nasal irritation and sneezing occur. Anxiety, mental confusion, lethargy, and in some cases seizures may happen. Skin reactions, which are reported in the majority (80% to 90%) of patients, include flushing, hives, itching, and angioedema. Throat tightening, chest tightness, bronchospasm, difficulty breathing, rhinitis, voice hoarseness, and irritated eyes might occur but may be absent in some cases. The pulse may be rapid, weak, irregular, and difficult to detect.

In severe cases, these symptoms are rapidly followed by loss of consciousness, and death may occur from suffocation (due to edema of the larynx, epiglottis, and pharynx) or from shock and cardiac arrhythmia. Death may occur within minutes of ingesting the offending food and is often a result of respiratory failure. People who have asthma are at greatest risk for severe reactions.[10]

Not all of these symptoms occur in each case of anaphylaxis, and they may appear in any order. The previous description refers to the response most commonly experienced.

Patterns of Anaphylactic Reactions

Severe reactions occur within minutes and up to 1 hour after food ingestion, but the onset of a reaction may be delayed for up to 2 hours. Attempts at delineation of reaction patterns and prediction of outcomes for anaphylactic reactions suggest that the reaction may be divided into uniphasic and biphasic reactions:[11]

▪ *Uniphasic* reactions are described as occurring immediately after an encounter with the allergen and resolve within a few minutes or hours. They do not recur within that anaphylactic episode.

▪ *Biphasic* reactions refer to a recurrence of symptoms after the initial response seems to have abated. Such reactions typically occur from 8 to 72 hours after the first reaction. The incidence of biphasic reactions has been documented as 1% to 20% in different reports.[12]

▪ A *protracted* reaction is defined as a reaction that persists for hours or days following the initial reaction.[13]

Unfortunately, it is not easy to predict the outcome of any anaphylactic reaction to food, so practitioners need to be aware of the different patterns of response that may appear and be ready to respond both initially and to a biphasic reaction should it occur. In a significant number of reported cases of anaphylactic reactions to foods, the person was asthmatic, indicating that people with asthma are more likely than the general population to experience anaphylactic reactions to foods.[14] This potential for an anaphylactic reaction increases when the patient is receiving desensitization injections and is allergic to wasp and bee venom. In most cases, the later the onset of symptoms following food ingestion, the less severe the reaction is likely to be.

Foods Responsible for Anaphylactic Reactions

Almost any food can cause an anaphylactic reaction (see Box 4.2), but the foods most commonly responsible include peanuts, nuts, shellfish, fish, cow's milk, and eggs.[15] Anaphylactic reactions to cow's milk, egg, wheat, and chicken have most often occurred in children under the age of 3 years.

Food-Dependent Exercise-Induced Anaphylaxis

Food-dependent exercise-induced anaphylaxis (FDEIA) is rare and occurs only when an individual eats a food that contains an allergen to which he or she is hypersensitive and exercises within 3 to 4 hours after eating. Consuming the same food without exercise does not elicit any symptoms.

FDEIA is considered to be a subtype of exercise-induced anaphylaxis (EIA), which is characterized by airway obstruction, urticaria, and hypotension following exercise.[16] Other symptoms may include angioedema, gastrointestinal symptoms, bronchial constriction, and vascular collapse.[17]

In most cases, specific foods cause anaphylaxis when exercise follows ingestion but are tolerated when ingestion of these foods is not followed by exercise (specific FDEIA). In other cases, EIA results from exercise following consumption of any meal, regardless of the food eaten (nonspecific FDEIA).

BOX 4.2 Examples of Foods Specifically Reported to Cause Anaphylactic Reactions[a]

Nuts
- Pecan
- Pistachio
- Cashew
- Brazil

Legumes
- Peanut

Seeds
- Millet
- Sunflower
- Sesame
- Flax
- Psyllium

Shellfish
- Crab
- Shrimp
- Lobster
- Limpet

Fish
- Cod
- Halibut
- Fish gelatin
- Seal meat
- Whale meat

Grains
- Wheat
- Rice
- Quinoa

Vegetables
- Potato
- Celery
- Pea
- Pinto bean
- Soy
- Chickpea
- Corn

Fruit
- Orange
- Tangerine
- Mango
- Banana
- Kiwi fruit

Milk products
- Cow's milk (usually in children under 5 years)
- Milk products such as cheese, ice cream

Poultry
- Chicken

Egg
- Chicken egg

Beverages
- Chamomile tea
- Wine

[a]This list gives examples only and does not include every food that is capable of inducing an anaphylactic reaction. Anaphylactic reactions are entirely individual.

In specific FDEIA, an IgE-mediated mechanism is usually responsible; skin-prick tests are positive and IgE food-specific antibodies can be detected in the patient's serum.[5] Serum histamine and tryptase levels are increased during symptomatic attacks, indicating the release of inflammatory mediators from mast cells induced by IgE-mediated degranulation.[18]

Incidence of FDEIA

Only rare epidemiological data about the frequency of FDEIA are available, but case reports of incidents of the condition have increased over the past 20 years, possibly reflecting an increased popularity of exercise in the general population[19] as well as an increased awareness of the condition.

The first published case report of FDEIA appeared in 1979. A 31-year-old male developed anaphylaxis after consuming shrimp or oysters up to 24 hours before long-distance running events. Since then, numerous other case reports of FDEIA have been published.[20]

FDEIA seems to be twice as common in females than in males and is especially prevalent in individuals 25 to 35 years of age. Individuals experiencing this type of reaction typically have asthma and other allergic conditions.[21]

Foods Associated with FDEIA

Although any food may contribute to this form of anaphylaxis, foods that have been reported most frequently as triggers of FDEIA include wheat, shellfish, fruit, milk, celery, and fish. However, the frequency that specific foods have been reported indicates that there may be differences in eliciting factors among countries. For example, European and Japanese reports indicate wheat to be the most common food involved in FDEIA,[16] whereas wheat accounts for only 5% of cases in the United States, with shellfish being highest at 16%, followed by alcohol (11%), tomato (8%), cheese (8%), celery (7%), strawberries (5%), wheat (5%), peach (5%), and milk (4%).[22] A list of foods reported to trigger FDEIA is provided in Box 4.3.[23,24]

Allergens in Food Associated with FDEIA

A few recent studies have sought to identify the specific allergens in foods that trigger FDEIA. It seems that the allergens in the foods associated with FDEIA may differ from those previously identified as causing other forms of allergy, including anaphylaxis. For example, soluble proteins in wheat have been identified as allergens in baker's asthma, whereas insoluble proteins (gluten) are allergens for wheat-dependent exercise-induced anaphylaxis.[22] Wheat-gamma-gliadin was determined to be the presumptive allergen in two cases of wheat-associated exercise-induced anaphylaxis (WAEIA)[25] and wheat-omega-5-gliadin in four cases of WAEIA[26] in separate Japanese studies. There is increasing evidence for the important role of omega-5-gliadin in WAEIA to the extent that the allergen is being promoted as a marker in the differential diagnosis of the condition.[25]

In addition to the native allergen, the antigenicity of gluten seems to be increased during digestion in individuals with WAEIA. When the wheat was digested with pepsin, the antigenicity of the gluten was increased, but it decreased when digested with trypsin. This suggests that the antigenicity of gluten is enhanced in the stomach and attenuated in the duodenum. Based on these observations, it is hypothesized that

---

BOX 4.3 Frequently Reported Foods Associated with FDEIA, by Food Group

Grains
Barley
Buckwheat
Corn
Oats
Rice
Rye
Wheat

Shellfish and seafood
Crab
Cuttlefish
Octopus
Oyster
Shrimp
Squid

Poultry
Chicken

Nuts and seeds
Hazelnut
Almond
Mustard
Poppy seed
Walnut

Legumes
Soy bean
Peanut

Fruit
Apple
Grape
Kiwi
Lychee
Orange
Peach
Pear
Strawberry

Vegetables
Cabbage
Celery
Fennel
Garlic[23]
Lettuce
Matsutake mushroom
Onion[24]
Potato
Tomato

Egg
Chicken egg

Milk
Cheese
Milk

Beverages
Alcohol

Other
Snail

---

exercise might induce an increase in mucosal absorption of food peptides, including pepsin-digested gluten, in the small intestine before trypsin in the duodenum has an opportunity to act on the protein. This situation would then result in an enhanced allergen entering the circulation and triggering IgE-mediated allergy in sensitized individuals.[27]

Mechanism Responsible for FDEIA

The physiological and immunological mechanisms responsible for FDEIA are presently only partially understood. It seems that exercise triggers an anaphylactic reaction in those who have IgE-mediated allergy specific for certain foods. In addition to the presence of the allergen, several other factors may be involved in the reaction:[28]

- Involvement of the autonomic nervous system
- Intake of certain drugs
- Weather conditions
- Humidity
- Stress
- Inherited factors
- Menstruation cycle
- General physical condition of the individual
- Concomitant intake of aspirin, nonsteroidal anti-inflammatory drugs (NSAID), and some other medications[29]

It has also been suggested that exercise might change the efficiency of absorption of the allergen as a result of changes in blood flow through the major vessels and organs.[30] A dysfunction of the autonomic nervous system and the ability of gastrin to increase cutaneous mast cell mediator release have also been hypothesized as contributing to the onset of symptoms.[30]

Diagnosis of FDEIA

The diagnosis of FDEIA is usually made on the basis of the individual's history. Development of signs of anaphylaxis during exercise, often starting with urticaria (hives), pruritus (itching), and erythema (reddening) that may be followed by breathing difficulty, and/or digestive tract symptoms in a food-allergic individual suggests FDEIA.[30]

Some studies have attempted to identify individuals who are likely to develop FDEIA by determining their sensitization to specific foods by allergen-specific IgE and skin tests and subjecting the test-positive individuals to treadmill stress tests. However, because other variables not included in the test protocols may be contributing to the development of symptoms, most studies have been only partially successful in predicting which food-allergic subjects are likely to develop anaphylaxis while exercising.[31]

Directives for People Who Exhibit Anaphylactic Reactions to Foods

The most important preventive measure is to take every precaution possible to avoid exposure to the anaphylaxis-inducing food. The first requirement for prevention is accurate identification of the food trigger. People who have experienced an anaphylactic reaction or who are deemed at risk as a result of their reaction to highly allergenic foods in the past are prescribed a kit for use when accidental exposure to the allergen occurs. The kit contains injectable adrenaline (epinephrine) and sometimes an oral antihistamine. The directives include:

- Inject the adrenaline.
- Take the antihistamine if available.
- Proceed immediately to the nearest hospital emergency department.

After the injection of the adrenaline, it is extremely important that the person is taken to the hospital, even if the symptoms appear to be improving; it is sometimes a secondary phase of the response that can prove fatal. Specific instructions for the use of injectable adrenaline (epinephrine) should be obtained from the allergic person's doctor or health care provider.

Anaphylaxis-prone individuals are also advised to wear a medic-alert bracelet to expedite appropriate treatment if they become unconscious. People most at risk for anaphylaxis include:

- Adolescents and young adults
- Individuals with known food allergy, especially those with a prior history of anaphylaxis
- People with asthma, especially severe asthma
- Individuals with cardiovascular disease
- People with mastocytosis

General Guidelines for Avoiding Food Allergens Associated with Anaphylaxis

- Avoid all sources of the offending food; become familiar with all potential sources of the food, especially when eating in restaurants and other places where ingredients may not be obvious.
- Become familiar with every term on food labels that indicates the presence of the allergen. Many terms bear little resemblance to the original name of the food, so there must be careful education about these terms, especially with children of reading age.
- Make sure that the food does not enter the home, and make as many meals as possible from scratch from basic ingredients.
- When manufactured foods are used, make sure that *all* ingredients are known.
- When eating outside the home, make sure that the ingredients in every meal are known.
- Inquire about ingredients in recipes used in restaurants.

Factors That Contribute to the Expression of Allergy to Foods

Merely inheriting the appropriate genes for allergy will not necessarily lead to their expression as clinical symptoms. Several environmental and lifestyle factors will determine which allergies are experienced. Some of these factors include increased permeability of the digestive tract lining, combined allergic reactions, enhanced uptake of food allergens, exercise, changes in hormone levels, and stress.

Increased Permeability of the Lining of the Digestive Tract

Increased permeability of the digestive tract lining allows food allergens to contact cells of the immune system, whereas the intake, less permeable mucosa may exclude the larger (and therefore potentially allergenic) molecules. Increased permeability can be from numerous causes, including:

▨ Immaturity: The digestive lining is hyperpermeable in the early months of life and gradually matures over the first 3 to 4 years. Children younger than 5 years are particularly vulnerable to food allergies. Most sensitization to food allergens occurs within this period, particularly during the first year.

▨ Inflammation: An inflammatory reaction in the digestive tract (enteritis) can compromise the integrity of the lining of the digestive tract and give food allergens more ready access to cells of the immune system. Inflammation can result from infection, an autoimmune process, or some other pathology.

Combined Allergic Reactions

When more than one allergic reaction takes place at the same time, inflammatory mediators from each of the reactions tend to add up and reach a level greater than any single reaction alone. For example, a respiratory allergy to airborne, inhaled allergens combined with a food allergy may result in symptoms, whereas the level of inflammatory mediators from the food alone might be insufficient to cause clinical expression of the reaction. This may also explain the observation that certain foods eaten in combination result in an allergic reaction, while either eaten alone may not.

Enhanced Uptake of Food Allergens

Any process that promotes the absorption of food allergens through the epithelium lining the digestive tract has the potential to increase the allergic response. Any process that weakens the tight junctions between the epithelial cells in the digestive mucosa will allow food molecules to bypass the immunological processing of the gut-associated lymphoid tissue (GALT) and encounter reactive cells unimpeded.

Alcohol can increase the rapidity of uptake from the digestive tract, as much as halving the time it normally takes for absorption of certain food components. It is also theorized that alcohol may weaken the tight junctions by dehydration. Thus, taking an alcoholic drink at the same time as an allergenic food will cause a dramatic rise in the level of a food allergen at a reaction site. This may result in allergic symptoms, when taking the food alone does not.

Exercise

Vigorous exercise after eating an allergenic food sometimes results in an allergic reaction when eating the food without exercise does not. The physiological mechanism responsible is presently unknown. It may result from an enhanced rate of uptake of the food or may be a result of increased body temperature during exercise. (Please see earlier discussion for details of food-associated exercise-induced anaphylaxis.)

Changes in Hormone Levels

Changes in the levels of hormones such as estrogen, progesterone, and testosterone appear to affect the responsiveness of the immune system to allergens.[31] It has been suggested that this effect is expressed at the level of the T-suppressor cells, which apparently regulate the degree of the immune system's response. Clinically, the symptoms of food allergy have been observed to fluctuate, depending on the level of estrogen and/or progesterone during the menstrual cycle (symptoms appearing more frequently at ovulation and just prior to and at the onset of the menstrual period) and during pregnancy. Both boys and girls sometimes change their reactivity to allergens at puberty. Women's allergic responses sometimes change at menopause, and men seem to experience a change in their allergic reactivity in their mid-30s.

The possibility that the level of other hormones, particularly thyroid hormones, may influence the degree of the immune system's reactivity has been considered.[32] Anecdotal reports suggest that this may result in food allergy or intolerance. It is known that an important link between the endocrine and immune systems exists, but the clinical significance of these findings has yet to be determined.

Stress

Many allergy sufferers notice that their symptoms appear or worsen during periods of stress. This could be from the release of "stress hormones," which affect the degree of the immune system's responsiveness. The production of neuropeptides such as vasoactive intestinal protein (VIP) and substance P, which can release inflammatory mediators from intestinal mast cells, may be triggered by stress.[33]

References

1. Sampson HA. Food allergy part 2. Diagnosis and management. *J Allergy Clin Immunol.* 1999;103:981-989.
2. Sampson HA, Munoz-Furlong A, Campbell RL, et al. Second Symposium on the Definition and Management of Anaphylaxis: Summary Report—Second National Institute of

Allergy and Infectious Disease/Food Allergy and Anaphylaxis Network Symposium. *Ann Emerg Med.* 2006;47(4):373-380.

3. Simons FER. Anaphylaxis: recent advances in assessment and treatment. *J Allergy Clin Immunol.* 2009;124(4):625-636.

4. Lieberman P. Epidemiology of anaphylaxis. *Curr Opin Allergy Clin Immunol.* 2008;8(4):316-320.

5. Neugut AI, Ghatak AT, Miller RL. Anaphylaxis in the United States: an investigation into its epidemiology. *Arch Intern Med.* 2001;161(1):15-21.

6. Decker WW, Campbell RL, Manivannan V, et al. The etiology and incidence of anaphylaxis in Rochester, Minnesota: a report from the Rochester Epidemiology Project. *J Allergy Clin Immunol.* 2008;122(6):1161-1165.

7. Webb LM, Lieberman P. Anaphylaxis: a review of 601 cases. *Ann Allergy Asthma Immunol.* 2006;97(1):39-43.

8. Oswalt ML, Kemp SF. Anaphylaxis: office management and prevention. *Immunol Allergy Clin North Am.* 2007;27(2):177-191.

9. Boyce JA, Assa'ad A, Burks AW, et al. Guidelines for the diagnosis and management of food allergy in the United States: report of the NIAID-sponsored expert panel. *J Allergy Clin Immunol.* 2010;126(6):S1-S58 (section 6.2.2).

10. Keet CA, Wood RA. Food allergy and anaphylaxis. *Immunol Allergy Clin North Am.* 2007:193-212.

11. Boyce JA, Assa'ad A, Burks AW, et al. Guidelines for the diagnosis and management of food allergy in the United States: report of the NIAID-sponsored expert panel. *J Allergy Clin Immunol.* 2010;126:S1-S58.

12. Tole JW, Lieberman P. Biphasic anaphylaxis: review of incidence, clinical predictors, and observation recommendations. *Immunol Allergy Clin North Am.* 2007;27:309-326, viii.

13. Sampson HA, Mendelson L, Rosen JP. Fatal and near-fatal anaphylactic reactions to food in children and adolescents. *New Eng J Med.* 1992;327(6):380-384.

14. Bock SA, Munoz-Furlong A, Sampson HA. Further fatalities caused by anaphylactic reactions to food 2001–2006. *J Allergy Clin Immunol.* 2007;119(4):1016-1018.

15. Kemp SF, Lockey RF. Anaphylaxis: a review of causes and mechanisms. *J Allergy Clin Immunol.* 2002;110(3):341-348.

16. Chong SU, Worm M, Zuberbier T. Role of adverse reactions to food in urticaria and exercise-induced anaphylaxis. *Int Arch Allergy Immunol.* 2002;129:19-26.

17. Aihara M, Miyazawa M, Osuna H, et al. Food-dependent exercise-induced anaphylaxis: influence of concurrent aspirin administration on skin testing and provocation. *Br J Dermatol.* 2002;146:466-472.

18. Castells MC, Horan RF, Sheffer AL. Exercise-induced anaphylaxis. *Curr Allergy Asthm R.* 2003;3:15-21.

19. Aihara Y, Kotoyori T, Takahashi Y, Osuna H, Ohnuma S, Ikezawa Z. The necessity for dual food intake to provoke food-dependent exercise-induced anaphylaxis (FEIAn): a case report of FEIAn with simultaneous intake of wheat and umeboshi. *J Allergy Clin Immunol.* 2001;107:1100-1105.

20. Perkins DN, Keith PK. Food- and exercise-induced anaphylaxis: importance of history in diagnosis. *Ann Allergy Asthma Immunol.* 2002;89:15-23.

21. Shadick NA, Liang MH, Partridge AJ, et al. The natural history of exercise-induced anaphylaxis: survey results from a 10-year follow-up study. *J Allergy Clin Immunol.* 1999;104(1):123-127.

22. Morita E, Yamamura Y, Mihara S, Kameyoshi Y, Yamamoto S. Food-dependent exercise-induced anaphylaxis: a report of two cases and determination of gamma-gliadin as the presumptive allergen. *Br J Dermatol*. 2000;143:1059-1063.

23. Perez-Pimiento AJ, Moneo I, Santaolalla M, de Paz S, Fernandez-Parra B, Dominguez-L. Anaphylactic reaction to young garlic. *Allergy*. 1999;54(6):626-629.

24. Perez-Calderon R, Gonzalo-Garijo MA, Fernandez de Soria R. Exercise-induced anaphylaxis to onion. *Allergy*. 2002;57:752-753.

25. Jacquenet S, Morisset M, Battais F, et al. Interest of ImmunoCAP system to recombinant omega-5 gliadin for the diagnosis of exercise-induced wheat allergy. *Int Arch Allergy Immunol*. 2009;149:74-80.

26. Matsuo H, Morita E, Tatham AS, et al. Identification of the IgE-binding epitope in omega-5 gliadin, a major allergen in wheat-dependent exercise-induced anaphylaxis. *J Biol Chem*. 2004;279:12135-12140.

27. Romano A, Di Fonso M, Giuffreda F, et al. Food-dependent exercise-induced anaphylaxis: clinical and laboratory findings in 54 subjects. *Int Arch Allergy Immunol*. 2001;125:264-272.

28. Chong SU, Worm M, Zuberbier T. Role of adverse reactions to food in urticaria and exercise-induced anaphylaxis. *Int Arch Allergy Immunol*. 2002;129:19-26.

29. Aihara M, Miyazawa M, Osuna H, et al. Food-dependent exercise-induced anaphylaxis: influence of concurrent aspirin administration on skin testing and provocation. *Br J Dermatol*. 2002;146:466-472.

30. Hosey RG, Carek PJ, Goo A. Exercise-induced anaphylaxis and urticaria. *Am Fam Physician*. 2001;64(8):1367-1372.

31. Chen W, Mempel M, Schober W, Behrendt H, Ring J. Gender difference, sex hormones, and immediate type hypersensitivity reactions. *Allergy*. 2008;63:1418-1427.

32. Klecha AJ, Genaro AM, Gorelik G, et al. Integrative study of hypothalamus-pituitary-thyroid-immune system interaction: thyroid hormone-mediated modulation of lymphocyte activity through the protein kinase C signaling pathway. *J Endocrinol*. 2006;189(1):45-55.

33. Joneja JM. Psychological factors and stress in IBS. In: *Digestion, Diet and Disease: Irritable Bowel Syndrome and Gastrointestinal Function*. New Brunswick, NJ. Rutgers University Press; 2004:195–206.

CHAPTER **5**

Diagnosis of Food Allergy

Restrictive diets place both physical and emotional stress on food-allergic individuals and their families. No food should be restricted unless there is a good reason for doing so. Elimination of large numbers of foods from the diet is rarely necessary. Every effort should be made to diagnose food allergy and food intolerances correctly, and each food eliminated from a person's diet must be replaced with one of equivalent nutrient value. Merely avoiding the culprit food(s) is not sufficient to maintain health. A well-balanced and nutritionally complete diet is essential.

Determining the cause of a reaction requires a careful and systematic approach. Any number of foods or food additives could be responsible for the reactions, and clinical presentation can involve an array of symptoms. Food allergy and intolerance symptoms, especially those occurring in the gastrointestinal tract, can be caused by a variety of other clinical entities, so before food allergy is considered as the reason for a person's symptoms, all other causes must be ruled out. The process of determining the specific foods responsible for a person's adverse reactions can sometimes prove challenging and is optimally achieved by a collaborative team approach involving the person's family physician or pediatrician, a certified allergist, a registered dietitian, and other health care professionals as appropriate.

The Importance of Correct Identification of Foods Responsible for Adverse Reactions

There are several reasons why the correct identification of the food(s) responsible for symptoms should be made:

- Symptoms can only be controlled when all the foods and food additives responsible for symptoms are removed from the diet: This requires accurate identification of the culprit foods.
- It is particularly important that the food responsible for an anaphylactic reaction be correctly identified, because all forms of the food must be strictly avoided to prevent a potentially life-threatening situation.

- Restriction of foods that do not elicit symptoms is unnecessary and may be detrimental to health in many ways. For example:
  - Serious nutritional deficiencies and disease in people following overly restricted diets have been reported, especially in children.[1]
  - Because food plays such an important and integral role in normal family and social life, over-restriction of the diet may seriously threaten a person's quality of life and emotional health.[2]
  - Inappropriate reinforcement of food avoidance may lead to obsessions with food as a "threat"; in extreme cases this may lead to food phobia and possible anorexia nervosa in vulnerable people.

Unnecessary Food Avoidance

In the past, whole groups of foods have been restricted unnecessarily because of the perception that botanical, or zoological, relatedness implied antigenic relatedness or cross-reactivity. The first classification of foods into botanically related families for the purpose of diagnosing food allergy was published in 1929. To this day, many allergists continue to advise their food-allergic patients to avoid all members of a botanic family when allergy to one representative is demonstrated. In fact, many allergy textbooks still perpetuate this myth. It is common to see statements to the effect that if peanut allergy is diagnosed, avoidance of all members of the *Leguminosae* (legume family) should be carefully avoided.[3]

Modern research in molecular immunology has demonstrated that a person is typically allergic to only a small number of foods and that there is often a greater degree of antigenic relatedness between nonbotanically related plants than between those within the same botanic family. Research into oral allergy syndrome and latex allergy has helped greatly in expanding our knowledge in this area (see Chapters 33 and 34).

The most recent guidelines (2010) for the diagnosis and management of food allergy in the United States states that "patients at risk for developing food allergy do *not* need to limit exposure to foods that may be cross-reactive with the eight major food allergens in the United States (milk, egg, peanut, tree nuts, soy, wheat, fish, and crustacean shellfish)."[4] This means that a person allergic to peanut or soy does not need to avoid all members of the legume family. Each food must be assessed individually before it is identified as allergenic for a food-sensitive person.

Laboratory Tests for Food Allergen Identification

Considering the wide range of immunological and physiological mechanisms that are responsible for the clinical symptoms of adverse food reactions, it is unrealistic to expect a single test to be able to identify the specific food components responsible for all types of reactions. Laboratory tests are of little value on their own and can lead to a misleading diagnosis if the patient's clinical history is not considered at the same time. All tests must be confirmed by carefully eliminating the suspect foods for a specified time period and reintroducing each eliminated food individually while monitoring any adverse reactions. This procedure, known as "elimination and challenge," is discussed in detail in Chapters 6 and 7.

The following is a summary of the tests most commonly employed in the diagnosis of food allergy, with a brief appraisal of their diagnostic value.

Tests for Food-Specific IgE

Most tests used by allergists in the diagnosis and treatment of food allergy are designed to detect the presence of antibodies against foods—in particular, food-specific IgE. They depend on the immunological concept that when antibodies specific to food antigens are present, an allergic state exists. Tests for allergen-specific antibodies work well for respiratory allergy to inhaled allergens such as plant pollens, animal dander, dust, dust mites, and mold spores because the allergen is not changed in the encounter with the immune system and the response is unambiguous. Antigens are continuously entering the respiratory tract in each breath. The inhaled antigens in their natural state encounter cells of the immune system and are recognized as foreign. The immune system is able to distinguish between "foreign and a threat" (potentially pathogenic microorganisms) and "foreign but safe" (inhaled allergens). In atopic individuals, the former situation may trigger a TH1 response (protection) and the latter may trigger a TH2 response (allergy); in both situations, the foreign antigen is rejected (see Chapter 1). However, the immune system of the digestive tract is complex and has diverse functions, so tests depending on the response of the GALT and the subsequent systemic immune response as antigens pass into the body are not reliable in delineating each reaction.

Skin Tests

The skin test is often the first step taken in diagnosing an allergy. It is designed to reveal the IgE, which is fixed to the skin mast cell. When the allergen bridges two IgE molecules on the surface of the cell, inflammatory mediators (particularly histamine) are released that cause edema (swelling) and erythema (reddening)—the "wheal and flare reaction."

The allergen may be introduced into the skin by several methods:

▪ Prick test: A drop of commercial allergen extract is placed onto the skin's surface and the skin underneath is pricked with a lancet.
▪ Scratch test: The skin is scarified and a drop of allergen is deposited onto the site.
▪ Intradermal test: The allergen is injected into the skin from a syringe.

In each case, two controls without allergen are included: (a) the positive control is a measured amount of histamine and (b) the negative control is the medium in which the allergen is suspended, usually saline. If the negative control triggers a reaction, or if the response to the histamine control is less than 3 mm in diameter, all of the tests are invalid. A wheal at least 3 mm larger than the negative control is considered positive.[5]

A positive skin test is indicated by the development of a raised central area (blister) at the site of the reaction (the wheal), surrounded by a flattened reddened area (the flare). The diameter of each area is measured in millimeters and is graded on a reaction scale:

- The most common measurement indicates the diameter of the total reaction, usually on a scale of 1+ (mild) to 4+ (strong reaction).
- Other practitioners consider a wheal that is 3+ mm in diameter (not including the erythema, or flare) greater than the negative control to be positive; anything less is considered negative.
- Some practitioners favor different scales of measurement, resulting in values of 30, 40, or higher.
- Others measure both wheal and flare and report the numbers separately (eg, 15 × 10; 8 × 12).

Although some practitioners consider intradermal tests to be slightly more sensitive than prick tests, they also cause more nonspecific positive responses and may induce systemic reactions. For the latter reason, most allergists strongly advise against using the intradermal test because of the danger of inducing a potentially fatal anaphylactic reaction.[6]

Estimated Accuracy of Skin Tests

Negative skin tests for IgE-mediated allergy to the highly allergenic foods such as egg, peanut, wheat, milk, fish, and tree nuts are considered by some practitioners to be accurate about 95% of the time.[7] However, negative reactions to other food allergens, such as soy, apparently have a significantly reduced rate of accuracy.

Positive skin tests have an even lower predictive value. The most optimistic clinicians rate positive skin tests to foods at less than 50% accuracy.[8]

In 2010, a British practice group issued guidelines for managing egg allergy in which they state, "Skin testing should only be carried out if there is clinical suspicion of egg allergy and has poor predictive value as a screening tool."[9] This opinion is becoming more widely applied in food allergy diagnosis, as the accuracy of skin tests in predicting clinical reactivity on ingestion of the food is being questioned due to an increasing number of published reports of evidence-based research on the topic. The current guidelines for diagnosis of food allergy in the United States recommend "performing an SPT (also known as a skin puncture test) to assist in the identification of foods that may be provoking IgE-mediated food-induced allergic reactions" but "the SPT alone cannot be considered diagnostic of FA."[10]

Prick-to-Prick Tests for Raw Foods

Because the allergens used in skin testing tend to be unstable (see discussion beginning on page 64) and many individuals react to the raw food, especially in cases of oral allergy syndrome (see Chapter 33), a prick-to-prick test is sometimes employed to determine reactivity to the undegraded allergen.[11] The usefulness and accuracy of such tests in food allergy diagnosis remains to be determined by well-controlled trials. The procedure is as follows:

- A sterile needle is inserted into the raw fruit or vegetable.
- The patient's skin (usually of the arm or back) is pricked with the same needle.
- The native antigen is transferred to the skin.
- The site of antigen application is observed for the wheal and flare response characteristic of an IgE-mediated reaction for up to half an hour.
- A positive response (graded from 1+ to 4+) indicates degranulation of mast cells and histamine release.

Patch Tests for Delayed Hypersensitivity Reactions

There are two types of patch tests in general use for the identification of allergens responsible for distinct types of allergic reactions:

- Delayed T-cell-mediated (type IV) hypersensitivity reactions in contact dermatitis
- Delayed reactions in which prick and scratch tests for food-specific wheal and flare reactions may or may not be positive

Delayed T-Cell Mediated (Type IV) Hypersensitivity

Reactivity to chemicals such as nickel and other metals; preservatives such as thimerosal, benzalkonium chloride, and parabens; constituents of medications and cosmetics, such as balsam of Peru; cinnamaldehyde; detergents; perfumes; latex; and any number of materials that trigger dermatitis on the skin after contact are commonly tested by this method, which involves the following steps:

- The test material is applied to the skin's surface, either in an impregnated patch or in an adhesive bandage that is placed over the material applied directly onto the skin surface.
- The skin is not abraded.
- The site is examined for an inflammatory response, typically 24 and 48 hours after application of the allergen.
- The patch usually remains in place for up to 72 hours; no response after this time is considered as negative.

Some of the materials testing positive for contact allergy by this method may trigger an IgE-mediated allergy when the material is ingested in the form of food or a food additive. Nickel sensitivity (Chapter 22) is an example of a nonprotein food component that may trigger an allergic reaction when consumed in food.

Atopy Patch Tests (APT) for Delayed Reactions to Foods

Atopy patch tests (APTs) have been in use since the 1970s in situations where conventional skin tests (prick, scratch, or intradermal) are negative but symptoms occur after consumption of a food. One method of performing the test is to suspend the allergen extract in a material that will enhance the uptake of the allergen through the skin. For example, in the DIMSOFT test, the food extract is suspended in 90% dimethyl sulfoxide, which is thought to aid in skin penetration by the food antigen. It has been suggested that the DIMSOFT allows detection of all types of hypersensitivity reactions (for a discussion of these reactions, see Chapter 1).

APTs have been employed especially with symptoms in the skin (atopic dermatitis) and in the digestive tract.[12] Such tests have proven useful in identifying the role of foods such as cereal grains and milk in childhood gastroenteritis and eczema. The results of a study reported in 1996[13] represented the type of responses seen. In a study of cow's milk allergy in 183 children ranging in age from 2 to 36 months, the following was observed:

■ 54% of children developed symptoms following ingestion of milk, either immediately or after several hours.
■ Skin prick tests were positive in 67% of the cases with acute onset of symptoms after milk challenge, while patch tests were generally negative.
■ Patch tests were positive in 89% of children with delayed onset symptoms, and skin prick tests were mostly negative in this group.

The clinical significance, mechanism of activity, and reliability of such patch tests in the diagnosis of delayed-onset food allergy remain to be confirmed by well-controlled investigations.[14] The current guidelines in the United States suggest that "the APT should *not* be used in the routine evaluation of non-contact FA" (Guideline 8).[15]

Blood Tests for Food-Specific Antibody

Numerous tests for the detection of antibodies in blood against food allergens are being used extensively for the diagnosis of food allergy. A variety of detection methods are being employed, including various versions of the radioallergosorbent test (RAST) and fluorescent allergosorbent test (FAST) for allergen-specific IgE; and the enzyme-linked immunosorbent assay (ELISA) for allergen-specific IgE and IgG, particularly IgG4. The basic method of testing is as follows:

■ A patient's blood serum is tested for the presence of antifood antibodies.
■ Because antifood antibodies are frequently present in normal blood, the level of antibody to each food is graded according to the laboratory standards, usually on a scale of nonreactivity, low reactivity, moderate reactivity, and high reactivity.
■ The patient is usually instructed to avoid the foods in the moderate and high categories.

Some laboratories use the Phadebas scoring method for IgE, in which case a score of 3 or greater is considered as positive.

Value of Blood Tests in Practice

Practitioners debate the degree of reliance that should be placed on blood tests in identifying allergenic foods. The question centers on the argument that the tests will not determine which foods will lead to clinical symptoms when consumed by an individual and must be followed by careful elimination and challenge of the test-positive foods before a definite diagnosis can be made. Laboratory tests for specific antibodies are considered to be of little if any practical value in the management of food intolerance unless considered together with a careful medical history and examination, and followed by confirmation with provocation of symptoms by the suspect food.[16]

A recent (2010) retrospective study[17] of 125 children aged 1 to 19 years demonstrated that 84% to 93% of the foods being avoided as a result of positive skin and serum allergen-specific IgE test results did not trigger an allergic reaction when reintroduced by oral challenge. The authors concluded that, "In the absence of anaphylaxis, the primary reliance on serum food-specific IgE testing to determine the need for a food elimination diet is not sufficient, especially in children with atopic dermatitis" and recommend oral food challenges to confirm food allergy status.

Blood tests have traditionally been considered to be slightly less accurate than skin tests in determining IgE-mediated food reactions; however, some practitioners rate the two types of test about the same. Newer methods, such as Phadebas (www.phadebas .com) and ImmunoCAP (www.phadia.com/en/allergens), are considered to be much more sensitive than the older blood tests, and practitioners are now relying more frequently on these tests to identify their patients' food allergies, especially those of children.

Comparison of skin prick tests and blood tests, both of which detect food-specific antibodies, often leads to inconsistent results and can be confusing when conducted simultaneously in a patient. The inconsistency stems from the fact that the skin prick test detects IgE linked to mast cells in the skin; the blood test identifies food-specific IgE in serum.[a] Although several practitioners have estimated the percentage risk of allergy based on IgE levels, most authorities agree that many atopic individuals exhibit an IgE with normal values, so no IgE level, no matter how low, rules out the diagnosis of food allergy.[5]

Tests for Other Food-Specific Antibodies

IgG

Blood tests for other antibodies implicated in food allergy, such as IgG4, are even less reliable in diagnosis. Most people develop IgG antibodies to the foods that they eat, and this is a normal immune response indicating exposure to the food but not allergic sensitization.[18] The level of IgG4 falls as a person avoids the food to which the antibody is formed, which would be an expected outcome of any antigen withdrawal.

---

[a] IgE in serum is sometimes referred to as sIgE, a designation that can be misleading because it can be confused with *s,* meaning "secretory," in the designation of an antibody having a secretory component such as secretory IgA (sIgA) or sIgM.

IgG4 may be high in people with food allergy, but its detection has no diagnostic value on account of its being found frequently in individuals who tolerate these nutrients, and it might indicate only an increase in intestinal permeability. Furthermore, recent research reports indicate that food-specific IgG4 tends to rise as IgE to the same allergen declines due to the development of tolerance.[19] (Discussion of oral tolerance to foods can be found in Chapter 44.)

In summary, the majority of allergy practitioners consider the so-called food allergy profile with simultaneous IgE and IgG determination against numerous food material to be both uneconomical and of no value in the diagnosis of food allergy.[20,21]

Total Serum IgE

Elevated total serum IgE indicates atopy (when parasitic infection has been excluded) but does not incriminate any specific allergens and does not indicate the organ system in which symptoms (if any) are likely to occur.[22]

Other Circulating Antifood Antibodies

The presence of IgM, IgG, IgA, and IgE plasma cells can give rise to antibodies that can be detected by immunofluorescence techniques. However, because IgG, IgA, IgM, and sometimes IgE antibodies directed against food antigens can be found in the serum of food-tolerant subjects, the significance of both the plasma cells and the antibodies arising from them remains to be determined. At the present time, the presence of these cells is not considered to be of any diagnostic value.

Limitations of Skin and Blood Tests in the Diagnosis of Food Allergy

Overall, routine skin and blood tests for food allergens may be unreliable or misleading for a number of reasons. Some of the causes of false-positive tests include:

- Patients may have IgE antibodies but no symptoms. There is a positive skin test, but the food causes no symptoms when eaten. Some practitioners refer to this as "latent food allergy."
- The commercial allergen extract contains histamine, which elicits a positive response when introduced into the skin.[23] This would pose a particular problem with intradermal skin tests in which the histamine in the extract is actually injected into the skin and is thus more likely to elicit a wheal and flare response independent of the allergen.
- The food can cause a nonspecific ("irritant") positive skin reaction.
- Skin mast cells release inflammatory mediators in response to a much wider range of both immunologic and nonimmunologic stimuli compared to mast cells in other types of tissue, especially in the digestive tract. As a result, many positive skin test reactions are due to factors other than food allergen-specific IgE.
- In many cases, the food is eaten in a processed or cooked form that changes the nature of the proteins that constitute the allergen molecules. The form in

which food molecules encounter the immune system at the digestive tract's mucosal barrier (the gut-associated lymphoid tissue [GALT]) is in many ways quite different from that of the intact food from which allergen extracts used in tests are derived. For example, digestive processes start immediately as food enters the oral cavity and continue throughout the length of the digestive tract. This means that the food molecules are changed, and new potential antigens are uncovered, as the food progresses through the system where it encounters a variety of digestive secretions and is acted upon by digestive enzymes.

It is estimated that only about one-third of patients with positive skin prick tests or serum-specific IgE show clinical symptoms during food challenge. Intradermal skin tests in particular are considered to have little value when positive, with some clinicians, especially in Europe, rating their accuracy no higher than 30%.[24] Other practitioners, especially in the United States, rate the accuracy of skin tests higher.[4] Negative skin tests especially are considered to be of greater value than those testing positive. However, there are several reasons for false-negative skin tests, including:

▪ The reaction may not be mediated by IgE antibodies.
▪ The commercial allergen extract contains none of the specified allergen.
▪ The allergen has been denatured in the preparation of the extract.

The latter reason in particular poses a problem in identifying plant foods that are responsible for oral allergy syndrome (OAS). In OAS, people with known respiratory allergy to plant pollens (pollinosis) develop irritation, swelling, and reddening in oral and perioral tissues when eating certain raw fruits and vegetables, which, in most cases are botanically unrelated to their allergenic pollen-producing plants (see Chapter 33). Commercial allergen extracts were found to be unsuitable for skin tests of the culprit food in these cases for two important reasons:

▪ Unlike pollen allergens, glycoprotein food antigens are often denatured by treatment with heat, acid, and proteases.
▪ When plant tissues are crushed, phenols are released to prevent microbial invasion of the damaged tissues. This leads to rapid protein denaturation by oxidized polyphenols.

Consequently, during preparation of the antigen for tests, the antigen is no longer in its natural form and does not elicit an immune response. To try to overcome this problem, the prick-to-prick test was developed.

Any positive tests should always be followed by elimination and challenge of the incriminated foods, because everyone is likely to have circulating antibodies to food antigens, but only a few people will develop symptoms of allergy. Because anaphylactic reactions are mediated by IgE, many allergists believe that any food-specific IgE might presage a life-threatening situation. For this reason, consuming food in a challenge test to confirm allergy when moderate or high levels of IgE have been detected is always conducted under medical supervision in the United States.

In most other countries, if the food has been eaten in the past with only mild or no symptoms, and if there is no history of a tendency for severe or anaphylaxis-like symptoms in the individual, such precautions are considered to be excessively restrictive, as well as very expensive in terms of using hospital facilities and expert personnel. Nevertheless, in the interests of safety, most food challenges of the most highly allergenic foods, especially in infants and young children, should be carried out under medical supervision in an appropriately equipped facility.

Potential Risks of Skin Tests

Although historically skin tests for food allergy diagnosis have been generally regarded as safe, new information about the impact of food allergens entering the body by a route other than the digestive tract is giving rise to some questions about their safety.

Intradermal testing is contraindicated because of the risk of an anaphylactic reaction in an already sensitized individual (see earlier discussion). However, introducing food through the "unnatural" route of the skin, and bypassing the protective GALT has the potential to sensitize an otherwise nonallergic individual to the allergen. Several recent reports indicate that exposure to a food allergen through the skin may contribute to systemic allergic disease and that atopy may be secondary to skin barrier dysfunction from numerous causes,[25] especially atopic dermatitis (eczema).

An increasing number of research studies[26] are demonstrating that allergens pass readily through the skin and encounter immune cells that become reactive to them; indeed, this is the basis of the skin test. A 2003 study indicated that sensitization to peanut protein may occur in previously nonallergic children through the application to inflamed skin of peanut oil in skin preparations.[27] Some experts suggest that sensitization to allergens occurs through environmental exposure to the allergen through the skin and that consumption of food allergens actually induces oral tolerance more often than sensitization.[28] This hypothesis provides a possible explanation for the close link between eczema and the development of food allergies.

Diagnosis of Reactions to Foods Not Mediated by Antibodies

Several adverse reactions to foods are now included under the umbrella of "food hypersensitivity reactions" that do not involve the production of food-specific antibodies. Consequently, the diagnosis of such conditions does not involve detection of food-specific antibodies and the tests designed for identifying the offending foods discussed earlier cannot be employed.

Foremost among these nonantibody-mediated conditions are those that involve eosinophils. Eosinophils are granulocytes that contain intracellular granules that, like mast cells, release inflammatory mediators when activated. The mediators act on body tissues, resulting in symptoms typical of the disease. Granule release, or degranulation, occurs when the immunological response is triggered, often by a food. (Refer to

Chapter 39 for a detailed discussion.) The specific food responsible is often difficult to identify. Several tests are employed in the diagnosis of the eosinophilic diseases.

Eosinophil Count

The eosinophilic gastrointestinal diseases (EGID) are a diverse group of intestinal diseases that are diagnosed by detecting the presence of eosinophils by endoscopic analysis and mucosal biopsy. The most common form of EGID is eosinophilic esophagitis (EE), which is diagnosed by the presence of more than 15 to 20 eosinophils per microscope high-power field.[29]

About 50% of individuals with EGID show the presence of eosinophils in the peripheral blood. The presence of eosinophils in blood, tissue, or stool suggests that an immunological reaction is taking place but does not provide any clue as to the identity of the allergen or its role in the development of symptoms. Eosinophils may also be detected in the stool of patients with the following:

■ Dietary protein-induced enterocolitis
■ Dietary protein-induced proctocolitis
■ Eosinophilic gastroenteritis

Because food allergens are thought to play an important role in the pathogenesis of EGID, several tests such as skin prick, atopy patch, and allergen-specific IgE tests have been employed to try identifying the foods responsible for the reaction. However, there is little evidence to support their use in predicting EGID or the severity of the condition.[30] The only reliable method for determining the role of foods in EGID is resolution of symptoms and a significant drop in the eosinophil count following dietary elimination, and recurrence of the eosinophilia with reintroduction of the suspect food.[31]

Intestinal Sigmoidoscopy and Biopsy Before and After Food Challenge

These techniques are used to rule out gastrointestinal pathology unrelated to food allergy, such as celiac disease, colitis, and Crohn's disease. Inflammation, villous atrophy, and other injuries in the digestive tract lining can be identified and measured by these methods.

Microscopic examination of biopsy samples is often used in confirming a diagnosis but will not identify the foods responsible for the reaction. A variety of more sophisticated methods for measuring changes in intestinal cells and the products of their activity (such as intestinal manometric techniques and gastric juice analysis[32]) are being researched in an attempt to identify those that can be used to make a definitive diagnosis and identify the causative factors in pathology in the digestive tract. However, the value of these procedures has yet to be assessed; currently, they remain within the realms of research, not clinical practice. Their use in identifying food allergy has been investigated by a few researchers, but their value in diagnosis has yet to be determined.

Controversial Tests

Several scientifically unproven tests are becoming popular in the often-frustrating search for a diagnosis in adverse reactions to foods. In the absence of a definitive diagnosis, many people with chronic, recurrent complaints seek alternative care. A large number of scientifically unproven methods of detecting "food allergies" have been developed to satisfy the demand for a "quick and easy" diagnosis.[12] Three of the most popular noninvasive tests include electrodermal or electroacupuncture (Vega) test, the antigen leukocyte cellular antibody test (ALCAT), and biokinesiology.

Vega Test

Vega testing, or electrodermal screening, was originally developed in Germany in 1953 by Reinholdt Voll and was modified in 1978 by Dr. Helmut Schimmel. The test is a method of electrodermal testing that utilizes energy waves to indicate an individual's reactivity to foods and other allergens in a vial within a circuit that includes a meter to measure the degree of reactivity. The Vega machine detects changes in skin resistance on the skin surface in response to the food or environmental allergen in the test vial. Allergy to food or reactivity to environmental factors is measured by a drop in electric current when the detection device is applied to the skin at points considered suitable for detecting food allergy (usually on a finger). By this method, practitioners also attempt to measure the activity of organ systems and endocrine glands.[33]

Cytotoxicity Tests (Including ALCAT)

Cytotoxicity tests depend on the theory that "sensitized" white blood cells change their shape and size when in contact with the specific food antigen that induced the immune response, thus indicating a patient's allergy to or intolerance of the food. The antigen leukocyte cellular antibody test (ALCAT) is one of the best-known testing modalities of this type. Its manufacturer claims that the test identifies a patient's immunological response to a food, and thus his or her food allergies or intolerances. However, journal articles, reviews, and allergology associations' position papers have characterized the ALCAT as an "unproven method" for diagnosing allergies, advised against its use, and concluded that relying upon the results of this test may lead to inappropriate advice and treatments.[20,34]

Biokinesiology or Applied Kinesiology

The basis of the applied kinesiology test is the assumption that muscles become weak when influenced by the allergens that are causing the person's symptoms. The allergen, contained in a vial, is held in one hand while the practitioner tests the strength of the other arm in resisting downward pressure. A weakening of resistance indicates a positive (allergic) reaction.[35] However, no evidence-based research has been able to demonstrate the efficacy or accuracy of this method of testing for food allergies.[36]

Other Allergy Tests

In an effort to identify foods responsible for triggering symptoms rather than measuring a putative immunological change such as antibody production, a number of tests have been developed to measure the level of mediators released in the allergic response. Two of the most well known include the basophil histamine/release or activation test,[37] which measures histamine release from "sensitized" basophils, and the mediator release assay, which forms a basis for the LEAP (Lifestyle Eating and Performance) diet.[38]

Status of Tests for Food Allergy and Intolerance: Current Opinion

The current opinion about nonstandardized and unproven procedures for the diagnosis of foods responsible for allergies and intolerances is summarized in the 2010 guidelines for the diagnosis and management of food allergy in the United States: "The Expert Panel recommends *not* using any of the following nonstandardized tests for the routine evaluation of IgE-mediated food allergy:"[39]

- Basophil histamine release/activation
- Lymphocyte stimulation
- Facial thermography
- Gastric juice analysis
- Endoscopic allergen provocation
- Hair analysis
- Applied kinesiology
- Provocation neutralization
- Allergen-specific IgG4
- Cytotoxicity assays
- Electrodermal test (Vega)
- Mediator release assay (LEAP)

A similar opinion is held by European allergists, which is summarized in a position paper published in 1999.[36] In their extensive treatise, these clinicians and researchers indicate that many doctors rely on tests such as skin, blood (antibody) tests, and others for the diagnosis of adverse reactions to foods. They state, "In reality, no test designed to establish allergy/intolerance carried out on a patient (in vivo) or in the laboratory (in vitro) will of itself allow one to formulate this diagnosis with certainty. The diagnostic accuracy of currently available tests is low, and for some tests there are no studies on diagnostic sensitivity and specificity." They conclude that the only reliable way to determine that a person's symptoms are caused by an adverse reaction to a food, food component, or food additive is elimination and challenge. This conclusion is supported by American allergists,[40,41] who agree that diagnostic tests indicate which foods are likely to be the cause of the allergic symptoms, but elimination and challenge is necessary to support the diagnosis.

The only definitive diagnostic test presently available for detecting specific foods, food components, and food additives that are responsible for food sensitivity reactions is the elimination and challenge procedure.[42] The process involves creating a diet diary or food record, followed by exclusion diets and oral provocation. The oral provocation test is the "gold standard" due to the fact that we cannot make the diagnosis only with a skin test or a positive serological reaction, and even in the immediate-type allergies, both may be negative.

Elimination and Challenge Procedure

Suspected foods and additives are eliminated from the diet for a specific period of time. The restricted foods are selected on the basis of very careful food intake diaries, medical history, and appropriate tests. When improvement is achieved (usually within 4 weeks), a sequential incremental dose challenge is instituted to identify the specific food components responsible for the reactions. Figure 5.1 illustrates how the elimination and challenge procedure works. Finally, a diet is developed that restricts the intake of the reactive foods and provides complete, balanced nutrition from alternative sources. Detailed instructions for this procedure are provided in Chapters 6, 7, and 8.

FIGURE 5.1

Flowchart for elimination and challenge to identify foods responsible for adverse reactions. Solid arrows: If symptoms resolve after suspect foods are eliminated, foods are reintroduced individually (challenge). If symptoms recur, the food is confirmed as the cause of the reactions. Dotted arrows: If symptoms persist after suspect foods are eliminated, diagnosis is not confirmed. Food restrictions are increased and the process is continued as indicated. Dashed arrows: If symptoms resolve and symptoms do not recur on challenge, diagnosis is not confirmed.

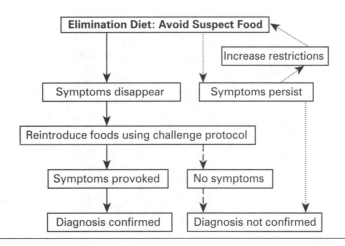

Ultimate Goal

The final goal is always the same: The food responsible for the symptoms must be correctly identified, avoided, and foods of equivalent nutrient value substituted. This may require major adjustments in lifestyle and certainly in food choices, but the ultimate reward of improved health and quality of life will justify all the time and effort that has gone into detecting the antagonistic foods and developing a nutritionally balanced and satisfying diet.

References

1. Christie L, Hine RJ, Parker JG, Burks W. Food allergies in children affect nutritional intake and growth. *J Am Diet Assoc.* 2002;102(11):1648-1651.
2. Ostblom E, Egmar AC, Gardulf A, Lilja G, Wickman M. The impact of food hypersensitivity reported in 9-year-old children by their parents on health-related quality of life. *Allergy.* 2008;63(2):211-218.
3. NIAID Task Force Report. *Adverse Reactions to Foods.* Bethesda, MD: National Institutes of Health; 1984. NIH publication 84-2442:7.
4. Boyce JA, Assa'ad A, Burks AW, et al. Guidelines for the diagnosis and management of food allergy in the United States: report of the NIAID-sponsored expert panel [Guideline 33]. *J Allergy Clin Immunol.* 2010;126(6):S1-S58.
5. Patriarca G, Schiavino D, Pecora V, et al. Food allergy and food intolerance: diagnosis and treatment. *Intern Emerg Med.* 2009;4:11-24.
6. Lockey RF. Adverse reactions associated with skin testing and immunotherapy. *Allergy Proc.* 1995;16:293-296.
7. Hill DJ, Heine RG, Hosking CS. The diagnostic value of skin testing in children with food allergy. *Pediatr Allergy Immunol.* 2004;15:435-441.
8. David TJ. Skin tests. In: *Food and Food Additive Intolerance in Childhood.* Oxford, UK: Blackwell Scientific Publishers; 1993:244-292.
9. Clark AT, Skypala I, Leech SC, et al. British Society for Allergy and Clinical Immunology guidelines for the management of egg allergy. *Clin Exper Allergy.* 2010;40:1116-1129.
10. Boyce JA, Assa'ad A, Burks AW, et al. Guidelines for the diagnosis and management of food allergy in the United States: report of the NIAID-sponsored expert panel [Guideline 4]. *J Allergy Clin Immunol.* 2010;126(6):S1-S58.
11. Webber CM, England RW. Oral allergy syndrome: a clinical, diagnostic, and therapeutic challenge. *Ann Allergy Asthma Immunol.* 2010;104(2):101-108.
12. Canani RB, Ruotolo S, Auricchio L, et al. Diagnostic accuracy of the atopy patch test in children with food allergy-related gastrointestinal symptoms. *Allergy.* 2007;62:738-743.
13. Isolauri E, Turjanmaa K. Combined skin prick and patch testing enhances identification of food allergy in infants with atopic dermatitis. *J Allergy Clin Immunol.* 1996; 97(1 pt 1):9-15.
14. Turjamma K, Darsow U, Nuggemann B, Rance F, Vanto T, Werfel T. EAACI/GA2LEN position paper: present status of the atopy patch tests. *Allergy.* 2006;61:1377-1384.
15. Boyce JA, Assa'ad A, Burks AW, et al. Guidelines for the diagnosis and management of food allergy in the United States: report of the NIAID-sponsored expert panel. *J Allergy Clin Immunol.* 2010;126(6):S1-S58.

16. Boyce JA, Assa'ad A, Burks AW, et al. Guidelines for the diagnosis and management of food allergy in the United States: report of the NIAID-sponsored expert panel [guideline 7]. *J Allergy Clin Immunol.* 2010;126(6):S1-S58.

17. Fleischer DM, Bock SA, Spears GC, et al. Oral food challenges in children with a diagnosis of food allergy. *J Pediatr.* 2011;158(4):578-583.

18. Gerez IFA, Shek LPC, Chng HH, Lee BW. Diagnostic tests for food allergy. *Singapore Med J.* 2010;51(1):4-9.

19. Patriarca G, Nucera E, Roncallo C, et al. Oral desensitizing treatment in food allergy: clinical and immunological results. *Aliment Pharmacol Ther.* 2003;17:459-465.

20. Wüthrich B. Unproven techniques in allergy diagnosis. *J Invest Allergol Clin Immunol.* 2005;15(2):86-90.

21. Antico A, Pagani M, Vescovi PP, Bonadonna P, Senna G. Food-specific IgG4 lack diagnostic value in adult patients with chronic urticaria and other suspected allergy skin symptoms. *Int Arch Allergy Immunol.* 2010;155(1):52-56.

22. Boyce JA, Assa'ad A, Burks AW, et al. Guidelines for the diagnosis and management of food allergy in the United States: report of the NIAID-sponsored expert panel [guideline 6]. *J Allergy Clin Immunol.* 2010;126(6):S1-S58.

23. Williams PB, Nolte H, Dolen WK, Koepke JW, Selner JC. The histamine content of allergen extracts. *J Allergy Clin Immunol.* 1992;89(3):738-745.

24. David TJ. Skin tests. In: *Food and Food Additive Intolerance in Childhood.* Oxford: Blackwell Scientific Publishers; 1993; 244-292.

25. Strid J, Strobel S. Skin barrier dysfunction and systemic sensitization to allergens through the skin. *Curr Drug Targets Inflamm Allergy.* 2005;4(5):531-541.

26. Saloga J, Knop J. The skin as target for IgE-mediated allergic reactions: Does sensitization through the skin occur? *Allergy.* 2000;55:905-909.

27. Lack G, Fox D, Northstone K, Golding J. For the Avon Longitudinal Study of Parents and Children Study Team. Factors associated with the development of peanut allergy in childhood. *New Engl J Med.* 2003;348(11):977-985.

28. Lack G. Epidemiological risks for food allergy. *J Allergy Clin Immunol.* 2008;121(6):1331-1336.

29. Furuta GT, Liacouras CA, Collins MH, et al. Members of the First International Gastrointestinal Eosinophil Research Symposium (FIGERS). Eosinophilic esophagitis in children and adults: a systematic review and consensus recommendations for diagnosis and treatment. *Gastroenterology.* 2007;133(4):1342-1363.

30. Spergel JM, Brown-Whitehorn T, Beausoleil JL, Shuker M, Liscouras CA. Predictive values for skin prick test and atopy patch test for eosinophilic esophagitis. *J Allergy Clin Immunol.* 2007;119(2):509-511.

31. Rothenberg ME. Biology and treatment of eosinophilic esophagitis. *Gastroenterology.* 2009;137(4):1238-1249.

32. Hwang JB, Song JY, Kang SP, Suh SI, Kam S, Choi WJ. The significance of gastric juice analysis for a positive challenge by a standard oral challenge test in typical cow's milk protein-induced enterocolitis. *J Korean Med Sci.* 2008;23(2):251-255.

33. Katelaris CH, Weiner JM, Heddle RJ, Stuckey MS, Yan KW. For the Australian College of Allergy. Position statement: Vega testing in the diagnosis of allergic conditions *Med J Aust.* 1991;155:113-114.

34. Potter PC, Mullineux J, Weinberg EG, et al. The ALCAT test—inappropriate in testing for food allergy in clinical practice. *S Afr Med J.* 1992;81(7):384.

35. Kinesiology Network Web site. www.kinesiology.net.

36. Ortolani C, Bruijnzeel-Koomen C, Bengtsson U, et al. Controversial aspects of adverse reactions to food. *Allergy.* 1999;54:27-45.

37. Wanich N, Nowak-Wegrzyn A, Sampson HA, Scheffler WG. Allergen-specific basophil suppression associated with clinical tolerance in patients with milk allergy. *J Allergy Clin Immunol.* 2009;123(4):789-794.

38. Signet Diagnostic Corporation. LEAP Disease Management Web site. www.nowleap.com.

39. Boyce JA, Assa'ad A, Burks AW, et al. Guidelines for the diagnosis and management of food allergy in the United States: report of the NIAID-sponsored expert panel [guideline 12]. *J Allergy Clin Immunol.* 2010;126(6):S1-S58.

40. Sampson HA. Food allergy part 2. Diagnosis and management. *J Allergy Clin Immunol.* 1999;103:981-989.

41. Boyce JA, Assa'ad A, Burks AW, et al. Guidelines for the diagnosis and management of food allergy in the United States: report of the NIAID-sponsored expert panel [guidelines 10, 11]. *J Allergy Clin Immunol.* 2010;126(6):S1-S58.

42. Nowak-Wegrzyn A, Assa'ad AH, Bahna SL, Bock SA, Sicherer SH, Teuber SS; Adverse Reactions to Food Committee of the American Academy of Allergy, Asthma and Immunology. Work Group Report: oral food challenge testing. *J Allergy Clin Immunol.* 2009;123(6):S365-S383.

CHAPTER 6

Elimination Diets

The aim of an elimination diet is to remove the food components that cause or exacerbate the clinical symptoms of concern. Elimination diets help determine the "culprit" food components by rendering the allergic person symptom-free when the foods are removed. When the culprit components are reintroduced during the "challenge" phase, they will trigger noticeable, and sometimes measurable, symptoms.[1]

In general, the elimination phase of the "elimination and challenge" process for identifying the foods responsible for food allergies and intolerances uses diets of three types: selective elimination diets, few foods elimination diets, and elemental diets. Each has a specific function in managing food sensitivity.

- Selective elimination diets: One or a small number of foods are eliminated for a specified period of time. For example, milk, eggs, and wheat, or a combination of these will be removed from the diet (see Chapters 10 through 19 for details).
- Few foods elimination diets (sometimes referred to as oligoantigenic diets): Only a few (usually less than 10) foods are allowed for a specified period of time (see discussion later in this chapter).
- Elemental diets: Only an amino acid–based formula is allowed for the duration of the elimination phase. No solid food is consumed. Sometimes an extensively hydrolyzed formula may be used, especially for babies and children.

To determine which elimination diet is appropriate, several pieces of information are required:

- A careful medical history. It is especially important that any *anaphylactic reactions* suspected to be due to food are recorded.
- Identification and exclusion of any other cause for the symptoms. This is determined by appropriate diagnostic tests and procedures.
- Results of any "allergy tests" previously carried out by qualified practitioners.

■ A careful record of all foods, beverages, supplements, and medications ingested during a 7-day period, together with details of symptoms experienced during this time. This record is called an *exposure diary*[2] (see Box 6.1).

The elimination diet is formulated to exclude all suspect allergens and intolerance triggers based on the preceding information, specifically:

■ The detailed medical history
■ Results of any previous allergy tests
■ Analysis of the exposure diary
■ Foods that the person suspects are causing their symptoms

Selective Elimination Diets

Selective elimination diets are usually used when ingesting a specific food causes an acute reaction and there is indication of an IgE-mediated hypersensitivity reaction based on tests for food-specific antibody (see Chapter 5). In the case of anaphylaxis or acute reactions, selective elimination diets can be considered therapeutic.

Selective elimination diets are also employed when food components are known or suspected to be the major factor in the etiology of defined conditions but where allergy or intolerance of a specific food is not the cause (eg, histamine sensitivity and tyramine sensitivity). These are dealt with in more detail later in the corresponding chapters.

Selective elimination diets may also be used to identify specific food triggers in chronic allergic disease, such as migraine headaches, atopic dermatitis (eczema),

---

BOX 6.1   Exposure Diary

Record for 7 days:
- All foods, beverages, medications, and supplements ingested
- Approximate quantities of each (teaspoons, tablespoons, cups, grams, ounces)
- Composition of compound dishes and drinks (ingredient list)
- The time at which each was taken
- All symptoms experienced, graded on severity: 1 (mild), 2 (mild to moderate), 3 (moderate), 4 (severe)
- Time of onset of the symptoms
- How long the symptoms last and whether medications were taken to control the symptoms
- Status on waking in the morning (symptom-free? type and severity of symptoms?)
- If sleep was disturbed during the night, whether this was due to specific symptoms

urticaria (hives) and angioedema (swelling), and some cases of eosinophilic gastro-intestinal diseases (EGID). In these cases, if the symptoms persist after specific foods have been eliminated, the assumption can be made that the foods avoided are not causing the reaction.

Selective and therapeutic diets are normally followed for 4 weeks. This allows sufficient time for recovery from the initial "withdrawal symptoms" and usually relief of all symptoms that are due to food components. It also allows enough time for people to adapt to the diet, both physiologically and psychologically, and to make the necessary adjustments in their lifestyle to accommodate the dietary restrictions.

Because selective elimination diets are nutritionally adequate, there is usually no risk associated with prolonged adherence to the diet. Taking into consideration the immunological response, 4 weeks' freedom from exposure to an allergen is also a suitable time to challenge the offending allergen. This interval of freedom allows symptom remission, but the level of antigen-specific IgE will not be reduced significantly, so during the challenge phase when each eliminated food is reintroduced, the person will experience a clear and sometimes enhanced response.

Specific Food Restrictions

The elimination of specific foods in preparation for challenge, or in situations where the culprit food component has been definitively identified, is a relatively straightforward process. The health care team should work with the food-sensitive individual to prepare three important written lists:

- The foods that must be avoided, and manufactured foods that commonly contain the subject food
- A comprehensive list of the terms that would identify the food in an ingredient list or on a food label
- Alternative food sources of all the nutrients that may be deficient when the subject food is eliminated, in order to reduce the risk of nutrient deficiency. If easily accessible food sources are limited, appropriate and specific supplements should be recommended.

Examples of selective elimination diets include diets free from:

- Milk
- Egg
- Wheat
- Peanut
- Soy
- Tree nuts
- Fish
- Shellfish

■ Food additives and naturally occurring chemicals such as:
  - Sulfites
  - Benzoates
  - Artificial food colors
  - Nickel
  - Monosodium glutamate (MSG)

Selective elimination diets are designed to remove all suspect allergens and intolerance triggers but include all foods that are not involved in the clinical condition or have tested negative on the diagnostic tests employed. Instructions for managing selective elimination diets for specific foods and details and discussion of therapeutic diets can be found in the relevant chapters in this book.

Nutritional Adequacy of Selective Elimination Diets

A person's nutrient needs can be adequately supplied by a selective elimination diet that incorporates alternative foods that are nutritionally equivalent to those removed. There is no reason why anyone should lose weight or fail to obtain all of his or her essential nutritional requirements on a selective elimination diet. If the allowed foods do not provide all the nutrients required, the health care professional should prescribe the appropriate dietary supplements to correct the deficit. The need for nutrient supplements is determined by the foods being eliminated from the diet (refer to specific chapters for details).

Duration of the Selective Elimination Diet

The selective elimination diet is usually followed for 4 weeks. In cases where the symptoms occur only intermittently (eg, migraine headaches), the diet should be extended to cover at least three or four episodes.

If the symptoms have not disappeared or greatly decreased after 4 weeks, either allergens or intolerance factors remain in the diet or the symptoms are unrelated to foods. To determine whether foods in the elimination diet are responsible for the remaining symptoms, another exposure diary should be recorded for 5 to 7 days while continuing with the elimination diet. Analysis of this second exposure diary should indicate if other foods or chemicals could be causing the remaining symptoms. A further elimination of foods can be carried out for 2 more weeks if indicated by the second food exposure diary. The new diet should be followed no longer than 2 weeks, and an exposure diary should be kept for the second week of the diet.

Follow-up to the Selective Elimination Diet

Following the 4 to 6 weeks on the selective elimination diet, the challenge phase should be initiated (see Chapter 7 for details). Even if the symptoms have only moderately improved, a specific challenge of food components may reveal adverse reactions that are not noticeable when the food is eaten frequently. Some practitioners refer to this as "unmasking a hidden food allergy."

Few Foods Elimination Diet

Sometimes it is difficult to determine the foods that should be excluded on a selective elimination diet. When there are multiple symptoms that do not fit into any perceivable pattern of reactivity that would suggest a reaction to food allergens, and when there are no indicators of food additive intolerance or sensitivity to natural components of foods, a few foods elimination diet is useful. Such diets are particularly valuable in managing chronic allergic conditions.

A few foods elimination diet differs from a selective elimination diet in that only a small number of foods are allowed. These are the foods that are considered to be the least likely to trigger an allergic reaction. Such diets are indicated when there are many symptoms with no clear relationship to specific foods.

Because an oligoantigenic diet is not nutritionally complete, it should never be followed for more than 14 days. Seven to 10 days is usually sufficient to show results, and this period *should not* be exceeded for children younger than 7 years of age. A role for foods in the etiology of symptoms should become apparent if symptoms disappear or improve significantly within this time period. Extending the few foods elimination diet beyond 14 days if the symptoms remain unchanged is fruitless and can be detrimental to the person's health, because the immune system may become depressed on this "semistarvation" regimen.

If symptoms do not clear within 14 days, two reasons should be considered:

- One or more of the foods included in the diet are allergenic for the person.
- Foods are not contributing to the symptoms.

To evaluate the first assumption: replace each food with one from the same food group and continue the elimination for an additional 7 days. To test the second assumption: initiate a sequential incremental dose challenge of each restricted food (see Chapter 7).

Pediatric Concerns

Young children are especially vulnerable to nutritional deficiency because all nutrients are needed in the years of maximum growth. When children are on the elimination diet, careful and frequent evaluation must be made to ensure that their nutritional needs are being met at each stage of the process of determining their allergenic foods. For this reason, a few foods elimination diet is rarely recommended before puberty. In most cases, a selective elimination diet is adequate for diagnosing food allergy in children.

If an extensive elimination diet is necessary to identify many suspected allergenic foods, the few foods elimination diet should not be followed for longer than 7 days for anyone younger than 13 years and must be done under the supervision of a suitably qualified health care practitioner. Sometimes an extensively hydrolyzed infant formula can be used alone or as a supplement to the few foods elimination diet to reduce the risk of nutrient deficiency during the elimination diet phase for children. Older children find consuming such a formula mixed in with the allowed foods more acceptable than drinking it alone.

Foods Allowed

There are many few foods elimination diets in use, and each practitioner tends to favor a particular diet.[3] Many so-called few foods diets contain too many different foods to be useful and could be considered selective rather than oligoantigenic diets. The few foods elimination diet provided in Box 6.2 includes foods that consistently prove low in allergenicity for the majority of the population and is the one most often followed.

Adjustments must be made for individuals with unusual reactions who might respond adversely to one or more of the foods included. The most effective oligoantigenic diets are individualized for each person, because the persistence of symptoms could be due to one or more foods left in the diet.

It is important that the foods selected are ones to which the person has shown no evidence of reactivity in the past. The diet contains no food additives, flavor enhancers, or modifiers, so both allergens and chemical food additives are minimized or eliminated.

Guidelines for the Few Foods Elimination Diet

It is wise to begin the diet trial during a quiet social season, not during Christmas, Hanukkah, or other religious holidays or around birthdays, weddings, or other important celebrations. If there is a social event during this diet, the person should be instructed to take his or her own food or hold the party in their home so that appropriate foods are available at all times.

It will be necessary to shop ahead to have plenty of appropriate foods on hand. The diet may be somewhat boring, but there is no need for anyone to go hungry. There is no restriction on calorie intake. Weight loss should not be a primary goal during this test period. It is important that the patient remain healthy and as well nourished as possible while investigating specific responses to foods. The issue of weight loss can be addressed later if necessary. The meals are simple, without spices, butter, or condiments. As many fresh food sources as possible should be used. Frozen is the next best alternative.

The duration of the elimination diet is usually 10 to 14 days. During the first 5 days, symptoms may seem to get worse or the person may feel unwell, even experiencing flulike symptoms. Lots of rest and drinking distilled or filtered water will help to minimize these symptoms. By the end of 4 days, some symptoms should start to clear, and most food reactions should have greatly decreased or disappeared by the fifth or sixth day. Because the diet is nutritionally inadequate, it must *not* be continued for more than 14 days.

BOX 6.2   Foods Allowed on the Few Foods Elimination Diet

Meat and alternates
- Lamb
- Turkey
- If lamb and turkey are not tolerated: fish (specifically perch, red snapper, sea bass)

Grains
- Whole grains, flours, and pure cereals made from rice, tapioca, or millet

Vegetables
- Squash (all kinds, including acorn, butternut, chayote, hubbard, winter squash, pattypan, spaghetti squash, yellow squash, summer squash, crookneck, zucchini, pure infant squash in jars)
- Parsnips
- Sweet potatoes (including pure infant sweet potatoes in jars)
- Yams
- Lettuce (iceberg [head lettuce] is the least tolerated of the lettuces. If it is not tolerated, other varieties may be acceptable.)

Fruits
- Pears (including pure bottled pear juice and pure infant pears in jars)
- Cranberries (fresh or frozen; homemade cranberry juice from cranberries)

Oils
- Canola
- Safflower

Condiments
- Sea salt

Desserts
- Pudding made from tapioca beads or rice; fruit and fruit juice of allowed fruits
- Agar-agar (seaweed) may be used as a thickener

Beverages
- Distilled water
- Juice from the allowed fruits and vegetables

A diary of the entire experience is very useful. The individual should keep a record of the date and time of eating and any reactions experienced. Food should be washed and cooked with distilled or filtered water if possible. Tap water and even bottled water may contain contaminants that could cause reactions.

Pots, pans, and containers made from iron, aluminum, or glass should be used in food preparation and cooking. Utensils made from stainless steel or that have nonstick coatings may add reactive chemicals to the foods being cooked in them.

The following should be avoided:

- Chewing gum
- Over-the-counter medications (unless they are essential)
- Breath mints
- Coffee
- Tea (including herbal tea)
- Diet drinks
- Mouthwash
- Cigarettes and other tobacco products

Necessary prescription medications should be continued as required and advised by the patient's physician.

Elemental Diets

When allergy to multiple foods is suspected, and when either selective or few foods elimination diets have failed to resolve a person's symptoms, an elemental formula alone for a short period of time should determine whether the illness is food related. An elemental diet supplies calories and all essential macro- and micronutrients in the form of an amino acid–based formula. Such diets are easy to maintain in infancy but are more difficult in adulthood. Most elemental formulas are unpalatable and may be better tolerated by nasogastric feeding, which is sometimes considered in extreme cases. Elemental formulas can be rendered more palatable by flavoring added by the manufacturer, but this adds the risk for adverse reactions to the chemicals in the flavoring compounds.

Elemental formulas are used only in rare cases in which all other elimination diets have failed to resolve symptoms, but the suspicion of an allergic etiology for the person's illness remains high. There are several elemental formulas available. None should be used without the knowledge and approval of the patient's physician, and none should be continued for any prolonged period of time. Formulas[a] such as Vivonex (Nestlé Nutrition) and Tolerex (Nestlé Nutrition) are examples of formulas suitable for adults. The elemental formulas Neocate (Nutricia) and EleCare (Abbott Nutrition) and extensively hydrolyzed casein formulas such as Enfamil Nutramigen (Mead-Johnson), Similac Alimentum (Abbott Nutrition), and Enfamil Pregestimil

---

[a] The brand names are included as examples only. The author and publisher do not recommend the use of any mentioned product in preference to another. Manufacturers often change their formulations. Always check current product information to ascertain the suitability of a product for a particular individual.

(Mead-Johnson), although not elemental, are usually tolerated by infants. The suitability for the individual should be ascertained before a specific formula is chosen. The number of daily calories supplied by the formula must be calculated for each person so that he or she consumes the required quantity of formula. In addition, the precise composition of each formula should be confirmed by asking the manufacturer, since sometimes the ingredients are changed without notice.

Summary: Expected Results of the Elimination Diet

If all or most of the major reaction triggers have been excluded, the person may actually feel *worse* on days 2 to 4 of the elimination diet. Theoretically, this may be due to a condition of antibody excess, causing a condition similar to serum sickness. By day 5 to 7 of exclusion, definite improvement should be evident if the allergens and intolerance triggers responsible for the symptoms have been eliminated. The symptoms should have improved significantly after 10 to 14 days of exclusion. If all allergens and antagonistic foods have been eliminated, all symptoms should have disappeared after about 3 weeks. If substitution of alternative foods for excluded nutrients is adequate, no weight loss should occur in the 2 or 4 weeks of the elimination diet. If symptoms have not improved significantly, it is likely that unidentified allergens or intolerance factors may still be present in the diet, or foods are not the cause of the symptoms.

The duration of the initial elimination phase will depend on the type of symptoms being managed. For example, reactions that appear only intermittently at widely spaced intervals (such as migraine headaches) or those that may be due to delayed reactions to foods and additives may require a longer elimination phase. However, gastrointestinal symptoms and skin reactions will usually respond promptly to appropriate dietary measures, and improvement may be experienced within 7 to 10 days.

Most selective elimination diets are followed for 4 weeks; few foods elimination diets are usually followed for 10 to 14 days. An elimination diet should never be followed for longer than 10 to 14 days if there is any danger of nutritional deficiency such as may occur on the few foods elimination diet.

The patient should be instructed to keep another food and symptoms record for the last week of the elimination phase. This will show whether symptoms have improved. If symptoms still persist, a clear pattern of occurrence might be obvious that could point to a specific food trigger that can be avoided for a longer trial period. Further elimination of foods can be carried out, in addition to the original list, for another 2 weeks, based on analysis of the second exposure diary. After 14 days on the few foods elimination diet or after 4 weeks on a selective elimination diet (or 6 weeks if more foods have been eliminated for 2 weeks after the original 4), a sequential incremental dose challenge should be started (see Chapter 7). Even if the symptoms do not seem to have improved a great deal, specific challenge of food components sometimes reveals adverse reactions that are not noticeable when the food is eaten continuously.

Reasons for Failure in Following an Elimination Diet

The following are among the several key reasons why a person may not adhere to dietary restrictions:

▪ Insufficient knowledge or understanding about the restrictions and why they are necessary.
▪ The diet is too intrusive to be acceptable (eg, too many restrictions or the prescribed diet plan does not take into account lifestyle and tastes).
▪ The diet fails to reduce or abolish symptoms. This can be due to a number of factors:
  • The diet is frequently abandoned during the first 2 to 4 days because symptoms may intensify or do not seem to be resolving.
  • The diet may have improved the symptoms for which food components are responsible, but the remaining symptoms are caused by factors other than foods, which will not improve by dietary manipulation.
  • Allergenic foods remain in the diet.
  • Some of the restricted ingredients might have been introduced during manufacture or serving of the allowed foods. For example, contamination of utensils and equipment in the processing of several different foods without adequate cleaning in between batches—this is a particular problem with ice cream and bakery products such as cookies.
▪ Excessive expectations of the diet have not been met (eg, a cure rather than mere improvement was expected).
▪ The diet is no longer needed because the symptoms abated spontaneously, or, in children, the child grew out of the symptoms.
▪ Cost should not be an important element in not adhering to a diet, because most of the initial elimination diets are followed for only a short period of time and the savings from those eliminated usually offset the cost of the substitute foods. A few comparison studies show that there is not a significant difference in cost between the regular diet and the elimination diet except in the cases where expensive elemental food replacements and supplements have been prescribed.

Follow-up to the Elimination Diet

Following the elimination diet, sequential incremental dose challenge should be initiated in order to identify the specific food(s) responsible for the patient's reactions (see Chapter 7). When the culprit food components have been identified, a selective elimination diet, now referred to as a *maintenance diet* (see Chapter 8), can be continued as long as necessary, without incurring any nutritional risk.

Therapeutic Diets

The information provided in this chapter is designed to manage the diet when food allergy or intolerance is the suspected cause of a person's symptoms. However, there is another type of selective elimination diet that is used in situations where a diagnosis has been made and the cause of the condition has been identified as a food component. Treatment for these conditions is strict avoidance of the causative food component, and carefully designed therapeutic diets are essential in managing the person's condition. Such diets are referred to as *therapeutic diets*. They are designed to remove all suspect allergens and intolerance triggers but include all foods that are not involved in the clinical condition as well as those foods that have tested negative on the diagnostic tests employed.

Therapeutic diets can be classified by the situations in which they are used. For example, some therapeutic diets address inborn errors of metabolism of various types, such as the following:

■ Errors in carbohydrate metabolism, such as galactosemia, hereditary fructose intolerance, and glycogen storage diseases
■ Errors in amino acid metabolism, of which the most well known is phenylketonuria, in which dietary phenylalanine must be restricted
■ Anomalies in lipid metabolism, of which hyperlipoproteinemia is probably the most frequently encountered example

Therapeutic diets are also used for metabolic anomalies that are more commonly referred to as *food intolerances*. Examples include disaccharide deficiency of several types, such as the following:

■ Lactose intolerance, caused by a deficiency in the enzyme lactase
■ Sucrose intolerance, usually a congenital condition caused by a deficiency in the production of sucrase
■ Glucose-galactose intolerance

In addition, therapeutic diets are used for conditions in which a component of food is inadequately absorbed, such as fructose intolerance, as well as conditions in which food components need to be restricted as a result of immunological processes other than allergy, such as the following:

■ Gluten-sensitive enteropathy (celiac disease), in which all gluten-containing foods must be avoided
■ Food protein enteropathy, most frequently seen in young infants, in which all the identified food proteins must be excluded
■ Eosinophilic gastroenteritis, esophagitis, and colitis

Finally, some types of therapeutic diets are used when specific food components are suspected to be a causative or exacerbating factor in a clinical condition in which all other causes have been ruled out. Most of the diets in this category are experimental, as further research still must confirm their utility and possibly define the physiological mechanism in which the suspect food component is adversely impacting the individual. Therapeutic elimination diets have been utilized successfully in the management of conditions such as:

- *Idiopathic urticaria and angioedema*, in which dietary sources of histamine are restricted
- *Irritable bowel syndrome*, in which the foods are modified to promote digestion and absorption in the small intestine and to reduce the residue of undigested food passing into the colon to act as a substrate for microbial fermentation
- *Migraine headache*, in which biogenic amines such as histamine, tyramine, phenylethylamine, and octopamine are restricted
- *Infant eczema*, in which the major food allergens and all artificial food additives are restricted

References

1. Sampson HA. Food allergy. Part 2: diagnosis and management [review]. *J Allergy Clin Immunol.* 1999;103(6):981-989.
2. Joneja, JMV. *Dealing with Food Allergies: A Practical Guide to Detecting the Culprit Foods and Eating a Healthy, Enjoyable Diet.* Boulder, CO: Bull Publishing Company; 2003.
3. Patriarca G, Schiavino D, Pecora V, et al. Food allergy and food intolerance: diagnosis and treatment. *Intern Emerg Med.* 2009;4:11-24.

CHAPTER **7**

Challenge Protocols

After a person completes the elimination test diet, the next step in identifying the foods and food additives associated with adverse reactions is to reintroduce each component individually so that those responsible for symptoms can be clearly identified. This is achieved by careful challenge with precise quantities of each food component and careful monitoring of symptom development, looking for immediate reactions (within a 4-hour period) or delayed reactions (from 1 to 4 days) following ingestion.[1]

Food Challenge Protocols

There are three basic methods of reintroducing the eliminated foods to determine those that are responsible for the adverse reactions:

- Double-blind placebo-controlled food challenge (DBPCFC) is usually employed in research studies or specialized clinics. Neither the patient nor the supervisor knows the identity of the test food component, and each test is compared to the patient's reaction to a placebo (usually glucose powder) enclosed within a gelatin capsule similar to that of the food.
- Single-blind food challenge is usually supervised by a physician or, more commonly, a dietitian or nurse in an office setting. The patient is unaware of the food's identity, but the supervisor knows. The food is disguised in another, stronger-tasting, food.
- Open food challenge is most frequently carried out by the allergic person at home. The person is aware of the identity of the food and the quantity being consumed in each test. This method is used for foods that have been eaten in the past without severe reactions and for foods that are considered unlikely to elicit an anaphylactic reaction.

Double-Blind, Placebo-Controlled Food Challenge

The double-blind, placebo-controlled food challenge (DBPCFC) is regarded as the "gold standard" by most traditional allergists. DBPCFCs are expensive and labor-intensive, so most are conducted either in a research setting or in specialized facilities such as allergy clinics or hospitals when knowing the identity of the culprit food is extremely important for the patient's health. The challenge is always conducted by a clinician or other qualified health professional (eg, a registered dietitian or nurse) in a medical or research facility.

In this procedure, described here, neither the patient nor the supervisor of the challenge knows the food's identity:

■   The food is lyophilized (freeze-dried) to a powder and a known quantity is enclosed in a gelatin capsule.

■   A known quantity of placebo, usually glucose powder, is enclosed within the same kind of capsule and is used as a negative control.

■   The patient is given a specific number of capsules, usually starting with one and increasing through the test. Thus the quantity of the food consumed is measured. The capsules are coded and contain either the test food or the placebo. Neither the supervisor of the test nor the patient is aware of the contents (ie, it is double-blind).

■   The patient's reactions are recorded.

■   Analysis of the patient's response with the code identifies the food and the dosage at which a reaction occurs.

■   A reaction after consuming the placebo indicates a nonfood (and likely nonallergic) response.

For IgE-mediated reactions, the method of administration tends to vary from clinic to clinic. Two examples are described in the following sections.[2,3]

Method 1

For *IgE-mediated reactions*, the challenge food is administered in the fasting state (a minimum of 4 hours since the last meal), starting with a dose unlikely to provoke symptoms (25 to 500 mg of lyophilized food). The dose is usually doubled every 15 to 60 minutes; the interval between doses is dictated by the reported course of the patient's symptoms. Two hours after the feeding, the patient is observed for the development of symptoms. If the patient tolerates 10 g of lyophilized food (equivalent to about one egg white, or one 4 oz glass of milk), clinical reactivity is considered to be unlikely. In most IgE-mediated disorders, challenges to new foods may be conducted every 1 to 2 days.

The methods for *non-IgE-mediated reactions* are as follows. In dietary protein–induced enterocolitis, allergen challenges require up to 0.3 to 0.6 g of food per kg of body weight given in one or two doses. The patient is usually observed for 24 to 48 hours for the development of symptoms. In eosinophilic gastroenteritis, several feedings over a 1- to 3-day period may be required to elicit symptoms; the patient is observed for up to 4 days for the development of symptoms. With most non-IgE-mediated reactions, challenges need to be at least 3 to 5 days apart.

Method 2

In this test, 8 to 10 g of the dry (lyophilized) food, 100 mL of wet food, or double these quantities for meat or fish are used. The dose is consumed at 10- to 15-minute intervals over a total of 90 minutes. A meal-sized portion of the food is consumed a few hours later. Symptoms are recorded and assessments made for reactions in the skin, gastrointestinal tract, and respiratory tract. Challenges are terminated when a reaction becomes apparent. However, all negative challenges need to be confirmed by an open feeding under observation to rule out false-negative responses.

Single-Blind Food Challenge

In this method of challenge, the test supervisor knows the suspect allergen but the patient does not. The food is disguised in a strongly flavored food such as one of the following:

- Fruit juice (cranberry, apple, or grape)
- Infant formula for babies and children
- Elemental formula appropriate for a child or adult
- Meat patties
- Cereals
- Added ingredients with strong flavors such as mint, fish, or garlic
- Lentil soup

Testing for most IgE-mediated reactions, and those resulting in severe allergic symptoms, is conducted under medical supervision, in appropriately equipped facilities. The majority of anaphylactic reactions to foods are not challenged because it is frequently possible to identify the food responsible based on the patient's history. If such challenges are necessary, they should only be conducted under the strictest medical supervision with appropriately qualified and equipped personnel in attendance.

Open Food Challenge: Sequential Incremental Dose Challenge (SIDC)

Open food challenges are considered a safe procedure in the office setting for those patients whose history and food-specific IgE approach negative predictive values,[4] especially if the food has been eaten in the past without overt reactivity.

Many adverse reactions to foods do not result in severe reactions and can be safely carried out in an office setting or at home.[5] It must be recognized that many people carry out such challenges on their own at home without professional knowledge, especially if the food has been eaten in the past and reactions are generally mild.

However, despite how mild the allergy symptoms appear to have been, it is important that some professional supervision be provided in the interests of safety, especially if the patient is a child. The methods described here for identifying foods that trigger adverse reactions would be more appropriately considered "reintroduction" rather than challenge and would be carried out on foods not deemed likely to cause a severe reaction. Because unnecessary restriction of foods can be detrimental to a person's nutritional health and emotional and social well-being, it is important that the foods responsible for adverse reactions be correctly identified, even though they do not threaten a person's life.

In many types of foods, several different components can be challenged individually. By separating those that can be tolerated from those that need to be avoided, a person's diet can include a wider range of safe food choices that ensure a more complete nutritional intake. Reactivity to a component of a food, but not the whole food, is well known in the case of lactose intolerance wherein only the milk sugar (lactose) needs to be avoided; the milk proteins are tolerated, so lactose-free milk and its products can be included in the diet to supply many essential nutrients. A similar liberalization of dietary restrictions can be achieved when individual food components are reintroduced separately. For example, in milk allergy/intolerance, challenge with casein, whey, and lactose individually will determine a person's reactivity to each; those that cause a reaction will be avoided; those that are tolerated can be included in the regular diet.

The initial selective elimination diet, few foods elimination diet, or elemental formula is continued for the duration of the challenge phase of the program. For adults, foods are not added back into the diet until all of the foods within a category have been tested separately, even if they produce no reaction during the challenge. This is to ensure that the quantity of each food component is consistent with the test directives. If foods are added back as they are tolerated, the quantity of a single component will be increased by inclusion of previously tested and tolerated foods containing that component. For example, while testing milk components, if Test 1 for casein proteins is tolerated, including cheese in the diet while the subsequent challenges are carried out will increase the quantity of casein in each test.

The instructions presented in Box 7.1 are designed to allow challenge with increasing doses of the test components, so that an idea of a person's limit of tolerance (ie, the point at which symptoms develop) and the individual food components that are safe can be determined. A chart is provided for recording the outcome of each challenge test. The initial selective elimination diet, few foods elimination diet, or elemental formula is continued for the duration of the challenge phase of the program.

BOX 7.1 General Instructions for Conducting the SIDC

IMPORTANT: Any foods that have caused an anaphylactic reaction, have been suspected to trigger an anaphylactic reaction, or have been or suspected to be the cause of a severe allergic reaction (especially in an asthmatic) should only be challenged under medical supervision in a suitably equipped medical facility.

- The selective or few foods elimination diet continues for all meals throughout the testing period.
- An initial screening challenge provides a measure of safety (labial food challenge):
  - The food is placed on the outer border of the lower lip for 2 minutes.
  - The site is observed for the development of a local reaction for 30 minutes.
- Signs of a positive reaction are:
  - Swelling, reddening, or irritation at the site of application
  - Development of a rash of the cheek and/or chin
  - Rhinitis or conjunctivitis
  - A systemic reaction
- Placing a sample of the food on the cheek and observing for a local reaction (reddening, blistering, or irritation) before the labial food challenge will add an extra margin of safety. This is especially useful when testing a child.
- If the labial food challenge is negative, the individual will consume each food component three times on the test day at four hourly intervals in increasing doses and will carefully monitor his or her response and the development of symptoms.
- The symptoms that develop will be the same as those that have been experienced in the past, but the intensity or severity may be significantly increased. Any new symptoms not previously experienced are unlikely to be due to the food; an unrelated cause should be investigated and the food challenge repeated after an interval of at least 2 weeks.
- If symptoms develop at any time, consumption of the food component being tested stops immediately. The basic elimination diet should be continued until the symptoms subside completely. Testing of the next food in the sequence can commence 48 hours *after the symptoms have resolved*. This interval allows sufficient time for all of the reactive food to be eliminated from the body before another is introduced.
- If the test food does not cause an immediate reaction on day 1 of its introduction, the next day (day 2) is a monitoring day for delayed reactions. The basic elimination diet is eaten at each meal, but none of the test food is eaten during day 2. Symptoms that appear on day 2 are usually due to a delayed-type hypersensitivity reaction to an antigen or to a nonimmune-mediated reaction to a food additive.
- If no symptoms develop on days 1 or 2 of the test, the food can be considered safe. On day 3, the next food in the sequence can be challenged.
- Under most circumstances, 2 days are adequate for reactions to the test food to become apparent. However, occasionally it is unclear whether the symptoms are due to the food or to some unrelated event, or the reaction may be extremely mild. In such cases, the same food is eaten on day 3 in larger quantities than on day 1, again in three increasing doses. Day 4 would then become a second monitoring day for delayed reactions. If the test food is responsible for the reaction, the symptoms will increase in severity on both day 3 and day 4. If the food is not responsible, the symptoms will diminish or remain unchanged over days 3 and 4.
- The food category selected for each test is an individual choice.

Challenge Tests for Food Additives

Testing for food additives is more difficult than testing for allergens because, in most cases, it is not easy to obtain the additive in its pure form or even to find it as a single additive in a manufactured food. Usually, several different chemicals, such as flavor and texture modifiers, color, preservatives, and so on, are added simultaneously.

Several research studies have reported testing adverse reactions to food additives. A variety of levels of the additives have been used in various challenge studies, depending on the condition being evaluated. For example, different protocols have been used in studies on additives in asthma with aspirin sensitivity,[6] atopic dermatitis and urticaria,[7] and hyperactivity,[8] among others. In the latter study, the following levels were added in their pure form to an orange drink:

- Tartrazine: 8.5 mg/250 mL
- Sunset yellow: 8.5 mg/250 mL
- Sodium metabisulfite: 12.5 mg/250 mL
- Sodium benzoate: 55 mg/250 mL

However, for home and office challenge tests, it is probably sufficient to test the foods containing additives in the context within which they would normally be eaten. Food with a high level of the suspect additive is consumed, and the reaction is compared with that experienced after eating the same food without the additive. For example:

- Many prepackaged macaroni-and-cheese dinners contain tartrazine. The manufactured product should be tested and compared to a similar homemade meal, using cheddar cheese, which has a similar color but contains the natural yellow color annatto and not tartrazine.
- Cinnamon contains a high level of naturally occurring benzoates. Eating applesauce with cinnamon and applesauce without the spice will indicate whether cinnamon, and therefore benzoate, is tolerated.
- Sulfite sensitivity can be tested by comparing the reaction after eating dried fruit without sulfite (available in many health food stores) to the reaction after eating regular (sulfited) dried fruit generally available in supermarkets.
- To test for nitrates, test additive-free beef in comparison to a beef to which nitrates have been added to preserve the color. The butcher or supermarket manager will be able to supply you with that information.
- MSG can be obtained as a flavor enhancer in most food stores. Test food with and without MSG to determine sensitivity.

References

1. Nowak-Wegrzyn A, Assa'ad AH, Bahna SL, Bock SA, Sicherer SH, Teuber SS, on behalf of the Adverse Reactions to Food Committee of the American Academy of Allergy, Asthma and Immunology. Work Group report: oral food challenge testing. *J Allergy Clin Immunol*. 2009;123(6):S365-S383.

2. Sampson HA. Food allergy part 2. Diagnosis and management. *J Allergy Clin Immunol.* 1999;103(6):981-989.
3. Sicherer SH. Food allergy: when and how to perform oral food challenges. *Pediatr Allergy Immunol.* 1999;10:226-234.
4. Mankad VS, Williams LW, Lee LA, et al. Safety of open food challenges in the office setting. *Ann Allergy Asthma Immunol.* 2008;100(5):469-474.
5. Patriarca G, Schiavino D, Pecora V, et al. Food allergy and food intolerance: diagnosis and treatment. *Intern Emerg Med.* 2009;4:11-24.
6. Corder EH, Buckley CE. Aspirin, salicylate, sulfite and tartrazine induced bronchoconstriction. Safe doses and case definition in epidemiological studies. *J Clin Epidemiol.* 1995;48(10):1269-1275.
7. Hannuksela M, Lahti A. Peroral challenge tests with food additives in urticaria and atopic dermatitis. *Int J Dermatol.* 1986;25(3):178-180.
8. Bateman B, Warner JO, Hutchinson E, et al. The effects of a double blind placebo controlled artificial food colourings and benzoate preservative challenge on hyperactivity in a general population sample of preschool children. *Arch Dis Child.* 2004;89:506-511.

CHAPTER **8**

Maintenance Diets

When all of the food components responsible for triggering an allergic or intolerance reaction have been identified, a diet is formulated that will allow the food-sensitive individual to remain symptom-free and be well nourished. This is an important step in the management program, because if it becomes difficult for a person to comply with the dietary strategies, lapses into eating the reactive foods will likely occur with increasing frequency. Eventually, the diet will likely be abandoned, and when symptoms recur, the patient will be convinced that the whole exercise was a waste of time. Therefore, the diet should aim to meet several important goals right from the beginning:

- The diet must *exclude* all foods and additives to which a positive reaction has been recorded.
- It must be nutritionally *complete*, providing nutrients from nonreactive sources.
- It must take into account the person's lifestyle, financial status, and taste.
- It should include sufficient flexibility to accommodate "unusual" situations such as religious festivals, celebrations (eg, birthdays and weddings), vacations, travel, and eating in social settings where obtaining substitute foods might be a problem.

If dose-related intolerances are an issue, a rotation diet might be beneficial. However, at the present time there is no good evidence-based research to support the claims of benefit of rotation diets,[1] although many practitioners seem to favor their use, and there are a number of popular books on the market that provide details about a variety of rotation diets and schedules. For more on rotation diets, see Box 8.1.[1-5]

The Final Diet

When people are focusing on the foods that are making them sick and following often complex restrictive elimination diets, it is easy to lose sight of the most fundamental

BOX 8.1   Rotation Diets

Rotation diets were developed as a theoretical way to give the body more variety in nutrients and to give a "rest" from each food family. This was thought to prevent the development of new intolerances or increased sensitivity to foods.[2] In addition, it was claimed that rotation diets achieved freedom from allergic symptoms for a longer period and facilitated the identification of offending foods. Unfortunately, there are no good evidence-based research studies to support these claims.[3] Furthermore, recent research has demonstrated that members of the same botanic food family are not necessarily related allergenically. In fact, there is often a closer antigenic association between unrelated foods than those within the same family. Oral allergy syndrome and latex allergy effectively demonstrate this (see Chapters 33 and 34 for details).

The structure of rotation diets varies between practitioners.[2] Some favor the 4-day rotation in which members of a food family eaten on one day of the rotation could not be consumed for another 3 days. People with more complex food allergies were recommended to widen the rotation to a 1 in 7-day, 1 in 14-day, or, at the most extreme, a 1 in 30-day rotation.[2] Rotations of 4, 5, 7, and 31 days have been advised by various practitioners. Since 2 to 4 days is the approximate gastrointestinal transit time, a 4-day rotation is considered to be the most effective schedule. After 4 days, the amount of a specific food in the body is considered to be sufficiently low that eating it again will not increase the level to a reactive threshold.

Rotation diets and food allergy

No well-designed controlled studies have been conducted on the efficacy of rotation diets based on food families. Most authorities consider rotation diets as a management strategy for food allergy and intolerance to be controversial and of little or no benefit.[1] Because cross-reactivity between foods within a food family is unusual, diets that are based on the avoidance of entire food families are illogical. Furthermore, following a strict rotation diet can be tedious and time-consuming and can cause unnecessary risk of nutritional deficiency.

Rotation diets and food intolerance

When an adverse response to foods is due to a nonimmunologically mediated reaction, limiting the quantity of all foods containing the reactive component might make sense. In situations of enzyme deficiency, such as lack of lactase, consuming a greater quantity of the enzyme substrate (in this case lactose) than the enzyme can process will lead to the development of intolerance symptoms. A diet that restricts the intake of all lactose-containing foods will ensure that the limit of tolerance is not exceeded, and the person can remain symptom-free. A similar situation probably exists for most food intolerances, so a type of "rotation diet" that restricts the number and quantity of foods known to contain the culprit component is necessary. Such diets need to be formulated on an individual basis to ensure that the "dose" of the reactive component is reduced to a minimum, while nutrients equivalent to those eliminated are supplied by alternative foods.[5]

principle of dietary practice: Good health can be achieved and maintained only by providing the body with all of the macro- and micronutrients essential for its optimal functioning. At each stage of the process of determining the foods that are responsible for a person's adverse reactions, complete balanced nutrition must be provided, preferably from foods, but if this is not entirely possible, then appropriate supplements must be added.

When the culprit food components and additives have been identified, a maintenance diet must be formulated that removes the reactive foods and supplies complete balanced nutrition from alternative sources. Because this diet will need to be followed for the long term, it is important that it supply every essential nutrient and that it is appropriate for the person's lifestyle and financial situation. If a diet is difficult to follow because of its emphasis on foods unacceptable to the individual; if it requires the expenditure of excessive time, money, and effort; or if it is inappropriate for the person's lifestyle, it will soon be abandoned. All of the effort and energy invested in identifying the culprit foods will have been for naught, and the sensitive individual will be left with the same degree of distress as before. Formulating the appropriate diet for each person individually requires a great deal of time and effort but is essential to a positive outcome. The tools provided here should make the process fairly straightforward.

Ensuring That All the Essential Nutrients Are Present

The process of devising the ideal diet for an individual starts with identifying the nutrients that may be deficient when specific foods are removed and correcting the deficiency by substituting different foods containing the same nutrients.

The most important directive is that a person must consume a nutritionally balanced diet that supplies all required macronutrients (protein, fat, carbohydrate) and micronutrients (vitamins and trace minerals) every day. To simplify the process, *each meal* should contain three components: (a) protein (PRO); (b) grain (GR) or starch (ST); and (c) fruit and/or vegetable (FR/VEG). See Boxes 8.2, 8.3, and 8.4 for detailed lists.

Micronutrients (Vitamins and Minerals)

In general, the foods grouped together in Boxes 8.2, 8.3, and 8.4 will provide equivalent nutrients to those within the same category (eg, all the meats provide roughly the same nutrients; one type of stone fruit is roughly the nutritional equivalent with any other type of stone fruit). Therefore, one food in a category can be substituted for any other within the same group. In most cases, very similar micronutrients will occur in the equivalent foods, so deficiency of vitamins and minerals will not be a problem.

However, there are a few foods that when removed from the diet require an additional source of the nutrient. Such foods are listed in Table 8.1 with indications of

BOX 8.2 Protein Foods (PRO)

Fresh meat
- Beef
- Bison
- Buffalo
- Deer
- Elk
- Lamb
- Moose
- Mutton
- Pork
- Rabbit
- Veal (beef)
- Venison (deer)

Processed meats
- Bacon
- Sausages
- Cured sausages, such as salami, pepperoni, bologna
- Luncheon meats

Poultry (all types)
- Chicken
- Duck
- Grouse
- Ostrich
- Partridge
- Pheasant
- Pigeon
- Quail
- Turkey

Eggs
- Chicken
- Duck
- Ostrich
- Plover
- Quail
- Turkey

Fish
- Anchovy
- Bass
- Cod
- Flounder
- Haddock
- Halibut
- Orange roughy
- Sardine
- Plaice
- Pollack
- Salmon
- Sardine
- Sea bass
- Smelt
- Sole
- Sturgeon
- Trout
- Tuna
- Whitefish

Shellfish
- Mollusks (bivalves): clam, cockle, mussel, oyster, scallop, whelk, winkle
- Crustaceans: Crab, crayfish (crawfish), lobster, prawn, scampi, shrimp

Milk[a]
- Cow
- Buffalo
- Goat
- Mare
- Sheep

Milk products (from above species of milk)[a]
- Cheese of all types: cheddar and other hard fermented cheeses, cottage cheese, cream cheese, ricotta
- Yogurt and lassi
- Kefir
- Buttermilk
- Paneer

Continues

BOX 8.2   Protein Foods (PRO) (*Continued*)

Nuts
- Almond
- Brazil nut
- Chestnut
- Coconut
- Hazelnut (filbert)
- Macadamia
- Mandalona (a peanut product)
- Peanut[b]
- Pecan
- Pine nut
- Pistachio
- Walnut

Seeds
- Melon
- Pumpkin
- Sesame
- Squash
- Sunflower

Legumes[c]
- Soybeans
- Soybean derivatives
- Tofu

Other
List any additional tolerated protein foods here.

---

[a]Milk is included as a protein because protein is the major nutrient. However, milk also contains the sugar lactose (4% weight in volume), so it is also a source of carbohydrate, a factor that should be considered in meal planning.

[b]Peanuts are actually legumes, but they have a nutritional composition similar to tree nuts, so for convenience are listed here.

[c]For a vegan diet, include legumes listed in Box 8.3 as a source of plant protein.

BOX 8.3   Grains (GR) and Starches (ST)

Grains (GR)
Choose whole grains as often as possible.

Wheat varieties and derivatives
- Wheat
- Spelt
- Kamut
- Bulgur
- Triticale
- Semolina

Other grains
- Rye
- Oats
- Barley
- Rice

- Corn
- Amaranth
- Quinoa
- Buckwheat
- Millet
- List any additional tolerated grains here.

Starches (ST)
Flours and starches derived from grains listed under "grains"
- Wheat flour
- Rye flour
- Rice flour
- Corn flour
- Millet flour

Continues

BOX 8.3   Grains (GR) and Starches (ST) (*Continued*)

Starches (ST; continued) *Legumes*[a]
- Broad beans (fava)
- Butter beans
- Dals
- Dried beans
- Dried peas
- Garbanzo beans (chickpeas)
- Lentils
- Lima beans
- Soybeans

High-starch root vegetables
- Beet
- Carrot
- Parsnip
- Potato
- Sweet potato
- Yam

Root-derived starches
- Arrowroot
- Tapioca (Cassava)
- Teff

Other
List any additional tolerated high-starch foods here.

---

[a]Legumes are eaten as plant-derived protein in a vegan diet. However, legumes provide more starch than protein. Therefore, when animal-source proteins are consumed in the diet, legumes are considered as starchy foods to provide balance.

BOX 8.4   Vegetables (VEG) and Fruits (FR)[a]

Vegetables (VEG)
Green leafy vegetables
- Beet greens
- Broccoli
- Brussels sprouts
- Cabbage (all types)
- Celery
- Chard
- Chinese greens
- Lettuce (all types)
- Spinach
- Turnip greens

Beans
- French
- Green beans
- Runner
- Snap beans
- String
- Yellow wax

Other nonstarchy vegetables
- Asparagus
- Cauliflower
- Cucumber
- Eggplant (aubergine)
- Garlic
- Green, red, yellow peppers
- Onions
- Radishes
- Tomatillo
- Tomato

Peas
- Green peas
- Sugar peas
- Snow peas
- Snap peas

Continues

BOX 8.4   Vegetables (VEG) and Fruits (FR)[a] (*Continued*)

Vegetables (VEG; continued) *Squashes (all types)*
- Acorn squash
- Ambercup squash
- Banana squash
- Buttercup squash
- Butternut squash
- Hubbard squash
- Spaghetti squash
- Turban squash
- Zucchini

Other
Add any additional tolerated vegetables here. Do not include high-starch vegetables or legumes (see Box 8.3). Do not include grains eaten as vegetables (eg, corn).

Fruits (FR)
Citrus fruits
- Grapefruit
- Kumquat
- Lemon
- Lime
- Mandarin orange
- Orange
- Tangelo
- Tangerine

Vine fruits
- Grapes
- Raisins
- Gourds
- Cantaloupe
- Honeydew
- Melon
- Watermelon

Fruits (FR; continued) *Seed fruits and berries*
- Blackberry
- Blueberry
- Boysenberry
- Cranberry
- Fig
- Gooseberry
- Kiwi fruit
- Mulberry
- Raspberry
- Strawberry

Tropical fruits
- Date
- Dragon fruit
- Guava
- Longan
- Lychee
- Mango
- Papaya (pawpaw)
- Pineapple
- Star fruit

Stone fruits
- Apple
- Apple pear
- Apricot
- Cherry
- Nectarine
- Peach
- Pear
- Plum
- Prune
- Quince

Other
List any additional tolerated fruit.

---

[a]The categorization of fruits and vegetables used here is for convenience in identifying the foods and indicating their approximate nutritional equivalence. It is not meant in any way to reflect botanical families, genera, or species.

TABLE 8.1
Important Micronutrients in Common Allergens

Nutrient	Milk	Egg	Peanut	Soy	Fish	Wheat	Rice	Corn
Vitamins								
A	+	+			+			
Biotin	+	+				+		
Folacin (folate; folic acid)	+	+	+		+			
B-1 (thiamin)			+		+	+	+	
B-2 (riboflavin)	+	+		+		+	+	+
B-3 (niacin)		+		+	+	+	+	
B-5 (pantothenic acid)	+	+	+					
B-6 (pyridoxine)		+	+	+	+			
B-12 (cobalamin)	+	+			+			
C								
D	+	+			+			
E (alpha-tocopherol)	+	+	+		+			
K	+	+		+				
Minerals								
Calcium	+			+	+			
Phosphorus	+		+	+	+	+		
Iron		+		+	+	+	+	+
Zinc		+		+	+			
Magnesium				+	+	+		
Selenium		+			+	+		
Potassium	+		+		+			
Molybdenum						+		
Chromium			+			+		+
Copper		+						
Manganese			+					

TABLE 8.2
Alternative Food Sources of Micronutrients When Certain Allergens Need to Be Avoided

Micronutrient	Alternative Food Sources
Vitamins	
Vitamin A	Liver, fish liver oils, dark green and yellow vegetables, tomato, apricots, cantaloupe, mango, papaya
Vitamin D[a]	Liver, fish liver oils
Vitamin E (alpha-tocopherol)	Liver, legumes, green leafy vegetables, tomato, whole grains, vegetable oils
Vitamin B-1 (thiamin)	Meats, especially pork; dried and green peas; legumes; whole grains; nutritional yeast
Vitamin B-2 (riboflavin)	Organ meats, legumes, green vegetables, whole grains, nutritional yeast

Continues

TABLE 8.2

Alternative Food Sources of Micronutrients When Certain Allergens Need to Be Avoided (*Continued*)

Micronutrient	Alternative Food Sources
Vitamin B-3 (niacin)	Organ meats, poultry, beef, legumes, whole grains, nutritional yeast
Vitamin B-6 (pyridoxine)	Meats especially organ meats, legumes, whole grains, green vegetables, carrots, potato, cauliflower, banana, prunes, avocado, sunflower seeds, nutritional yeast
Vitamin B-12 (cobalamin)	Meats, especially organ meats; poultry
Biotin	Organ meats, nutritional yeast, mushrooms, banana, grapefruit, watermelon, strawberries
Pantothenic acid	Organ meats, chicken, beef, fresh vegetables, whole grains, nutritional yeast
Folacin	Organ meats, legumes, green leafy vegetables, asparagus, beets, broccoli, avocado, oranges, bananas, strawberries, whole grains, nutritional yeast
Minerals	
Calcium	Amaranth, baked beans, rhubarb, green leafy vegetables, broccoli, dates, molasses
Phosphorus	Meats, poultry, legumes, whole grains, seeds, green peas, artichokes, potato, brussels sprouts
Iron	Meats, liver, legumes, raisins, dried apricots, prunes, pumpkin, asparagus, broccoli, chard, green peas, spinach, molasses
Zinc	Meat, liver, green leafy vegetables, beets, green peas, oranges, strawberries, prunes, chocolate syrup
Magnesium	Legumes, whole grains, meat, poultry, dark green vegetables
Selenium	Whole grains, meat, broccoli, onions, tomato
Potassium	Meats, oranges, banana, dried fruits, cantaloupe, honeydew melon, nectarines, papaya, tomato, avocado, dark greens, sweet potato, winter squash, potato, molasses
Molybdenum	Meat; legumes; whole grains; green vegetables, especially spinach; lettuce; brussels sprouts; carrots; squash; tomatoes; apple juice
Chromium	Vegetable oils, meats, liver, nutritional yeast, whole grains
Copper	Liver, meat, whole grains, green leafy vegetables, broccoli, potato, pears, banana, apple juice
Manganese	Sunflower seeds, whole grains, legumes, nutritional yeast, green beans, broccoli, cranberry, grape, pineapple

[a]Vitamin D also becomes bioavailable through the action of sunlight on skin.

the micronutrients in the food that may become deficient if nutritionally equivalent alternatives are not found. Table 8.2 provides information of food sources of the potentially deficient nutrients in some common allergens. Information on the daily requirements for all nutrients for each age category can be obtained from the Dietary Reference Intake tables.[5]

Supplements

When a food category supplying essential micronutrients (vitamins and minerals) needs to be restricted, and no nutritionally equivalent food sources are available or the alternatives may not provide adequate levels of the nutrients, nutritional supplements are advisable. A health care provider may, for example, recommend a multivitamin/mineral once a day, with the following considerations:

■ The supplement should be free of artificial color, flavor, preservatives, and any additional ingredients that are restricted in the diet, such as wheat, yeast, corn, lactose, sugar, and salt.

■ If the individual has histamine sensitivity, the multivitamin should also be free from niacin. Multivitamins that replace niacin with niacinamide are readily available.

Supplements of specific vitamins and minerals should be advised on an individual basis as required.

References

1. Teuber SS, Porch-Curren C. Unproved diagnostic and therapeutic approaches to food allergy and intolerance. *Curr Opin Allergy Clin Immunol*. 2003;3(3):217-221.
2. Monro J. Food families and rotation diets In: Brostoff J, Challacombe SJ. *Food Allergy and Food Intolerance*. London, Philadelphia, Toronto: Bailliere Tindall; 1987:303-343.
3. Ortolani C, Bruijnzeel-Koomen C, Bengston U, et al. Controversial aspects of adverse reactions to food. European Academy of Allergology and Clinical Immunology (EAACI) Reactions to Food Subcommittee. *Allergy*. 1999;54:27-45.
4. Joneja JMV. *Dealing with Food Allergies: A Practical Guide to Detecting Culprit Foods and Eating a Healthy, Enjoyable Diet*. Boulder, CO: Bull Publishing Company; 2003.
5. U.S. Department of Agriculture (USDA). Food and Nutrition Information Center. Dietary Guidance: DRI Tables. http://fnic.nal.usda.gov/nal_display/index.php?info_center=4&tax_level=3&tax_subject=256&topic_id=1342&level3_id=5140. Accessed February 17, 2012.

CHAPTER **9**

Labeling of Foods

When a person's food allergies and intolerances have been accurately identified, it is important he or she avoid every food or beverage containing the offending allergen or intolerance trigger. This is fairly easy to do if everything is consumed in its natural state, or "cooked from scratch," as each ingredient is obvious and can be readily avoided. The person with food allergies, especially one at risk for anaphylaxis, is strongly advised to implement the necessary lifestyle and diet changes in the interest of safety and good health.

However, in our modern world, much of the food we eat and the beverages we drink are manufactured and delivered to us in cans, bottles, and packages or prepared and served to us in restaurants. In these cases, we have little control over the ingredients, so it is particularly important for individuals who consume such convenience foods to ensure the product is free from problem ingredients. This is especially important for anyone who is at risk for anaphylaxis.

By law, all manufactured foods and beverages, apart from a few exceptions discussed later, must display an easily understood food label. Many regulations govern the way that labels are displayed and the information required to be included. However, the laws regarding labeling of foods containing potential food allergens are fairly new and still require careful scrutiny. People with food allergies must learn how to interpret ingredient lists on food labels and how to recognize labeling of the food allergens used as ingredients in foods.[1]

The Food Allergen Labeling and Consumer Protection Act

Current requirements under the U.S. Food Allergen Labeling and Consumer Protection Act (FALCPA) require food labels to disclose the presence of any of the eight major food allergens (or proteins derived from them) in clearly understood, simple language. FALCPA was passed by Congress in 2004 and became effective in law in

January 2006.[2] It identified the eight major food allergens that are responsible for at least 90% of serious adverse reactions to foods in the United States:

- Milk
- Egg
- Peanut
- Tree nuts
- Soy
- Wheat
- Fish
- Crustacean (shellfish)

FALCPA applies to packaged foods subject to Food and Drug Administration (FDA) regulation, including foods both domestically manufactured and imported. A food product may be subject to recall if it contains a major food allergen that is not declared on the food label in accordance with FALCPA requirements. FALCPA also requires the label to specify the type of tree nut (eg, almonds, pecans, walnuts), the type of fish (eg, bass, flounder, cod), and the type of crustacean shellfish (eg, crab, lobster, shrimp).

Exceptions to FALCPA

The labeling requirements do not apply to the following:

- Foods that are placed in a wrapper, a carryout box, or other container after being ordered by a consumer. For example, a sandwich ordered at a delicatessen that is wrapped, boxed, or put in a container is not subject to FALCPA labeling requirements.
- Raw agricultural commodities (including fresh fruits and vegetables)
- Meat, poultry, and egg products regulated by the U.S. Department of Agriculture (USDA) Food Safety and Inspection Service
- Highly refined oils (or ingredients derived from them) made from one of the eight foods or food groups identified in the law

While FALCPA attempts to be clear and comprehensive, several concerns exist with regard to the allergen labeling of manufactured foods.

The Safety of Oils Derived from Allergenic Foods

Some oils including less well-refined oils and cold-pressed oils may contain protein from the allergenic source and can be hazardous for individuals with food allergy, especially for those at risk for anaphylaxis.[3] The amount of the protein within the oil can now be measured with a great deal of sensitivity, and oils previously thought to be completely protein-free have been shown to contain minute quantities of the protein, making them potentially hazardous for consumption by highly sensitive individuals. The current recommendation is for individuals to avoid oils derived from their allergenic foods.[1]

Precautionary Labeling of Products

Precautionary labeling of a product is not regulated under FALCPA. Precautionary statements—such as "this product may contain trace amounts of [*named allergen*]" or "this product does not contain [*named allergen*] but was prepared in a facility that makes products containing [*named allergen*]"—are voluntary and used at the manufacturer's discretion. This type of labeling is designed to protect consumers with allergies, but unfortunately it is difficult to interpret and leaves the individual with inadequate knowledge with which to make an objective decision.[4] In informal surveys, a surprising number of consumers admit to purchasing and consuming products with precautionary labeling indicating the possible contamination by their allergenic ingredient.[5] The 2010 guidelines for managing food allergy in the United States[1] recommend that products with precautionary labeling be avoided.

Labeling of Food Additives in the United States

The FDA regulates food additives such as colors, flavors, and preservatives under the U.S. Federal Food, Drug, and Cosmetic Act (FD&C Act; www.fda.gov/RegulatoryInformation/Legislation/FederalFoodDrugandCosmeticActFDCAct/default.htm). Some of the labeling regulations pertinent to food allergies and intolerances are briefly described here.

Colors

In 1990, the Nutrition Labeling and Education Act (NLEA) (www.fda.gov/Food/GuidanceComplianceRegulatoryInformation/GuidanceDocuments/FoodLabelingNutrition/FoodLabelingGuide/default.htm) amended the FD&C Act. Under NLEA, a certifiable color additive (ie, a manufactured food dye) used in food must be listed in the ingredient label by its common or usual name. All labels printed after July 1, 1991, must comply with this requirement. Colors exempt from certification are derived from natural sources. Box 9.1 provides examples of these colors and their designations.

Sulfites

U.S. labeling regulations do not require that products indicate the presence of sulfites in foods other than wine; however, many companies voluntarily label sulfite-containing foods. In the United States, wines bottled after mid-1987 must have a label stating that they contain sulfites if they contain more than 10 parts per million (ppm). In the European Union, an equivalent regulation came into force in November 2005.

U.S. regulations require that ingredient lists show sulfites if they were *added* to a product, but this requirement applies only if they were intentionally added in formulation and not if they are contained in an ingredient. For example, if a product

BOX 9.1 Color Additives Permitted for Direct Addition to Human Food in the United States[a]

Certifiable colors and European Economic Community (EEC) E numbers

Color	E Number
FD&C Blue No.1	E133
FD&C Blue No.2	E132
FD&C Green No.3	——
Orange B[b]	——
Citrus Red No.2[b]	——
FD&C Red No.3	E127
FD&C Red No.40	E129
FD&C Yellow No.5	E102
FD&C Yellow No.6	E110

Colors exempt from certification

Color	E Number
Annatto extract	E160b
Beet powder (dehydrated beets)	E126
Canthaxanthin	E161g
Caramel color	E150a-d
Beta-Apo-8'-carotenal[b]	E160e
Beta-carotene	E160a
Cochineal extract/Carmine	E120
Sodium copper chlorophyllin	E141
Toasted partially defatted cooked cottonseed flour	——
Ferrous gluconate[b]	——
Ferrous lactate[b]	——
Grape color extract[b]	E163
Grape skin extract (enocianina)[b]	E163
Synthetic iron	E172
Fruit juice	——
Vegetable juice	——
Carrot oil	——
Paprika	E160c
Paprika oleoresin	E160c
Mica-based pearlescent pigments[b]	——
Riboflavin	E101
Saffron	E164
Titanium oxide[b]	E171
Tomato lycopene extract and concentrate	E160
Turmeric	E100
Turmeric oleoresin	E100

[a]These regulations are located in Title 21 of the Code of Federal Regulations Parts 73, 74, 81, and 82. For approved conditions of use, the reader should refer to the regulation for the specific color additive of interest.

[b]These food color additives are restricted to specific uses.

Source: Adapted from US Food and Drug Administration. Summary of Color Additives for Use in the United States in Foods, Drugs, Cosmetics, and Medical Devices. www.fda.gov/ForIndustry/ColorAdditives/Color AdditiveInventories/ucm115641.htm#table1A. Accessed April 19, 2012.

includes an ingredient that contains sulfites, such as dried fruit, then the ingredients label will list only "dried fruit" and is not required to indicate whether the dried fruit contains sulfites. Furthermore, the products most likely to contain sulfites (dried fruits and alcoholic beverages containing less than 10 ppm of sulfites) do not require ingredient labels, so the presence of sulfites is usually undisclosed. In many countries, including Canada, the European Union, Australia, and New Zealand, sulfites are required to be listed on food and beverage labels if the level is at or exceeds 10 ppm. Detailed information on sulfites in foods is provided in Chapter 21.

Allergens Not Recognized as Major Food Allergens

Although more than 90% of individuals with food allergies react to one or more of the eight major food allergens, many consumers need to avoid ingredients not on this list. These individuals must be especially diligent in reading food labels and inquiring about the presence of their allergen or intolerance trigger in a food product. Often the ingredient may be listed under an unfamiliar name.

If there is any doubt regarding the presence of a person's allergen in a food, the consumer is strongly advised to contact the manufacturer, the restaurant chef, or food preparation staff in order to ensure that the food they are about to consume is safe for them.

Food Allergen Labeling Laws in Other Countries

Food eaten in foreign countries, or manufactured foods imported to the United States, may pose additional problems for individuals with food allergies. Although most Western countries have laws similar to those in the United States in which the major allergens must appear clearly on the food label, the lists of the major allergenic foods tend to differ slightly from country to country.[6,7] It is wise for travelers to become familiar with food labeling of products in the country in which they intend to travel.

In Canada, food labels are required to list the priority allergens,[8] which include:

■ Peanuts
■ Tree nuts (almonds, Brazil nuts, cashews, hazelnuts [filberts], macadamia nuts, pecans, pine nuts, pistachios, walnuts)
■ Sesame seeds
■ Milk
■ Eggs
■ Fish
■ Shellfish (clams, mussels, oysters, scallops, and crustaceans [eg, crab, crayfish, lobster, shrimp])
■ Soy

- Wheat
- Sulfites
- Mustard is currently being added to this list

In the European Union, the following allergens are required to be listed in addition to the eight major allergens listed in the United States:

- Celery
- Mustard
- Sesame
- Lupine
- Molluscan shellfish (eg, bivalves: clams, scallops, mussels, oysters; edible snails; squid; octopus)

In the European Union, identification of food intolerance triggers is facilitated by E number designations, which are applied to almost all food additives, including sulfites. The E numbers appear on ingredient labels, making it easy for consumers to avoid their particular sensitivity.

In South Africa, food allergens required on food product labels include:

- Milk
- Egg
- Fish
- Shellfish
- Tree nuts
- Peanuts
- Soybeans
- Gluten

In Japan, buckwheat is a major allergen in addition to the top eight listed for the United States. Australia and New Zealand require the following to be declared on a food label, however small the amount:

- Peanuts
- Tree nuts (eg, cashews, almonds, walnuts)
- Shellfish
- Finned fish
- Milk
- Eggs
- Sesame
- Soybeans
- Cereal grains containing gluten

At the present time, many countries seem to be experiencing similar difficulties in the interpretation of food labels for the presence of allergens. Each of the chapters on managing specific foods and food additives in this book provides information on where the ingredient is found and the names on food labels that indicate its presence. However, it is the consumer's responsibility to become fully informed about the terms on labels that indicate the presence of allergens and to be diligent in determining the safety of food by contacting the food manufacturer or food preparer for full disclosure of their ingredients; this is especially important for caregivers of children and for those at risk for food-associated anaphylaxis.

References

1. Boyce JA, Assa'ad A, Burks AW, et al. Guidelines for the diagnosis and management of food allergy in the United States: report of the NIAID-sponsored expert panel [guideline 24]. *J Allergy Clin Immunol*. 2010;126(6):S1-S58.
2. U.S. Department of Agriculture. Food and Nutrition Service: The FALCPA Act. www.fda.gov/food/labelingnutrition/FoodAllergensLabeling/GuidanceCompliance RegulatoryInformation/ucm106187.htm. Accessed April 19, 2012.
3. Hefle SL, Taylor SL. Allergenicity of edible oils. *Food Technol*. 1999;53:62-70.
4. Pieretti MM, Chung D, Pacenza R, Slotkin T, Sicherer SH. Audit of manufactured products: use of allergen advisory labels and identification of labeling ambiguities. *J Allergy Clin Immunol*. 2009;124(2):337-341.
5. Vierk KA, Koehler KM, Fein SB, Street DA. Prevalence of self-reported food allergy in American adults and use of food labels. *J Allergy Clin Immunol*. 2007;119(6):1504-1510.
6. Noimark L, Gardner J, Warner JO. Parents' attitudes when purchasing products for children with nut allergy: a UK perspective. *Pediatr Allergy Immunol*. 2009;20(5):500-504.
7. Cornelisse-Vermaat JR, Voordouw J, Yiakoumaki V, Theodoridis G, Frewer LJ. Food-allergic consumers' labeling preferences: a cross-cultural comparison. *Eur J Public Health*. 2008;18(2):115-120.
8. Canadian Food Inspection Agency. Food Allergies and Allergen Labelling Information for Consumers. www.inspection.gc.ca/english/fssa/labeti/allerg/allerge.shtml. Accessed April 19, 2012.

PART III

Management of Adverse Reactions to Specific Foods and Food Components

CHAPTER 10

Milk Allergy

Cow's milk is the most frequently encountered allergenic food in infancy, and milk allergy is often the earliest indicator that a baby is atopic. The exact incidence of cow's milk allergy (CMA) is difficult to determine for several reasons: the difficulties in obtaining an accurate diagnosis, differences in the populations used for research studies, and disagreement about the clinical criteria (symptoms) for the condition.[1] However, all studies agree that CMA is most prevalent in early childhood with an incidence of 2% to 7.5% being reported in different research studies.[2] Almost all infants develop their milk allergy within the first year of life.[3] Many children outgrow their early CMA with a good percentage likely to develop tolerance by their fifth birthday. The incidence of CMA in adults is reported to be about 0.1% to 0.5% of the population.[4]

Milk is a complex food with multiple proteins, many of which have the capacity to act as an allergen and elicit an immunological response in a sensitized individual. Furthermore, different individuals react to different proteins, and their immunological response to each can vary considerably as well, resulting in several quite distinct clinical presentations of CMA. These factors often lead to problems in diagnosing the condition.

Symptoms of Milk Allergy

Symptoms are most common in the skin and gastrointestinal (GI) tract. Skin symptoms include eczema, urticaria (hives), and angioedema (swelling). Among the gastrointestinal (GI) tract symptoms are abdominal bloating, pain, gas, diarrhea, constipation, nausea, vomiting, and occasionally blood loss in the stool (occult blood), especially in infants. In some individuals, upper respiratory tract symptoms and asthma may be caused or exacerbated when milk or dairy products are consumed.[1]

Blood in the stool that is associated with CMA is often difficult to see because it is hidden within the feces (occult blood loss). It can cause iron-deficiency anemia, especially in children, because blood is the most important source of iron in the body.

Chronic constipation, often refractory to laxative treatment, may result from cow's milk allergy or intolerance in children.[5] In a study of 65 children with refractory chronic constipation (one bowel movement every 3 to 15 days), 44 experienced a resolution in the constipation after milk was removed from their diet. The constipation recurred on challenge with cow's milk.[6] An inability to fall asleep and restless, disturbed sleep in children is also under investigation as a possible effect of CMA.

In an infant, inadequate growth and weight gain (failure to thrive) may be a result of milk allergy: the allergic reaction results in inflammation in the intestines, and absorption of nutrients may be impaired as a result of damage to the transport mechanisms that reside in the intestinal cells.

In very rare cases, milk allergy can cause fatal anaphylaxis. A 2000 study from the United Kingdom[7] reported eight fatal cases of anaphylaxis from food allergy in children younger than 16 in the 10 years between 1990 and 2000. None died from eating peanuts. Four children died from milk allergy, and one from the inappropriate use of injectable adrenaline to treat a mild reaction to a food. This report emphasizes the fact that milk allergy in early childhood cannot be taken lightly and should always be treated with the utmost care and caution.

Diagnosis of Milk Allergy

The diagnosis of milk allergy is not simple. A 2010 report by Vieira et al[1] states, "The diagnosis of cow's milk allergy is difficult even with the use of several diagnostic tests. Therefore, elimination diets and challenge tests are essential for the diagnosis and treatment of this disorder." Elimination and challenge in the management of food allergies were discussed in detail in Chapters 6 and 7.

Several practitioners have attempted to classify CMA on the basis of immunological mechanism and clinical presentation to aid in diagnosis. A 1995 report identified three distinct types of infant CMA with different symptoms and laboratory findings:[8]

- Type 1: Symptoms developed within minutes of ingestion of small volumes of cow's milk. Symptoms included urticaria (hives), angioedema (tissue swelling), eczema, gastrointestinal (GI) and respiratory symptoms that were part of a generalized anaphylactic reaction, which varied in severity from person to person. Skin prick tests to milk allergen were positive.
- Type 2: Symptoms were confined to the digestive tract. Vomiting and/or diarrhea developed several hours after ingestion of modest volumes of cow's milk. Skin prick tests to milk allergen were mostly negative. Those in this group were described as having cow's milk protein enteropathy.
- Type 3: Symptoms developed in the GI tract more than 20 hours after ingestion of large volumes of milk. Sometimes the GI tract symptoms were accompanied by respiratory symptoms and eczema. Skin prick tests to milk allergen were less marked than the patients in type 1 and usually occurred only in those with eczema.

BOX 10.1   Milk Allergy vs. Lactose Intolerance

If an individual ingests milk and experiences localized adverse effects in the GI tract, the problem may be lactose intolerance, not an immunologically mediated allergy to milk proteins. Whereas milk allergy is caused by an immune reaction against milk *proteins*, lactose intolerance is caused by the body's inability to produce sufficient quantities of the digestive enzyme lactase, which splits lactose into its constituent monosaccharides (single sugars), glucose and galactose. Note that some symptoms, such as abdominal pain, diarrhea, and vomiting, may be common to both conditions. Additionally, milk protein allergy can cause inflammation of the GI tract and may then trigger a lactase deficiency. Therefore, it is possible for both conditions to exist together.

Symptoms in other organ systems, such as the respiratory tract and the skin, are not symptoms of lactose intolerance. If an individual has these adverse effects after ingesting milk, it is an indication that milk allergy is a problem. Management of lactose intolerance is discussed in detail in Chapter 11.

This report highlights some important factors in CMA diagnosis:

- After ingestion of cow's milk, symptoms might develop in minutes or could occur more than 20 hours later.
- Skin prick tests are of limited value in diagnosing the condition.
- The prevalence of gastrointestinal symptoms makes the distinction between CMA and lactose intolerance difficult to determine on clinical signs alone (see Box 10.1 and Chapter 11).

For additional information on the various presentations of milk allergy and algorithms for suggested diagnosis and management, see Caffarelli et al.[9]

Mechanisms of Milk Allergy

Milk allergy results when the immune system produces antibodies against milk allergens. (For a discussion of the immunology of allergy, see Chapter 1.) More than 25 distinct milk proteins have been identified in the various fractions of milk. The fractions include casein, whey, serum, and other ingredients (see Box 10.2). Most milk-allergic individuals (children and adults) react to more than one milk protein.

The potential of individual milk proteins to cause allergy has been studied by skin tests and oral challenge, but the results obtained from the two types of tests may not agree. For example, casein proteins produce the highest number of positive skin tests in children with milk allergy, whereas beta-lactoglobulin produces the highest number of positive oral challenges.

Heat will change the nature of some milk proteins (heat labile), but others remain unaffected (heat stable). Serum proteins, beta-lactoglobulin and alpha-lactalbumin are the most labile and are readily decomposed by heat, whereas the caseins are the most heat stable. This means that people who are allergic to the heat-labile

---

BOX 10.2   Major Proteins in Cow's Milk[a]

Whey

Major proteins:

- Beta-lactalbumin
- Alpha-lactoglobulin

Serum proteins:

- Proteose peptones
- Serum albumins
- Immunoglobulins

Transportation proteins:

- Lactoferrin

Enzymes:

- Lactoperoxidase
- Alkaline phosphatase

Catalase

Casein

Alpha-caseins:

- Alpha s1
- Alpha s2

Beta-caseins

Kappa-caseins

Gamma-caseins

---

[a]Caseins, beta-lactalbumin, and alpha-lactoglobulin are produced by epithelial cells in the mammary gland. Serum proteins in whey are absorbed from the blood.

proteins can consume boiled or cooked milk; those who are allergic to proteins unaffected by heat (heat-stable proteins) cannot consume either boiled or unboiled milk. However, in many cases, a person may be allergic to both heat-labile and heat-stable proteins, in which case milk must be avoided in all forms.

Antibodies produced against milk proteins may be IgE, IgM, IgG, or sometimes IgA (see Chapter 1 for a discussion of antibodies). Coupling of the milk protein antigen with its homologous (matching) antibody leads to the release of inflammatory mediators, which act directly on body tissues. The tissues may be in the digestive tract, the skin, or the respiratory tract. Symptoms typical of allergy result in the affected systems.

To successfully manage adverse reactions to cow's milk constituents, whether it is an allergic or hypersensitivity reaction to cow's milk proteins or an inability to tolerate lactose, a diet free from all sources of milk proteins and lactose is necessary initially. When the culprit components have been identified by appropriate challenge,[10] the tolerated milk fractions can be reintroduced and the diet liberalized.

Feeding the Milk-Allergic Infant

Mother's Milk

Without question, the best nutrition for the newborn and young infant is the mother's breastmilk. Babies will not be allergic to their mother's milk but may react to allergenic proteins that gain access to her milk from her diet. If the baby is definitely showing signs of allergy and is being exclusively breastfed, then the mother's diet must be investigated for the presence of allergenic foods to which her baby is reacting.

Detecting Milk Allergy in Breastfed Babies

If the exclusively breastfed baby is exhibiting the type of symptoms previously discussed, a mother will inevitably question whether foods in her diet are responsible. However, the baby's physician should be consulted to rule out any other cause for the symptoms before allergy is considered.

When CMA is suspected or proven to be causing the baby's symptoms, it is essential for the mother to remove all sources of milk from her diet while she is breastfeeding. Molecules of milk from the maternal diet pass into her milk and will cause distress in her baby. The mother should carefully follow the milk-free diet and make sure that she takes supplemental calcium and vitamin D in addition to any vitamin and mineral supplements she needs.

The most common allergenic foods that seem to cause symptoms at this early life stage are eggs and milk and sometimes soy. The mother should avoid these and any other foods suspected to be causing a reaction in her infant for at least 4 weeks to determine if these are causing the baby's symptoms. The mother should follow a milk- and egg-free diet for a trial period of at least 2 weeks. She should also exclude any other suspect food while continuing to breastfeed her baby. Most importantly, the mother must be provided with information to obtain complete balanced nutrition from alternative sources while following these restrictions. Each of the diet plans in this book provides many alternatives to eliminate the risk of a nutritional deficiency, as long as the directives are closely and completely followed.

After 2 to 4 weeks on a restricted diet, the mother should consume each food individually and monitor the baby's reactions from 2 to 4 hours after she eats the food. She should be instructed to consume a good quantity to ensure that enough of the food molecules pass into her breastmilk to trigger a response in her baby. This means at least one serving (more if possible) of each food avoided (as long as the mother is not allergic to it). To determine whether the baby is allergic to milk, for example, the mother should drink a cup or more of whole milk.

If the baby reacts adversely to the food, the mother must avoid that particular food as long as she is breastfeeding her baby.

This is also a good way to determine whether a baby is still allergic to a food after the mother has avoided it for 4 or 6 months. Sometimes babies outgrow their food allergies early, which means that both mother and baby can relax their food restrictions, to the relief of all concerned.

Feeding Lactose-Intolerant Baby

If the breastfed baby is lactose intolerant (often a temporary condition following intestinal infection at this age), the mother can continue to breastfeed or pump her milk and treat it with lactase enzyme until the baby's symptoms resolve. Details concerning feeding the lactose-intolerant infant are provided in Chapter 11. There is no point in the mother eliminating milk and milk products from her diet to treat lactose intolerance in her baby, because her milk will contain 6% lactose (per weight in volume; w/v) regardless of whether she consumes milk.

Milk-Free Infant Formulas

If the milk-allergic baby cannot be breastfed, extensively hydrolyzed formulas (EHF) are the best alternative. Hydrolyzed casein formulas such as Similac Alimentum (Abbott Nutrition), Enfamil Nutramigen (Mead-Johnson), and Enfamil Pregestimil (Mead-Johnson), in which the proteins have been broken down extensively into peptides that are usually too small to be allergenic, are usually tolerated by the milk-allergic infant.

In a few unusually sensitive infants, the small peptides in EHF may still trigger a reaction. In such cases, an elemental formula such as EleCare (Abbott Nutrition) or Neocate (Nutricia), in which the milk proteins are broken down into their constituent amino acids, is likely to be tolerated. The greatest disadvantage of EHF and elemental formulas is their high cost.

Partially hydrolyzed milk-based formulas, such as partially hydrolyzed whey (eg, Good Start [Nestlé]), are not suitable for an infant with suspected or diagnosed cow's milk protein hypersensitivity. The protein molecules are incompletely hydrolyzed and are capable of initiating an allergic reaction in a baby allergic to milk. These formulas are suitable for babies who have no signs of milk allergy. Some studies have suggested that these types of formula may be effective in reducing the risk of a nonallergic baby developing milk allergy.[11-13] However, a research study in 2011 stated that "despite current dietary guidelines, we found no evidence to support recommending the use of pHWF (partially hydrolyzed whey formula) at weaning for the prevention of allergic disease in high-risk infants."[14]

Introducing Formula to Breastfed Babies

Changing from breastfeeding to bottle-feeding can at first be confusing to the exclusively breastfed baby, but eventually most babies will adjust. However, mothers who wish to continue breastfeeding at the same time as supplementing with a formula often prefer to give the formula in a nursing cup rather than using a feeding bottle. Babies use less energy in feeding from a bottle compared with extracting milk from a breast, so over time they tend to reject the breast for the easier option. Using a cup for the formula avoids this problem.

The hydrolysis process in a hydrolyzed formula (EHF) radically changes the taste of milk, so there will be a period when the baby adjusts to the taste. Nevertheless, over time, all babies seem to accept the taste; taste preferences are not well established at such an early age, and even if the parents find the taste of the hydrolyzed formula unappealing, babies usually have no such prejudices.

A further difference between an extensively hydrolyzed formula, a cow's milk–based formula, and breastmilk is the osmotic pressure of the EHF. EHF requires adaptation of the digestive tract to avoid the transient abdominal distress that accompanies a sharp change in osmotic pressure within the colon. This is best achieved by gradually introducing the formula over time. The following is a replacement schedule that seems to work well for a breastfed baby:

- Replace one nursing per day with formula, at first mixed with breastmilk for a week.
- Replace two nursings per day with formula for the next week.
- Continue replacing one extra nursing period with formula per week until all feedings are replaced with formula, without mixing with breastmilk.

For a cow's milk formula–fed baby, start by diluting the EHF by half with sterile (boiled and cooled) water, and gradually increase the strength of the formula over a week (or two if the baby is fussy) until the baby is taking the EHF at full strength.

Children should continue the hydrolysate or amino acid formula until they are eating a range of solid foods sufficient to supply all their nutritional needs. After the age of 12 months, or when they are eating a good range of solid foods, children allergic to milk may do well on milk substitutes (eg, calcium and vitamin D–fortified soy or rice milks) and other calcium-fortified foods, if allergy to these foods is not suspected. For more details on feeding the baby with allergies, refer to Chapter 44.

Soy-Based Formulas and the Allergic Baby

Soy-based infant formulas have frequently been fed to non-breastfed babies with milk allergy or intolerance. Many practitioners recommend a soy-based formula as a substitute for a cow's milk–based formula for infants allergic to milk because of the high cost of EHF, which many families cannot afford.

Furthermore, soy-based formulas have been recommended in the past as a substitute for cow's milk–based formulas as a preventative measure for infants considered to be at high risk for allergy. However, recent professional guidelines for diagnosis and management of food allergies in the United States[15] do not recommend using soy infant formula instead of cow's milk formula as a strategy for preventing the development of food allergy in high-risk infants. Although the guidelines state that "there appears to be neither long-term harm nor significant benefit in using soy infant formula,"[15] there are a few potential risks that should be considered before using a soy-based formula to manage an established cow's milk allergy:

- About 50% of babies with IgE-mediated cow's milk allergy develop an allergy to soy (see Chapter 17).
- Soy can cause a non-IgE-mediated reaction that is separate from allergy. The effects are localized in the digestive tract, where symptoms such as colicky pain, abdominal bloating, gas, and diarrhea are apparent. This is sometimes referred to as *soy protein enteropathy* (see Chapter 39).
- Both cow's milk and soy proteins have been strongly implicated in eosinophilic conditions of the digestive tract (EGID; eg, eosinophilic esophagitis,

gastroenteritis, and proctocolitis). In these conditions, all tests for allergy (presence of allergen-specific IgE) are negative. The conditions involve infiltration of eosinophils, which release inflammatory mediators into the local tissues. These conditions are discussed in more detail in Chapter 39.

Development of Tolerance to Cow's Milk

Although cow's milk allergy is generally reported to resolve in 85% of children by the age of 3 to 5 years,[3,16] a 2007 study indicates that fewer children outgrow their allergy as early as previously thought.[17] In that study, 19% of milk-allergic children outgrew their milk allergy by 4 years of age, 42% by 8 years, 64% by 12 years, and 79% by 16 years. It is important that children with a milk allergy be evaluated at regular intervals to determine their allergic status. Research indicates that once tolerance to an allergen has developed, it is essential that the person continues to consume the food regularly in order to maintain tolerance (see Chapter 44 for more details).

The Importance of Milk in the Human Diet

Milk is a unique food in human nutrition for several important reasons:

- It is the indispensable first food of the newborn infant. Ideally the first milk the baby ingests is its own mother's milk; if this is not possible, human milk may be available from a donor. In the absence of either of these sources, cow's milk–based infant formulas are usually provided. Manufacturers of infant formula try to simulate human milk as closely as possible in order to supply all the known nutrients required for the baby's optimal growth and development. Of course, infant formulas lack the biological agents required for optimal development that are present in human milk.
- Milk is considered to be so unique that it is given its own "food group" in most countries whose governments have developed guidelines for adequate nutrition for the population.
- Milk provides some essential nutrients, especially calcium and vitamin D, which are not so readily available, nor so well absorbed, from any other source.

For these reasons, an allergy to milk, especially in the young, can make it harder to ensure complete nutrition than when milk and milk products can be consumed with impunity. When milk allergy is an issue, it is essential to obtain alternate sources of all the nutrients in milk.

Management of Cow's Milk Allergy

When milk allergy has been diagnosed, a milk-free diet needs to be carefully followed to ensure symptom resolution. It is particularly important that all sources of milk proteins are avoided when there is a risk of anaphylaxis. Because there is no real guarantee that CMA may not progress to anaphylaxis, it is important for people allergic to milk, especially children and adolescents, who are considered at highest risk for anaphylaxis avoid all sources of milk and become informed as to where milk proteins may be encountered, particularly in manufactured foods and when eating foods with unknown ingredients.

Another important use of the milk-free diet is when milk is suspected to be a trigger for a patient's symptoms but tests are equivocal or of no clinical value, such as with milk protein enteropathy or other non-IgE immunologically mediated conditions (see Chapter 39). In the latter case, a milk-free diet is often used in diagnosis: The diet is usually followed for 4 weeks, and then challenge with milk components is implemented to determine the role of milk in the disease. Refer to Chapters 6 and 7 for details of these diagnostic tools.

The Milk-Free Diet

On the milk-free diet, all milk and milk-containing foods—including liquid and evaporated milks; fermented milks (yogurt, buttermilk); cheeses (hard cheeses, cottage cheese, cream cheese); ice cream; ice milk; and any foods containing milk solids such as cream, butter, and margarines containing whey—must be avoided. In addition, all foods or beverages containing components of milk such as casein, whey, lactoglobulin, and hydrolyzates of these must not be consumed.

Alternatives to Milk on the Milk-Free Diet

Heating and Processing of Milk

Heating or boiling milk will not make it nonallergenic, although a few of the proteins may be decomposed, reducing their allergenicity to some extent. Only people who are allergic to heat-labile proteins (see earlier discussion) will tolerate boiled milk and canned milk (evaporated milk) that has been extensively heated.

The cow's milk in common infant formulas has the same allergenicity as milk and will induce an allergic reaction in milk-allergic babies.

Milk from Other Animals

Goat's Milk   Goat's milk may be tolerated by a small number of people allergic to cow's milk for a time. However, goat's milk allergy often develops quickly in children who are allergic to cow's milk. In one study, 24 out of 26 children allergic to cow's milk had an allergic reaction to goat's milk.[18] Also, immunological studies have indicated that proteins in cow's milk and goat's milk are antigenically very similar. The chances of developing an allergy to goat's milk if a person is allergic to cow's milk is high, and authorities agree that "the milk of goat and sheep harbor an allergic potential and is not suitable for the nutrition of milk-allergic patients."[19]

If goat's milk is used as a replacement for cow's milk, it is important to make sure that there are adequate sources of folate in the diet, because compared to cow's milk, goat's milk is deficient in this vitamin.

Mare's Milk   Only a few proteins in mare's milk are similar to cow's milk proteins. In a 2000 research study, only 1 out of 25 children allergic to cow's milk were allergic to mare's milk,[20] so mare's milk may be a good substitute for cow's milk for these children; however, it is an expensive product and difficult to obtain. For more information on mare's milk, visit www.burleson-arabians.com/horse_milk.htm.

Donkey's Milk   Donkey's milk has also been considered as an alternative to cow's milk. A report from Italy[21] indicated that donkey's milk was a viable alternative to both IgE-mediated and non-IgE-mediated cow's milk protein allergy in terms of palatability and weight–height gain. Again the problem is obtaining a supply. Most of the donkey's milk suppliers are in countries such as Greece, Morocco, or Israel. For more information, visit www.alibaba.com/showroom/donkey-milk.html.

No doubt future research will identify the most appropriate species of alternative milks for use in cow's milk allergy, and possibly domestic suppliers will move to fill the need should there be sufficient demand for the product.

Important Nutrients in Milk and Their Alternative Sources

Milk is an important source of protein in the diet. Fortunately, adequate protein is readily available from meat, poultry, eggs, fish, shellfish, soybeans and other legumes, nuts, and seeds.

Milk and milk products are an important source of calcium, phosphorus, vitamin D, vitamin B-12, riboflavin, pantothenic acid, potassium, vitamin A, and vitamin E (vitamin D and A are added as fortification during processing). Most of these nutrients can be obtained from other foods and supplements when all milk is removed from the diet (details about alternative sources of micronutrients are provided in Chapter 8). However, sufficient calcium and vitamin D are often difficult to obtain from food sources alone, so in many cases supplements of these micronutrients will be required to ensure optimum nutrition.

Calcium

Milk is the most abundant and readily available source of calcium in the normal diet. One cup of milk contains 290 mg calcium. Calcium is essential for many important body functions, including bone. It is important that sufficient calcium be consumed daily. Consult the Dietary Reference Intakes (DRIs) for calcium to determine requirements for healthy individuals.[20]

Some foods other than milk contain calcium, but the mineral may not be absorbed as efficiently as the calcium in milk. Box 10.3 lists foods containing significant quantities of calcium. These should be included in a milk-free diet.

BOX 10.3 Nondairy Sources of Calcium (Ca)

NOTE: Any allergenic foods on the list must be avoided.

More than 300 mg Ca
Collards, frozen, cooked, 1 cup (170 g)
Rhubarb, frozen cooked, 1 cup (240 g)[a]
Sardines, with bones, canned, 3 oz (85 g)
Wheat flour, enriched and calcium-fortified, 1 cup (125 g)

250 to 300 mg Ca
Rhubarb, cooked, fresh, 1 cup (240 g)[a]
Soy beans, green, cooked, 1 cup (180 g)
Soymilk, calcium-fortified, 1 cup (243 g)
Spinach, cooked, 1 cup (180 g)[a]
Tofu, firm, ½ cup (126 g)

200 to 250 mg Ca
Oysters, raw, meat only, 1 cup (248 g)
Salmon, pink, with bones, canned, 3 oz (85 g)
Salmon, sockeye, with bones, canned, 3 oz (85 g)
Turnip greens, cooked, 1 cup (144 g)[a]

150 to 200 mg Ca
Almonds, ½ cup (72 g)
Beans, white, cooked, 1 cup (179 g)
Beet greens, leaves, and stems, cooked, 1 cup (144 g)[a]
Chinese cabbage (bok choy), shredded, cooked, 1 cup (170 g)[a]

100 to 150 mg Ca
Amaranth, cooked, 1 cup (246 g)
Brazil nuts, ½ cup (67 g)
Cereal, All-Bran Original, ½ cup (31 g)
Cereal, Cheerios, 1 cup (28 g)
Greens, dandelion, cooked, 1 cup (105 g)[a]
Greens, mustard, 1 cup (140 g)[a]
Molasses, cane, blackstrap, 1 Tbsp (20 g)
Okra pods, cooked, 1 cup (160 g)
Shrimp, meat only, 4 oz (113 g)
Tofu, soft, ½ cup (124 g)

50 to 100 mg Ca
Baked beans, vegetarian or plain, canned, 1 cup (254 g)
Beans, garbanzo (chickpeas), cooked, 1 cup (164 g)
Beans, green, cooked, 1 cup (125 g)
Beans, kidney, cooked, 1 cup (256 g)
Beans, lima, cooked, 1 cup (170 g)
Beans, yellow or wax, cooked, 1 cup (125 g)
Broccoli, cooked, 1 cup (156 g)
Brussels sprouts, cooked, 1 cup (156 g)[a]
Cabbage, fresh, cooked, 1 cup (150 g)[a]
Cereal, 100% Bran, 1 cup (87 g)
Cereal, granola, ⅔ cup (80 g)
Chili con carne with beans, 1 cup (242 g)
Kale, frozen, cooked, 1 cup (130 g)
Parsnips, cooked, 1 cup (156 g)
Sauerkraut, undrained, 1 cup (235 g)[a]

Continues

BOX 10.3   Nondairy Sources of Calcium (Ca) (*Continued*)

50 to 100 mg Ca (continued)
  Sesame seeds, 1 Tbsp (9 g)
  Tomatoes, canned, solids and liquid,
    1 cup (240 g)
  Turnip, mashed, 1 cup (230 g)
  Orange, raw, 1 medium (131 g)
  Orange sections, 1 cup (180 g)
  Soymilk, unfortified, 1 cup (243 g)

15 to 50 mg Ca

Cereals
  Branbuds, 1/3 cup (30 g)
  Bran flakes and raisins, 1 cup (59 g)
  Oatmeal, cooked, 1 cup (234 g)
  Shredded wheat, 2 biscuits (46 g)

Bread
  Multigrain, 1 slice (26 g)
  Rye, light, 1 slice (32 g)
  Tortilla, corn (24 g)
  White, 1 slice (28 g)
  Whole wheat 100%, 1 slice (28 g)
  Whole wheat 60%, 1 slice (29 g)
  White bun, hamburger or hot dog,
    1 (42 g)

Vegetables
  Arugula, raw, 1 cup (32 g)
  Asparagus, fresh, cooked, drained, 1 cup
    (180 g)

Cabbage, raw, shredded, 1 cup (70 g)
Carrot, raw, 1 medium (61 g)
Carrots, cooked, 1 cup (156 g)
Cauliflower, cooked, 1 cup (124 g)
Cauliflower, raw, 1 cup (107 g)
Celery, diced, raw, 1 cup (101 g)
Lentils, cooked, 1 cup (200 g)
Olives, black, 5 large (42 g)
Olives, green, 5 medium (14 g)
Onions, cooked, 1 cup (210 g)
Parsley, raw, chopped, 2 Tbsp (8 g)
Peas, green, cooked, 1 cup (160 g)
Spinach, raw, chopped, 1 cup (30 g)

Fruit
  Fig, dried, uncooked, 1 medium (9 g)
  Grapefruit, raw, 1 medium (256 g)
  Kiwi, 1 large (69 g)
  Pear, raw, 1 medium (178 g)
  Raisins, 1/2 cup (82 g)

Other
  Chocolate, 1 square (30 g)
  Egg, whole, cooked, 1 large (50 g)
  Hazelnuts, chopped, 1 oz (28 g)
  Maple syrup, 1 Tbsp (20 g)
  Peanuts, oil roasted, 1/4 cup (33 g)
  Sunflower seeds, kernel, 1/4 cup (35 g)

*Contains oxalic acid, which impairs calcium absorption. Although the calcium is present in the food at the given level, the actual amount absorbed is significantly less.

Source: US Department of Agriculture, Agricultural Research Service. 2011. USDA National Nutrient Database for Standard Reference, Release 24. http://www.ars.usda.gov/ba/bhnrc/ndl. Accessed April 20, 2012.

Calcium Absorption

The percentage of the calcium contained in foods that is actually absorbed, used, and retained by the body is variable, depending on age, level of calcium intake, type of food eaten, and other nutrients eaten at the same time. Average adults will absorb approximately 40% of the calcium in their diet. This is increased during growth, pregnancy, and lactation and reduced during aging. In general, the lower the intake, the more calcium is retained in the body (ie, less calcium is excreted when intake is low).

Some nonmilk foods contain varying levels of calcium (see Box 10.3). However, because it is often difficult to obtain sufficient calcium on a milk-free diet, a manufactured supplement is often required.

In order to efficiently absorb calcium, an adequate level of vitamin D in the body is necessary. Use the DRIs for vitamin D to determine daily requirements for healthy individuals. Vitamin D is obtained from some foods (eg, milk, liver, egg yolk), but the best source is the action of sunlight (UV light) on the skin. A diet high in phosphorus and protein (a traditional high-protein American diet) tends to reduce the amount of calcium retained in the body. Most people require supplemental vitamin D up to the level for their age and life stage (see discussion on Vitamin D below).

Calcium Supplements

There are many calcium supplements available commercially. Calcium carbonate is usually the most economical form of calcium supplement but should be taken with a meal to ensure optimal absorption. Calcium citrate can be taken without food and is the supplement of choice for individuals with achlorhydria or who are taking histamine-2 blockers or protein-pump inhibitors. Calcium lactate, calcium malate, and calcium gluconate are less concentrated forms of calcium and are not usually taken alone as oral supplements. They may be present together with calcium carbonate or citrate. Research on hydroxyapatite as a source of calcium is limited, so this form of calcium is not presently recommended.[22]

Calcium supplements contain varying amounts of elemental calcium. For example, calcium carbonate is 40% calcium by weight, whereas calcium citrate is 21% calcium. The amount of elemental calcium will be listed on the label. For instance, calcium carbonate provides 625 to 750 mg elemental calcium per 2.5 mL (½ teaspoon).

The percentage of calcium absorbed depends on the total amount of elemental calcium consumed at one time; as the amount increases, the percentage absorption decreases. Absorption is highest in doses at or less than 500 mg.[23] The maximum dose of elemental calcium that should be taken at a time is 500 mg. So, for example, a person who takes 1,000 mg of calcium from supplements per day might split the dose and take 500 mg at two separate times during the day.

The choice of a supplement is often bewildering because of the number of products available in the North American marketplace. In general, it is a good idea to choose supplements with familiar brand names that have the USP (United States Pharmacopeia) symbol. Supplements made from unrefined oyster shell, bone meal, or dolomite that do not have the USP symbol are not recommended, because they may contain high levels of lead or other toxic metals. If adverse side effects are experienced, try different forms of calcium in a supplement. Some individuals who take calcium supplements might experience gastrointestinal symptoms, including gas, bloating, constipation, or a combination of these symptoms. Calcium carbonate appears to cause more of these side effects than calcium citrate.

The use of calcium-based antacids as a source of calcium is not recommended. These antacids are designed to neutralize stomach acid in cases of heartburn and acid reflux or indigestion. However, stomach acid is essential for the first stage of protein digestion (acid hydrolysis) and neutralizing this acid reduces the digestion of proteins in food. In addition, the antacid produces an alkaline environment that may reduce the uptake of a variety of minerals, such as iron, zinc, copper, and calcium, that require an acidic medium for efficient absorption.

Vitamin D

Vitamin D promotes calcium absorption in the gut and maintains adequate serum calcium and phosphate concentrations to enable normal mineralization of bone. It is a fat-soluble vitamin that is naturally present in very few foods, added to others, and available as a dietary supplement. It is also produced endogenously when ultraviolet rays from sunlight strike the skin and trigger vitamin D synthesis.[24]

Very few foods in nature contain vitamin D. The flesh of fatty fish (eg, salmon, tuna, and mackerel) and fish liver oils are among the best sources.[24] Fortified foods provide most of the vitamin D in the American diet.[25] For example, almost all of the U.S. milk supply is voluntarily fortified with 100 IU/cup. In Canada, milk is fortified by law with 35 to 40 IU/100 mL, as is margarine at 530 IU/100 g or higher.[26] Therefore, anyone consuming a milk-free diet will lose this source of vitamin D. Some manufacturers add vitamin D to their food products. For example, some ready-to-eat breakfast cereals, some brands of orange juice, margarine, and others may be fortified with vitamin D. Reading food product labels for vitamin D content is recommended for anyone requiring vitamin D supplementation.

In supplements and fortified foods, vitamin D is available in two forms, D_2 (ergocalciferol) and D_3 (cholecalciferol), that differ chemically in the structure of their side chains. The two forms have traditionally been regarded as equivalent and most steps involved in the metabolism and actions of vitamin D_2 and vitamin D_3 are identical.[26] Both forms (as well as vitamin D in foods and from cutaneous synthesis) effectively raise serum 25(OH)D levels.[27] However, it appears that at nutritional doses, vitamins D_2 and D_3 are equivalent, but at high doses vitamin D_2 is less potent.

References

1. Vieira M, Morais MB, Spolidaro JVN, et al. A survey on clinical presentation and nutritional status of infants with suspected cow' milk allergy. *BMC Pediatr.* 2010;10:25-31.
2. Host A. Frequency of cow's milk allergy in childhood. *Ann Allergy Asthma Immunol.* 2002 Dec;89(6):33-37
3. Sampson HA. Food allergy part I: immunopathogenesis and clinical disorders. *J Allergy Clin Immunol.* 1999;103(5 part 1):717-728.
4. Crittenden RG, Bennett LE. Cow's milk allergy: a complex disorder. *J Am Coll Nutr.* 2005;24(6):582S-591S.
5. Carroccio A, Iacono G. Review article: chronic constipation and food hypersensitivity—an intriguing relationship. *Aliment Pharmacol Ther.* 2006;24:1295-1304.

6. Iacono G, Cavataio F, Montalto G, et al. Intolerance of cow's milk and chronic constipation in children. *N Engl J Med*. 1998;338:1100-1104.
7. Pumphrey RS. Lessons for management of anaphylaxis from a study of fatal reactions. *Clin Exper Allergy*. 2000;30:1144-1150.
8. Hill DJ, Hosking CS. The cow milk allergy complex: overlapping disease profiles in infancy. *Eur J Clin Nutr*. 1995;49(suppl 1):1S-12S.
9. Caffarelli C, Baldi F, Bendandi B, Calzone L, Marani M, Pasquinelli P, on behalf of EWGPAG Ital. Cow's milk protein allergy in children: a practical guide. *J Pediatr*. 2010;36:5-12.
10. Correa FF, Vieira MC, Yamamoto DR, Speridião Pda G, de Morais MB. Open challenge for the diagnosis of cow's milk protein allergy. *Pediatr (Rio J)*. 2010;86(2):163-166.
11. Hays T, Wood RA. A systematic review of the role of hydrolyzed infant formulas in allergy prevention. *Arch Pediatr Adolesc Med*. 2005;159:810-816.
12. von Berg A, Koletzko S, Filipiak-Pittroff B, et al; German Infant Nutritional Intervention Study Group. Certain hydrolyzed formulas reduce the incidence of atopic dermatitis but not that of asthma: three-year results of the German Infant Nutritional Intervention Study. *J Allergy Clin Immunol*. 2007 Mar;119(3):718-725.
13. vonBerg A, Koletzko S, Grubl A, et al for the German Infant Nutritional Intervention Study Group. The effect of hydrolyzed cow's milk formula for allergy prevention in the first year of life: The German Infant Nutritional Intervention Study, a randomized double-blind trial. *J Allergy Clin Immunol*. 2003 Mar;111(3):533–534.
14. Lowe AJ, Hosking CS, Bennett CM, et al. Effect of a partially hydrolyzed whey infant formula at weaning on risk of allergic disease in high-risk children: a randomized controlled trial. *J Allergy Clin Immunol*. 2011;128(2):360-365.
15. Boyce JA, Assa'ad A, Burks AW, et al. Guidelines for the diagnosis and management of food allergy in the United States: report of the NIAID-sponsored expert panel. *J Allergy Clin Immunol*. 2010;126(6):1S-58S.
16. Sicherer SH. The natural history of IgE-mediated cow's milk allergy. *Pediatrics*. 2008;122(suppl 4):186S.
17. Skripak JM, Matsui EC, Mudd K, Wood RA. The natural history of IgE-mediated cow's milk allergy. *J Allergy Clin Immunol*. 2007;120(5):1172-1177.
18. Bellioni-Businco B, Paganelli R, Lucebti P, Giampietro PG, Perborn H, Businco L. Allergenicity of goat's milk in children with cow milk allergy. *J Allergy Clin Immunol*. 1999;103(6):1191-1194.
19. Spergin P, Walter M, Schiltz E, Deichmann K, Forster J, Mueller H. Allergenicity of alpha-caseins from cow, sheep and goat. *Allergy*. 1997;52(3):293-298.
20. Businco l, Giampietro P, Lucenti P, et al. Allergenicity of mare's milk in children with cow's milk allergy. *J Allergy Clin Immunol*. 2000;105(5):1031-1034.
21. Monti G, Bertino E, Muratore MC, et al. Efficacy of donkey's milk in treating highly problematic cow's milk allergic children: an in vivo and in vitro study. *Pediatr Allergy Immunol*. 2007;18(3):258-264.
22. Straub DA. Calcium supplementation in clinical practice: a review of forms, doses, and indications. *Nutr Clin Pract*. 2007;22(3):286-296.
23. United States Department of Agriculture. National Agricultural Library. Food and Nutrition Information Center. Dietary Guidance. DRI Tables. Washington, DC: http://fnic.nal.usda.gov/nal_display/index.php?info_center=4&tax_level=3&tax_subject=256&topic_id=1342&level3_id=5140. Accessed 4/19/2012

24. U.S. Department of Agriculture. Agricultural Research Service. 2010. USDA National Nutrient Database for Standard Reference, Release 23. http://www.ars.usda.gov/ SP2UserFiles/Place/12354500/Data/SR23/sr23_doc.pdf Accessed 4/19/2012

25. Calvo MS, Whiting SJ, Barton CN. Vitamin D fortification in the United States and Canada: current status and data needs. *Am J Clin Nutr.* 2004;80:1710S-1716S.

26. Cranney C, Horsely T, O'Donnell S, et al. *Effectiveness and Safety of Vitamin D.* Evidence Report/Technology Assessment No. 158 prepared by the University of Ottawa Evidence-Based Practice Center. Rockville, MD: Agency for Healthcare Research and Quality; 2007. AHRQ Publication No. 07-E013.

27. Holick MF. Vitamin D deficiency. *N Engl J Med.* 2007;357:266-281.

CHAPTER **11**

Lactose Intolerance

Lactose intolerance results from a deficiency in the production of the enzyme lactase, which splits lactose into its constituent monosaccharides glucose and galactose. Symptoms in the digestive tract develop from undigested lactose remaining in the large bowel (see Box 11.1). Several conditions are responsible for lactase deficiency and symptoms result from both maldigestion and malabsorption of lactose.[1]

Human milk contains 6% (weight in volume [w/v]) lactose compared to 4% in cow's milk. At birth, virtually every baby has adequate supplies of lactase to digest the lactose in its mother's milk, which is a primary source of energy for the developing child. The exception is the extremely rare medical condition called *congenital alactasia*, or *primary lactase deficiency*, in which the baby is born without the ability to produce the enzyme. Congenital lactase deficiency (CLD) is due to an autosomal recessive gastrointestinal disorder.[2] If breastfed infants or babies fed lactose-containing milks develop watery diarrhea in the first 1 to 10 days of life, this could indicate CLD.

A temporary lactase deficiency can develop in babies when the inflammation associated with a bacterial or viral infection in the digestive tract damages the cells that produce the enzyme. This is known as *secondary lactase deficiency*, to distinguish it from primary congenital alactasia. In secondary lactose intolerance, the cells rapidly return to normal when the infection abates, and the usual level of lactase production is quickly reestablished.

The majority of adults have some degree of lactase deficiency due to a natural reduction in the level of the enzyme's production, which in certain populations can start in childhood after weaning. This type of lactose intolerance is termed *primary adult-onset lactase deficiency*. The characteristics of the different types of lactase deficiency are summarized in Table 11.1.

In certain ethnic groups, such as Asians, Africans, Native Americans, and people of Middle Eastern, Arctic, or Mediterranean descent, lactose intolerance may be as high as 80% of the population. In contrast, only about 20% of people of northern European origin lose the ability to produce lactase. Table 11.2 provides a summary

BOX 11.1   Lactose Intolerance at a Glance

- Lactose is the major sugar in the milk of all mammals.
- Lactose intolerance is caused by a lack of the enzyme lactase.
- Lactase splits lactose into its constituent sugars, glucose and galactose.
- Undigested lactose moves into the large bowel.
- Symptoms result from the change in osmotic pressure and the products of microbial fermentation of lactose within the colon.
- Lactose intolerance does not involve the immune system, and it is not an allergic reaction to milk.

TABLE 11.1
Summary of Types of Lactase Deficiency

Condition	Cause	Effects
Congenital alactasia	Autosomal recessive disorder	Baby experiences intestinal symptoms from birth whenever lactose (in the mother's milk or formula) is ingested.
Primary adult-onset lactase deficiency	Reduction in lactase enzyme determined by genetic inheritance, often starting in late childhood or adolescence	Individual experiences dose-related symptoms of lactose intolerance when consuming milk and milk products. The dosage of lactose ingested and the quantity of lactase produced determines the onset and severity of symptoms.
Secondary lactase deficiency	Damage to brush-border cells due to a variety of insults, such as: • Infection in the digestive tract (eg, rotavirus) • Parasite infestation in the GI tract (eg, *Giardia; Cryptosporidium; Blastocystis*) • Celiac disease • Inflammatory bowel diseases (eg, Crohn's disease) • Trauma or surgery that damages the intestinal epithelium	There is an intolerance of lactose with typical symptoms as long as the damage persists. When the brush border cells heal, enzyme production resumes, the person becomes tolerant of lactose, and symptoms remit.

of the prevalence of primary adult-onset lactase deficiency in several populations worldwide.[3,4] Table 11.3 indicates the incidence and age of onset of primary adult onset lactase deficiency in a variety of ethnic groups.[1,4,5]

In most cases of adult onset lactase deficiency, complete loss of lactase production does not occur, but the enzyme is produced at such a low level that consumption of large quantities of milk and milk products with normal levels of lactose leads to the uncomfortable symptoms of lactose intolerance.

TABLE 11.2
Prevalence of Primary Adult-Onset Lactase Deficiency in Populations

Country or Region	Percentage Lactase Deficient
Scandinavia	3%–5%
Finland	17%
Great Britain	5%–15%
Germany	15%
Austria	15%–20%
Northern France	17%
Southern France	65%
Italy	20%–70%
Balkans	55%
Africa (continental)	70%–90%
African Bedouin	25%
African Tuareg	13%
African Fulani	22%
Central Asia	80%
Eastern Asia	90%–100%
Northern India	30%
Southern India	70%
North American whites	15%
North American blacks	80%
North American Hispanics	53%
South America	65%–75%

Source: Data are from references 3 and 4.

TABLE 11.3
Age of Onset of Primary Adult-Onset Lactase Deficiency in Populations

Ethnic Group	Onset at 2–3 years	Onset at 6 years	Onset at 9–10 years
White American	0%	0%	6%
Americans of Mexican descent	18%	30%	47%
Black South Africans	25%	45%	60%
Chinese and Japanese	30%	80%	85%
Mestizos of Peru	30%–55%	90%	> 90%

Source: Data are from references 1, 4, and 5.

Secondary lactase deficiency can occur in adults and children. Bacterial and viral infections and sometimes the use of strong medications taken by mouth (eg, antibiotics) may damage the fragile digestive tract epithelial cells. If lactose was tolerated prior to the epithelial damage, regular lactase activity will usually resume as soon as the cells return to normal.

Symptoms of Lactose Intolerance

The most common symptoms of lactose intolerance include abdominal pain, diarrhea, and excessive flatulence. Less commonly, abdominal bloating, abdominal distention, and nausea may occur. The symptoms develop after consuming milk or a milk product containing lactose and may not appear immediately after consumption, as in an allergy, but may take minutes to hours to develop.

The severity of the symptoms is related to the quantity of lactose consumed and the person's level of tolerance to it. A person's tolerance level (limit of tolerance) is determined by the amount of lactase available and the efficiency of absorption of the products of lactose metabolism (glucose and galactose). Additional factors also influence the rate of onset and severity of the symptoms:

- A person's sensitivity to pain in the digestive tract
- The rate at which the contents of the stomach empty into the small intestine
- The speed at which food moves along the digestive tract
- The type of microorganisms colonizing the large intestine

Mechanism of Lactose Intolerance

Lactose is a sugar that occurs only in milk. It is found in the milk of all mammals and is the most important source of immediate energy for the immature infant of all species from birth until weaning.

Lactose is a disaccharide.[a] The complete lactose molecule is too large to pass through the layer of cells that line the digestive tract (the epithelium), so it must be broken down into its constituent monosaccharides,[b] glucose and galactose. The digestive enzyme that performs this breakdown is *lactase*. The monosaccharides are transported across the cells that line the digestive tract and enter into circulation, where they are an important source of energy for many body functions.

The normal diet usually contains 10% lactose. When this is digested in the small intestine by the lactase enzyme, it produces 5% glucose and 5% galactose, both of which are carried into circulation by an active transport system across the epithelium.

Lactase is a beta-galactosidase (β-galactosidase) enzyme synthesized within brush border cells in the digestive epithelium. If these cells are damaged, they are unable to produce adequate amounts of lactase. As a result, lactose is incompletely broken down into glucose and galactose. The remaining undigested lactose stays in the intestines and eventually finds its way into the large bowel. Here, millions of microorganisms metabolize any undigested food, multiplying rapidly and producing a large number of by-products. Usually a variety of gases, organic acids, and other fermentation products result from the activity of these microorganisms. Symptoms of excessive flatus, abdominal bloating, pain, loose stool, or diarrhea result.

---

[a] Disaccharide: double sugar (*di* = two; *saccharide* = sugar)

[b] Monosaccharide: single sugar (*mono* = one or single; *saccharide* = sugar)

Lactase is produced in quite small amounts compared to the other enzymes that digest disaccharide sugars in the diet, such as sucrose, maltose, and others derived from starches. For example, lactose is broken down at only half the rate of sucrose (see Chapter 23 for more details). This means that if a large dose of lactose is consumed, there may not be enough lactase present to digest it all at once. As a result, some of the undigested lactose finds its way into the colon, where it causes osmotic imbalance and provides a substrate for microbial fermentation.

Distinguishing Between Milk Allergy and Lactose Intolerance

It is sometimes difficult to distinguish milk allergy from lactose intolerance on the basis of clinical symptoms alone, because some of the symptoms, such as abdominal pain, diarrhea, nausea, vomiting, gas, and bloating, are common to both conditions. However, milk allergy often results in symptoms in other organs, such as the upper respiratory tract (eg, a stuffy, runny nose), or skin reactions (such as eczema or hives), which does not occur with lactose intolerance.

Since secondary lactase deficiency is a consequence of inflammation in the digestive tract, the intestinal inflammation caused by milk allergy can sometimes result in lactase deficiency. Thus, both milk allergy and lactose intolerance can exist together. Because milk is the only source of lactose in the normal diet, eliminating milk from the diet will cure both conditions but will not distinguish which was the cause of the symptoms.

It is important to determine which condition is causing the problem, because milk and milk products are a significant source of nutrients, especially for infants and young children, and should not be eliminated unless it is absolutely necessary to do so. Furthermore, completely eliminating milk from the diet is not easy, because so many different foods, such as baked goods, soups, salad dressings, gravies, desserts, and so on, contain milk, and avoiding them can make meal planning very difficult.

Diagnosis of Lactose Intolerance

There are several laboratory tests that are often used to identify lactose intolerance.

Fecal Reducing Sugar Test

Many clinicians consider the *fecal reducing sugar test* to be the most reliable way to diagnose lactose intolerance. After the patient consumes a drink containing lactose, the feces is collected and Fehling's solution added. The presence of lactose is indicated by a change in color, from blue to red. The lactose "reduces" the chemical in the solution. Thus, a change in color indicates that a deficiency of lactase has led to undigested lactose being excreted in the feces.

Hydrogen Breath Test

The *hydrogen breath test* is a more common test for lactose intolerance. In this test, the patient ingests a quantity of lactose and after a prescribed interval, a breath sample is analyzed for the presence of hydrogen. If hydrogen is detected, it indicates that bacteria in the digestive tract have acted on undigested lactose and produced hydrogen as one of their metabolic by-products. The hydrogen is absorbed, taken to the lungs, and excreted in the breath. Lactose intolerance is defined by a level of breath hydrogen of more than 20 parts per million (ppm) after ingestion of 1 g of lactose per kg of body weight or 50 g of lactose. Unfortunately, this test is not specific for lactase deficiency, because any sugar remaining in the digestive tract will be metabolized by bacteria, which then produces hydrogen. Undigested sucrose, maltose, or a starch will give a similar result.

Blood Glucose Test

The *blood glucose test* involves measurement of the level of glucose in the blood after taking a drink containing 50 g of lactose. An increase in blood glucose concentration indicates that lactose has been broken down to glucose and galactose, the levels of which rise in the blood as the monosaccharides are absorbed into circulation. An increase of less than 1.12 mmol/L indicates that lactose has not been digested, and suggests a diagnosis of lactose intolerance. Measuring the level of galactose would be equally informative. Blood glucose reference levels after 50 g of lactose are as follows: (a) Normal: greater than 1.7 mmol/L (lactose is digested); (b) borderline: 1.1 to 1.7 mmol/L (a small amount of lactose is digested); (c) abnormal: less than 1.1 mmol/L (lactose remains undigested).

If the feces collected after the lactose drink is acidic, with a pH of 6 or lower (the *fecal pH test*), it indicates that microorganisms in the large bowel have fermented the undigested lactose. The microbial activity results in the production of acids, which lower the pH of the stool. Thus, the diagnosis of lactose intolerance is further reinforced.

Biopsy

A more invasive test involves taking a biopsy sample from the small intestine epithelium and examining the cells for lactase activity. This test is rarely considered necessary.

Lactose Malabsorption Versus Lactose Intolerance

Although it is well known that an inability to digest lactose is a result of the deficiency in the lactase enzyme, the fact that some people with such a deficiency do not manifest the typical symptoms of lactose intolerance has led to speculation about the nature of the disorder. The condition is frequently divided into two different types, possibly based on different genetic factors.[6]

Lactose intolerance is defined as a clinical syndrome of abdominal pain, diarrhea, flatulence, and bloating after the ingestion of a standard lactose tolerance test dose (2 g of lactose per kilogram of body weight or 50 g/m² of body surface area, maximum 50 g in a 20% water solution). *Lactose malabsorption* refers to the state in which dietary lactose remains unhydrolyzed and subsequently unabsorbed from the gastrointestinal tract; symptoms may or may not result from lactose malabsorption.

Data[6] seem to suggest that a third of malabsorbers are tolerant of lactose, while a much smaller proportion of absorbers are intolerant of lactose. This conclusion was based on the observation that a third of the people who showed less than 20 mg/100 mL rise in blood glucose after a 50 g dose of lactose (clinical test positive) showed no signs of gastrointestinal distress, while a small percentage of people who showed an increase in blood glucose (indicating a negative test) did show gastrointestinal distress. The authors of the study[10] point out that most reports of the incidence of lactose intolerance are based on clinical test results and therefore are reports of lactose malabsorption rather than lactose intolerance. They further suggest that lactose tolerance (defined as lack of lactase but having the ability to tolerate lactose) is high among people of European ancestry and isolated pockets of individuals in ethnic groups where tolerance is usually low (eg, Punjabis, cattle-herding African peoples).

Management of Lactose Intolerance

Lactase deficiency is easier to manage than cow's milk protein allergy, because any milk or milk product free from lactose can be consumed with impunity. Lactose-free milk is available or a commercial form of lactase can be added to the milk before consumption. After 24 hours in the refrigerator, the lactose is split into its two component sugars, glucose and galactose, which the body can absorb and use without harm. All of the nutrients and proteins in milk are thus available to the body, eliminating the risk of nutritional deficiency as a result of long-term avoidance of milk.

It is more difficult to avoid lactose in prepared foods; anything containing milk or milk solids is likely to also contain lactose. Some people can consume lactose-containing foods with impunity if they take lactase in the form of a tablet before eating.

Lactose intolerance is dose-related. Usually the cells produce a limited amount of the enzyme lactase, and small doses of foods containing lactose can be processed. Problems occur when the amount of lactose in the food exceeds the capacity of the enzyme to digest it. The important thing is to determine tolerance levels. By remaining within personal limits, symptoms should not occur. Most individuals with presumed lactose intolerance or malabsorption can tolerate 12 to 15 g of lactose,[7] about 1 cup of milk, but will experience abdominal discomfort if they exceed this amount.

When lactose intolerance has been diagnosed, the degree of lactase deficiency can be assessed by taking increasing quantities of lactose in a variety of dairy products (Table 11.4) in a 24-hour period.[8] The level at which symptoms develop indicates the person's limit of tolerance.

TABLE 11.4
Lactose Content of Some Milk and Milk Products

Product	Lactose, g/100 g
Nonfat dry milk	50–52.3
Buttermilk powder	49–50
Condensed whey	38.5–39
Dry whole milk	35.9–38.4
Sweetened condensed milk	10–16.3
Evaporated milk (whole and fat-free)	9.7–11
American cheese, pasteurized, processed	1.9–14.2
Velveeta Cheese Food	9.3
Ice cream	3.1–8.4
Ice milk	7.6
Yogurt, low fat	1.9–7.7
Human milk	6.2–7.5
Fat-free milk	4.3–5.7
Low-fat milk	4.8–5.5
Reduced-fat milk	3.7–5.3
American cheese	1.6–5.2
Whole cow's milk	3.7–5.1
Ricotta cheese	0.2–5.1
Buttermilk	3.6–5
Chocolate milk	4.1–4.9
Goat's milk	4.1–4.7
Yogurt, whole milk	4.1–4.7
Sour cream	3.4–4.3
Feta cheese	4.1
Light cream (half-and-half) 10.5% milk fat	3.7–4
Parmesan cheese	2.9–3.7
Romano cheese	0–3.6
Cottage cheese, 2% milk fat	3.6
Cottage cheese, 3.25% milk fat	0–3.6
Swiss cheese	0.0–3.4
Mozzarella, part-skim cheese (15% milk fat)	0–3.1
Whipping cream (35% milk fat)	2.8–3
Cream cheese	0.4–2.9
Neufchatel cheese	0.4–2.9
Brick cheese	0–2.8
Cottage cheese, 1% milk fat	2.7
Blue cheese	0–2.5
Colby cheese	0–2.5

Continues

TABLE 11.4
Lactose Content of Some Milk and Milk Products (*Continued*)

Product	Lactose, g/100 g
Provolone cheese	0–2.1
Cheddar cheese	0–2.1
Gouda cheese	0–2.1
Orange sherbet	0.6–2.1
Roquefort cheese	0–2
Brie cheese	0–2
Camembert cheese	0–1.8
Edam cheese	0–1.4
Butter	0.8–1
Lactose-reduced yogurt	0.8
Lactaid milk	0–0.025

Source: From product labels, nutrient databases, and reference 8.

Not all foods derived from milk contain the same amount of lactose. In the process of making hard cheeses, whole milk is curdled, resulting in two distinct fractions: curds and whey. The curd is made up of solidified proteins known as *caseins*; the whey is the liquid from which the curds separate and consists of several soluble proteins that differ from the caseins. This liquid fraction also contains the lactose part of milk (see Chapter 10 for more details). The curds are used to make hard cheeses and are separated from the whey in the cheese-making process. This separation also removes the lactose from the curds, and therefore the hard cheeses made from the curds are virtually lactose free. Most lactose-intolerant people can eat almost any hard cheese without discomfort.

Butter contains virtually undetectable amounts of lactose. In making butter, the fat is removed from the rest of the milk and is churned in a process that results in a solid product. By separating the fat from the rest of the milk constituents, which include whey, lactose is also excluded, and hence the butterfat is lactose free.

Microorganisms and Lactose Intolerance

Fermented milk products such as yogurt may improve lactose digestion, and they are usually well tolerated by most lactose-intolerant people. Studies have shown that after eating unheated yogurt containing live bacteria, people with lactose intolerance have improved lactose digestion and consequently fewer and less severe symptoms than when they consume milk or pasteurized yogurt. These beneficial effects are due to the production of ß-galactosidase (the enzyme that digests lactose) by bacteria in the fermented milk product.[9] This microbial enzyme performs the same function as human lactase and therefore augments the lactase produced in the small intestine.

Another important effect of the intact microorganisms in a live culture is that the cell walls of the bacteria act as a mechanical protection of the lactase inside the cells during the movement of the food through the stomach; this allows the release of the enzyme into the small intestine, where it has the most effect on lactose breakdown. In addition, the more solid consistency of the yogurt or other fermented milk product delays the rate at which the food passes through the digestive tract (increased gastrointestinal transit time). This allows the digestive enzymes to act on the food for a longer period of time than if it were in a liquid form, such as milk, and thus digest more lactose than when the food passes through quickly.[9]

Other positive effects of fermented milk with live cultures include an improvement in intestinal functions, possibly associated with interactions with the immune cells of the mucous membranes of the digestive tract and a reduced sensitivity to symptoms in the region. Furthermore, the bacteria in the fermented product compete with those established in the colon and may replace them, thus leading to a more "friendly" microflora that has beneficial effects on health and digestion.[4] The bacterial culture that acts in this manner is known as a *probiotic* (see Chapter 47).

Can Continuing to Drink Milk Improve or Delay the Onset of Lactase Deficiency?

Lactase activity in humans and other mammals is not inducible. This means that it is not possible to increase the amount of lactase produced in the epithelial cell of the small intestine. Therefore, lactose digestion is not increased by consuming lactose. However, the ability for lactose-intolerant people to tolerate a higher level of lactose-containing foods can be improved by providing lactose to the bacteria that colonize the colon.

The continued presence of lactose in the colon contributes to the establishment and multiplication of bacteria capable of synthesizing the beta-galactosidase enzyme over time.[9] The undigested lactose enhances the fermentation capacity of bifidobacteria and other lactic acid bacteria, such as lactobacilli and certain strains of streptococci that metabolize lactose without the production of hydrogen gas. This process reduces the osmotic imbalance within the colon that causes much of the distress of lactose intolerance.

The number and types of lactose-metabolizing microorganisms in a person's colon may explain the observed difference between lactose intolerance and lactose malabsorption. Even though two people may have the same degree of lactase deficiency, if one has a microflora that produces a high level of β-galactosidase, lactose in the bowel will be broken down by the activity of these organisms and thus the symptoms of lactose intolerance will not be experienced.

Feeding the Lactose-Intolerant Baby[10]

The Breastfed Baby

A breastfed baby will ingest significant quantities of lactose in the mother's milk. The lactose composition of her milk will remain constant, regardless of whether she consumes milk and dairy products. The total amount of fat, protein, and lactose in breastmilk is relatively unaffected by the mother's diet and nutritional status. This is in contrast to the fatty acid profile and the concentrations of several micronutrients, particularly water-soluble vitamins, which are dependent to some extent on the composition of the maternal diet.

The symptoms of lactose intolerance in a young baby are liquid, frothy stools, frequent passage of gas, and irritability. The usual tests for lactose intolerance, especially the hydrogen breath test and tests for reducing sugars in the stools, are not good indicators in the young baby because these tests are positive in most normal babies under 3 months.[11]

If the lactose intolerance is secondary to a gastrointestinal tract infection or other condition that is expected to be transient, the usual advice[11] is to continue breastfeeding and expect the diarrhea to gradually diminish as the underlying inflammation disappears. Some authorities recommend placing a few drops of lactase directly into the baby's mouth before each feeding.[11] This may provide enough of the enzyme to break down the lactose in the breastmilk, and so reduce or eliminate the baby's digestive tract symptoms. Alternatively, mother can pump her breastmilk and treat the milk with lactase drops (5 drops per 250 mL milk) and allow the enzyme to act for 24 hours in the fridge. The baby is fed the lactose-free milk the next day. This is continued until the diarrhea abates, when the baby can be gradually put back to the breast.

Lactose Overload[11]

Lactose overload can mimic lactose intolerance and is frequently mistaken for it. An overload is commonly seen in babies consuming large amounts of breastmilk in mothers with an oversupply of milk. The baby is producing a normal amount of lactase, but the quantity of lactose entering the small intestine overwhelms the enzyme's capacity to break it down fast enough. This results in excess, undigested lactose passing out of the small intestine and into the colon. In the colon, the lactose causes osmotic imbalance with an increase in the amount of water in the bowel, and the resident microorganisms ferment the sugar with the production of gas, abdominal bloating, pain, and possibly diarrhea. Signs of this condition include:

- An unsettled or frankly distressed baby who shows signs of stomach pain (drawing up of the legs) with screaming or crying
- Adequate to large weight gains
- More than 10 wet and many dirty diapers in 24 hours
- Sometimes frothy, yellowish stool
- Baby needs to nurse frequently

Typically these symptoms occur in babies less than 3 months old.

Because of the baby's frequent need to nurse, a mother may mistakenly conclude that she has a low milk supply because her baby always seems to be hungry. However, the diaper count can be the biggest clue to what is actually happening—the large amount of milk the baby is consuming leads to a large production of urine and feces.

The real problem is that a large-volume, low-fat feed goes through the baby so quickly that not all the lactose is digested. The first milk produced in a feed is lower in fat than the hind milk that comes later as the baby continues to suckle. A higher fat content would slow the speed at which the milk moves through the digestive tract. The lactose reaching the lower bowel draws extra water into the bowel and is fermented by the bacteria there, resulting in gas and acid stools. Acid stool can cause diaper rash as the acid burns the baby's skin around the anus. Gas and fluid buildup in the bowel causes stomach pain and the baby appears to be hungry. Sucking is the best comfort the baby knows, and the milk helps move the gas along the bowel. This tends to ease the pain temporarily and may result in gas and stool being passed. Since the baby indicates that he or she wants to suck at the breast, the mother, logically, complies. Sometimes it is the only way to provide comfort. Unfortunately, this provides another large feed on top of the previous one. The amount of lactose consumed overwhelms the lactase available to digest it, and more lactose enters the colon, resulting in more gas and fluid accumulation. This creates a vicious cycle in which the milk seems to almost literally "go in one end and out the other."

A solution to the problem may be found by a strategy that increases the fat content of the mother's milk and thereby slows the speed at which the milk passes along the baby's digestive tract. This method consists of using the same breast for each feeding during a certain period of time.[12] For example, set aside a 3-hour period, and every time the baby wants to feed during this period, use the same breast. Then use the other breast for the next 3 hours. In this way, each time the baby returns to the already-used breast, there is a lower-volume, higher-fat feed that helps slow the system down. If there is still an oversupply of milk (indicated by a continuation of the abdominal symptoms), increase the one-breast feeding to 4 hours. When the baby's symptoms are relieved, the mother may go back to a normal according-to-need breastfeeding routine.

Some Important Facts About Lactose Intolerance and Breastfeeding

Contrary to some popular beliefs, lactose in the breastmilk will *not* be reduced if the mother stops eating dairy products. The nutritional composition of her breastmilk, especially with regard to lactose, is entirely unaffected by her diet (cows never consume milk—they eat only grass, and their milk contains about 4.8 g of lactose per 100 mL of milk). The typical lactose content of human colostrum (produced during days 1 to 5) is 5.2 g per 100 mL; mature milk (produced from day 15 onward) contains 7 g of lactose per 100 mL and remains at that level throughout lactation. Table 11.5 provides an idea of the amount of lactose, protein, and fat consumed by the breastfed baby from birth to 3 months.[12] See Box 11.2 for a summary of key points about lactose intolerance in breastfed babies.

TABLE 11.5
Typical Daily Intakes (g) of Selected Breastmilk Constituents

Age	Protein	Fat	Lactose
Day 1	5	< 1	1
Day 3	12	5	12
Day 8	9	22	40
3 mo	7.5	29	52

Calculated intakes assume the following daily milk volumes:

Day 1 (0–24 h), 40 mL

Day 3 (48–72 h), 200 mL

Day 8, 600 mL

3 months, 750 mL

Source: From Prentice A. Constituents of human milk. *Food Nutr Bull.* 1996;17(4):305-312. www.unu.edu/unupress/food/8F174e/8F174E04.htm. Accessed October 21, 2010.

BOX 11.2 Key Points Regarding Lactose Intolerance in the Breastfed Baby

- Lactose intolerance in other family members, including the mother, does not mean that the baby will be lactose intolerant. Different ethnic groups tend to lose the ability to produce a normal amount of lactase at different ages after infancy (see Table 11.3).
- Almost all babies produce adequate amounts of lactase in the first few years of life. The very rare exception is congenital alactasia, which is present and apparent from birth.
- Breastfeeding should not be discontinued if a baby develops lactose intolerance. Usually the condition is temporary, often associated with a gastrointestinal infection. Normal lactase production resumes once the tissues of the digestive tract have returned to normal, and the baby will then be able to tolerate lactose without any difficulty.
- Lactose intolerance is quite different from allergy to cow's milk protein. Milk protein allergy involves a complex series of events in the immune system; lactose intolerance is merely a deficiency in the enzyme that digests the milk sugar. The symptoms and management of the two conditions are quite distinct.

The Formula-Fed Baby

Infant formulas that are lactose free can be given to a lactose-intolerant infant. If the baby is not allergic to milk, the milk-based Enfalac Lactose-Free (Mead Johnson) or Similac Advance LF (Abbott Nutrition; *LF* means "lactose free"), which are free from lactose, are suitable.

If the infant is allergic to cow's milk, a casein hydrolysate formula such as Similac Alimentum (Abbott Nutrition), Enfamil Nutramigen (Mead Johnson), or Enfamil Pregestimil (Mead Johnson) may be tolerated. All are lactose free (see Chapter 44 for more details).

The Lactose-Restricted Diet

People differ in the amount of lactase they produce, which affects the quantity of lactose they can consume without symptoms. This amount varies not only between individuals but also in the same individual at different times. A recent study indicated that most adults with presumed lactose intolerance or malabsorption can tolerate 12 to 15 g of lactose.[7]

Lactose Restrictions

Foods, medications, and beverages containing milk and milk solids should be assumed to contain lactose, unless labeled "lactose-free." Products labeled as containing lactose, milk, milk solids, milk powder, cheese and cheese flavor, curd, whey, cream, and margarine containing milk solids should be avoided. Products containing lactic acid, lactalbumin, lactate, and casein *do not* contain lactose and can be consumed.

Acidophilus milk is milk to which the bacterium *Lactobacillus acidophilus* has been added. These bacteria do not break down lactose to any great extent, so the milk would not be tolerated by people with lactose intolerance.

Milk and Milk Products Suitable for a Lactose-Restricted Diet

Adding the enzyme lactase to liquid milk and allowing the enzyme to act for a minimum of 24 hours in the refrigerator will make it digestible, and no substitutes are then necessary. The amount of the enzyme that needs to be added will depend on the degree of lactase deficiency. Instructions are provided with the lactase product.

- 15 drops in 1 liter of milk will render it 99% lactose free.
- 10 drops reduces the lactose to 90%.
- 5 drops will provide a milk that is 70% lactose free.

Lactase tablets may be taken before eating or drinking lactose-containing products and may be sufficient to break down the amount of lactose consumed in the following meal. Lactase milks are 99% lactose free and are available in the dairy section of grocery stores. These are tolerated by lactose-deficient individuals but are more expensive than regular milk.

As discussed earlier, hard, fermented cheeses may be tolerated since most of the lactose is removed with the whey during their manufacture. Although butter and regular margarines contain a small amount of lactose (in whey), they are usually tolerated because the level of lactose is so low, and these products are eaten in small quantities.

Fermented milks such as yogurt and buttermilk may be tolerated because the level of lactose in these products is reduced (but not completely eliminated) by bacterial enzymes. Mixing lactase drops in the yogurt in the doses previously indicated and refrigerating the product for 24 hours may render it acceptable for the severely lactose-intolerant individual.

References

1. Gudmand-Høyer E. The clinical significance of disaccharide maldigestion. *Am J Clin Nutr.* 1994;59(3 suppl):735S-741S.
2. Järvelä I, Torniainen S, Kolho KL. Molecular genetics of human lactase deficiencies [review]. *Ann Med.* 2009;41(8):568-575.
3. Johnson JD. The regional and ethnic distribution of lactose malabsorption. Adaptive and genetic hypotheses. In: Paige DM, Bayless TM, eds. *Lactose Digestion. Clinical and Nutritional Implications.* Baltimore, MD: Johns Hopkins University Press; 1981:11-22.
4. De Vrese M, Stegelmann A, Richter B, Fenselau S, Laue C, Schrezenmeir J. Probiotics—compensation for lactase insufficiency. *Am J Clin Nutr.* 2001;73(suppl 1):421S-429S.
5. Sahi T. Genetics and epidemiology of adult-type hypolactasia. *Scand Gastroenterol.* 1994;202(suppl):7-20.
6. Jellema P, Schellevis FG, van der Windt DA, Kneepkens CM, van der Horst HE. Lactose malabsorption and intolerance: a systematic review on the diagnostic value of gastrointestinal symptoms and self-reported milk intolerance. *QJM.* 2010;103(8):555-572.
7. Shaukat A, Levitt MD, Taylor BC, et al. Systematic review: effective management strategies for lactose intolerance. *Ann Intern Med.* 2010;152(12):797-803.
8. Scrimshaw N, Murray E. The acceptability of milk and milk products in populations with a high prevalence of lactose intolerance. *Am J Clin Nutr.* 1988;48(4 suppl):1079-1159.
9. Montalto M, Curigliano V, Santoro L, et al. Management and treatment of lactose malabsorption. *World J Gastroenterol.* 2006;12(2):187-191.
10. Heyman MB, for the Committee on Nutrition, American Academy of Pediatrics. Lactose intolerance in infants, children and adolescents. *Pediatrics.* 2006;118(3):1279-1286.
11. Anderson J. Lactose intolerance and the breastfed baby. *Essence.* Australian Breastfeeding Association, August 2006. www.breastfeeding.asn.au/bfinfo/lactose.html. Accessed April 23, 2012.
12. Prentice A. Constituents of human milk. *Food Nutr Bull.* 1996;17(4):305-312. www.unu.edu/unupress/food/8F174e/8F174E04.htm. Accessed October 21, 2010.

CHAPTER **12**

Egg Allergy

Egg is a common cause of food allergy in children[1] and, along with milk, accounts for the majority of reactions to foods in children younger than 2 years of age.[2] Egg allergy typically develops before the child is 2 years old, and in many cases it disappears during the first 6 years.[3] Egg allergy has been estimated to affect 1% to 2% of children worldwide,[4] while reports from various countries indicate a prevalence of 0.5% to 2.5%, depending on the nutritional habits in different populations.[5] In contrast, about 0.1% of adults report egg allergy,[6] typically as a result of a persistent childhood egg allergy.

Most children allergic to egg develop tolerance to it by adulthood.[7] The age at which a child will outgrow an early egg allergy is difficult to predict. A 2007 study[4] indicated that 4% of children allergic to egg are likely to outgrow their allergy by the age of 4 years, 12% by 6 years, 37% by 10 years, and 68% by 16 years. Studies from Europe[8] indicated that 66% of children outgrew their allergy to egg by the age of 7 years. However, no tests or signs can predict which child will outgrow egg allergy or at what age eggs will be tolerated. Authorities suggest that children with the more severe allergy and higher egg-specific IgE levels will be less likely to outgrow their early allergy to eggs than those who experience only mild symptoms.[9] Egg allergy may persist into adulthood, especially when egg causes an anaphylactic reaction.

Symptoms of Egg Allergy

The most common sensitivity reaction to egg is an IgE-mediated allergy, and until recently IgE-mediated hypersensitivity was the most thoroughly researched aspect of adverse reactions to egg. However, more current information has indicated that egg can be an important trigger for eosinophilic diseases of the digestive tract and other immunologically mediated reactions[5] (for more details, see Chapter 39).

142

IgE-Mediated Allergy to Egg

The symptoms induced by an IgE-mediated allergic reaction to egg may involve the skin, with erythema (reddening), urticaria (hives), and angioedema (tissue swelling), especially of the face. Gastrointestinal reactions may include abdominal pain, nausea, vomiting, and diarrhea. Respiratory reactions include hay fever (rhinoconjunctivitis), throat tightening (laryngeal edema), wheezing, and asthma. Anaphylaxis may occur in rare instances.[9] Eating raw or undercooked egg may trigger more severe reactions than well-cooked egg.[10]

In the adult population, egg allergy may be associated with other types of IgE-mediated allergies. Bird-egg syndrome is an example. In this condition, the primary sensitization is to airborne bird allergens by inhalation, followed by secondary sensitization or cross-reactivity with albumin in egg. These individuals experience respiratory symptoms such as rhinitis and/or asthma on exposure to birds, and allergic symptoms, such as those previously mentioned, after ingesting egg.[11]

IgE-mediated egg allergy has also been reported as a trigger for food-dependent exercise-induced anaphylaxis (FDEIA).[12] (See Chapter 4 for details on FDEIA.)

In addition to IgE-mediated reactions, egg can be involved in mixed IgE and non-IgE-mediated reactions. The symptoms in these cases include atopic dermatitis and eosinophilic gastrointestinal diseases.[5]

Atopic Dermatitis (Eczema)

Egg allergy is closely associated with atopic dermatitis (eczema). A 1999 report indicated that two-thirds of children with atopic dermatitis in the study had a positive food challenge to egg,[13] and a 2008 multicenter study found a close association between egg sensitization and early onset, moderate to severe atopic dermatitis.[14] It has been suggested[15] that the reaction to egg in cases of eczema is probably a mixed IgE and non-IgE reaction; the onset of symptoms may be immediate or may be delayed for up to 48 hours after egg ingestion, suggesting that the latter are T cell–mediated reactions[16] (for details about the immunological response in allergy, see Chapter 1).

Non-IgE-Mediated Gastrointestinal Conditions

An immunological response to egg can result in eosinophilic esophagitis (EoE) in predisposed individuals in whom a large infiltration of eosinophils into the esophagus causes local inflammation with resultant difficulty in swallowing, regurgitation, and associated weight loss or failure to thrive in young children[16] (see Chapter 39 for more details). In a study of more than 600 people with EoE, egg was the second most common allergen that triggered symptoms, and eliminating egg from the diet was an effective treatment in these cases.[17] There have been reports of food protein enteropathy and food-protein-induced enterocolitis syndrome due to egg in babies,[18] but such conditions seem to be rare.

Diagnosis

Detection of egg-specific IgE antibodies is considered to be the earliest indicator that a baby is atopic.[19] However, several studies indicate that more babies and young children are skin-test positive to egg or have egg-specific antibodies in their blood than actually develop the symptoms of allergy when they consume egg. It is not unusual to see evidence of IgE sensitization to a food protein without symptoms being involved.[20] On the other hand, a negative skin test for egg is generally considered to be an accurate indicator of the *absence* of egg allergy, because skin tests for egg are considered to have a negative predictive value of 91%.[21]

As with any food allergy, diagnosis of egg allergy starts with a detailed history and physical examination. Typically skin tests and blood tests for egg-specific IgE are performed, followed by an elimination diet and oral food challenge.[5]

In many cases, loss of clinical reactivity (no symptoms) precedes loss of IgE antibodies, so skin tests and blood tests often may be positive while eating the egg causes no problem. Tolerance to egg may occur as a natural process of maturing. Some studies have indicated that ingesting a small quantity of egg over an extended period can induce tolerance in an allergic individual[22] (see Chapter 44 for more details). In 2008,[23] it was reported that ingesting extensively heated egg (eg, in baked products) can alter the immunological response in favor of tolerance in children allergic to egg. Continued ingestion of the egg altered the ratio of egg-specific IgE to IgG, with a decrease in IgE and a corresponding increase in IgG, indicating development of tolerance.[24]

Research indicates that once tolerance develops, it is important for a child to continue to eat the tolerated food to maintain tolerance to it;[24] therefore, it is advisable for the child to undergo a food challenge (eating a small quantity under close medical supervision) periodically to determine whether they continue to be allergic to the food. When children are older than 2 years, clinicians usually advise yearly challenge of foods to which the child is allergic and that have been avoided in the interim. In the case of egg allergy, it is important that such a challenge be undertaken under medical supervision because of the risk of anaphylaxis.

Mechanism of Egg Allergy

Eggs contain many different proteins that can lead to allergy.[1] Each individual is likely to be sensitized to more than one such protein. A person who has been proven to be allergic to eggs is usually advised to avoid egg in any form. This is particularly important in children younger than 7 years, because there is a higher risk of a severe or anaphylactic reaction to eggs in this age group. In general, children with egg allergy react principally to the ingestion of egg white. Although egg yolk contains several proteins, egg white contains the greatest number of *allergens*. Up to 24 different antigenic protein fractions have been isolated, although the *antigenicity* (ability to trigger an immunological reaction) of most of these is unknown. The main allergens are ovalbumin, ovomucoid, ovotransferrin, lysozyme, and α-livetin.

Because there is a great deal of difference between the proteins in egg yolk and egg white (as noted previously, the latter tend to be more allergenic than the former), it is sometimes useful to find out which of these egg components is causing the allergy so that the diet need not be so restricted. In addition, some egg proteins are destroyed by heat, which means that a person sensitized to heat-labile proteins can consume well-cooked eggs, especially in small quantities in baked goods, without any harmful effects. However, a person allergic to heat-stable proteins (those unaffected by heat) must avoid eggs in any form.

Egg Proteins

The typical chicken egg is composed of 51% to 61% egg white, 27% to 32% yolk, and 8% to 11% shell. The white of an egg contains about 10% protein and 80% water. The yolk is composed of 50% water, 34% fat, and 16% protein. Five specific proteins from the egg of the domestic hen (*Gallus domesticus*) have been studied extensively:

■ Gal d 1 (ovomucoid)
■ Gal d 2 (ovalbumin)
■ Gal d 3 (ovotransferrin)
■ Gal d 4 (lysozyme)
■ Gal d 5 (α-livetin)

Egg white is considered to be the source of the major egg allergens, which include *ovalbumin, ovotransferrin* (sometimes called *conalbumin*), *ovomucoid,* and *lysozyme* (Box 12.1).[25] Ovalbumin is present in the greatest quantity in an egg (54% of the protein); however, ovomucoid (11%) is the most frequent and persistent allergen triggering an egg allergy.[26] Research has demonstrated that children with egg allergy that persisted sometimes into adulthood had significantly higher levels of antibodies to ovomucoid than children who outgrew their egg allergy.[27]

Some egg yolk proteins, especially α-*livetin* (sometimes referred to as *chicken serum albumin*), may also induce the production of IgE antibodies, and there may be some degree of antigenic cross-reactivity between egg yolk and egg albumin proteins. Alpha-livetin is the allergen involved in the bird-egg syndrome (see the "IgE-Mediated Allergy to Egg" section earlier).[28] Several other allergens have been identified in egg yolk but have not been studied so extensively, and their role in egg allergy has not yet been elucidated. These proteins include vitellenin (apovitellenin I), apoprotein B (apovitellenin VI), and egg lecithin. Many manufactured food products contain egg lecithin in trace amounts, but in general the amount ingested from such a product is usually considered insufficient to induce symptoms.[29]

Although cooking may decompose many of the egg proteins (making cooked eggs more tolerated in cases where raw egg causes an allergic reaction), some egg proteins, especially ovomucoid, are heat-stable and people allergic to this component will react to cooked and raw egg. In most children, however, the small amount

---

BOX 12.1   Antigenic Proteins in Chicken Egg

Antigenic egg white proteins (known percentages of the total protein are given in brackets)
Major proteins
- Ovalbumin (54%)
- Ovotransferrin (conalbumin) (13%)
- Ovomucoid (11%)
- Ovomucin (1.5%)
- Lysozyme (3%-5%)

Trace amounts of
- Catalase
- Ovoflavoprotein
- Ficin inhibitor

- Ovoglycoprotein
- G2 and G3 globulins
- Ovomacroglobulin
- Ribonuclease
- Ovoinhibitor
- Avidin

Antigenic egg yolk proteins
Major proteins
- Lipovitellin
- Phosvitin
- Low-density lipoproteins
- Livetins

Source: From Langeland T, Aas K. Allergy to hen's egg white: clinical and immunological aspects. In: Brostoff J, Challacombe SJ, eds. *Food Allergy and Intolerance.* Philadelphia, PA: Bailliere Tindall; 1987:367-374.

of cooked egg in baked goods is usually tolerated unless there is risk of anaphylaxis. As a result of research indicating that ingestion of small amounts of an allergen over an extended period may lead to tolerance, some practitioners are suggesting that because extensively heated egg is tolerated by most people with egg allergy, incorporation of cooked egg in the diet may provide a natural form of oral tolerance induction (oral therapy) in such individuals.[5] Of course, anyone at risk of an anaphylactic reaction, or those allergic to cooked egg, must avoid all sources of egg in the interest of safety.

In some people, contact with egg can cause urticaria (hives), although they have no symptoms when they eat eggs. These individuals have IgE antibodies that recognize particular egg white molecules that are destroyed by the action of digestive enzymes.[30]

Egg Proteins and Chicken

In most cases of egg allergy, IgE antibodies are produced exclusively against the specific proteins associated with the egg, which differ from the proteins in chicken flesh. However, some livetins are derived from the blood of the hen. IgE antibodies to these proteins might result in allergy to both egg and chicken. In individuals who are allergic to egg white, skin tests often reveal sensitivity to chicken meat, but eating chicken does not lead to symptoms in most of these cases. Children with a positive skin test to egg need not avoid chicken unless they develop symptoms when they eat it.

Egg Proteins from Other Birds

Proteins in eggs from different bird species sometimes cross-react antigenically. In immunological studies, proteins in turkey, duck, goose, and seagull egg whites were shown to cross-react with chicken egg white proteins.[31] However, evidence from a single study indicates that people allergic to duck and goose eggs were not allergic to chicken eggs.[31] The subject of cross-reactivity between eggs from different bird species needs to be investigated further.

Based on our current knowledge, a person who is allergic to chicken eggs should treat eggs from different birds as if they were an entirely separate food, taking a small quantity at first and monitoring their reaction to it before consuming a whole egg. If the egg has been eaten without incident in the past, there is no reason to stop eating it. However, children younger than 7 years who have a known allergy to chicken egg should not eat eggs from other birds, because in this age group, egg allergy can lead to anaphylaxis in severe cases.

Egg as an Ingredient in Medications and Vaccines

Some medications and vaccines may include egg, or a derivative of egg, as an ingredient. It is important that people allergic to egg inform their clinician and pharmacist of their egg allergy, especially when taking a new medication or vaccine.

Vaccines That May Contain Egg Proteins

Viruses need living cells to grow in, so viruses used for vaccines are frequently grown in the chick embryo in an egg. Consequently, such vaccines may contain small quantities of the egg protein when the viruses are harvested. Vaccines that could potentially contain egg proteins include:

■ The triple virus vaccine of measles, mumps, and rubella (MMR)
■ Influenza viruses
■ Yellow fever

Small amounts of egg might also be found in the typhus and rabies vaccines, depending on the way they are prepared.

Anaphylactic reactions to vaccine components are rare. It is often difficult to determine whether a reaction has been caused by the vaccine antigens or by any of the vaccine components (neomycin, sorbitol, and gelatin) or whether the reaction is due to the egg protein it may contain.[32]

Triple Virus Vaccine

The triple virus vaccine (measles, rubella, mumps) does not contain significant amounts of egg proteins. Children who are allergic to egg, even those who are highly sensitive, are at very low risk for developing anaphylactic reactions to these vaccines,[33] although such reactions have occasionally been reported.[34] Skin tests with diluted vaccine preparations do not appear to be helpful in predicting possible allergic reactions after vaccine administration. In 1997, the Committee of Infectious Diseases of the American Academy of Pediatrics proposed routine administration of the vaccine without prior skin tests.[35] The committee recommends that people just vaccinated should be observed for 90 minutes by a team experienced in treating anaphylaxis.

Influenza Vaccine

The influenza vaccine has been reported to contain small quantities (1 to 7 mg/mL) of egg proteins. The actual measurable levels of the dominant protein, ovalbumin, vary between manufacturers and between batches of vaccine. Levels have been reported to vary from barely detectable on up to 42 µg/mL.[36] The Committee of Infectious Diseases of the American Academy of Pediatrics recommends that people with anaphylactic reactions or very severe reactions after egg ingestion should not be given this vaccine without prior skin testing with a diluted preparation of the vaccine.[35] The vaccine should not be given to anyone who is skin-test positive to it. The Committee states that children who react positively to the vaccine skin test should not undergo influenza vaccination because of the risk of a reaction and because yearly vaccinations, if required, might increase the child's allergic response.

If the person's clinical situation indicates that the protection of the influenza vaccine is essential and he or she has a negative skin test to the vaccine, the Committee recommends that the vaccine be administered under medical supervision in a facility equipped for anaphylactic emergencies.

H1N1 Influenza A Vaccine

In a controlled, prospective trial,[37] H1N1 skin testing and vaccination was compared between egg allergic (EA) individuals (n = 105) and non-EA controls (n = 19). All participants were skin tested with the vaccine prior to injection. Those with negative H1N1 skin test results received a full H1N1 dose; those with a positive skin test result received a graded challenge (10%, 90%). No significant allergic reactions resulted from either method of vaccination or from subsequent booster doses given as a single vaccine to all participants, including seven individuals with a history of egg-induced anaphylaxis. The authors conclude that H1N1 is safe for egg-allergic individuals.

Yellow Fever Vaccine

The yellow fever vaccine is also prepared in chicken embryo. Authorities recommend that skin tests with the vaccine should be carried out before yellow fever vaccination only in individuals with a history of systemic anaphylaxis after egg ingestion.[38] If immunization is required, the vaccine should be carefully administered at a medical center in multiple small separate doses.

Management of Egg Allergy

Management of egg allergy is similar to that of any other allergenic food. Avoidance of egg in all its forms is important, and especially so when there is a risk for anaphylaxis and in young children younger than 7 years in whom severe reactions are most likely to occur. Education regarding sources of egg and learning to read labels for the presence of egg in manufactured foods are essential.

As with any other allergenic food, maternal avoidance of eggs during pregnancy and lactation does not seem to be effective in preventing sensitization of the fetus to egg before birth, nor of the baby during breastfeeding. Of course, if the mother is allergic to eggs, she should avoid eating them. If the baby is diagnosed with egg allergy, the mother should avoid eggs in her diet while breastfeeding, because egg proteins will pass into her breastmilk and trigger symptoms in the baby. Timing of the introduction of allergenic foods in babies is discussed in detail in Chapter 44.

Avoiding egg as an individual ingredient in a meal (eg, omelet, scrambled, boiled, fried, etc) is relatively easy. However, eggs are often included as an ingredient in prepared foods, and as such may not be so easily recognized unless care is taken in reading food labels, becoming familiar with terms that indicate the presence of egg protein, and being aware of the foods that are traditionally made with eggs.

If egg is included as an ingredient in a manufactured food regulated by the Food and Drug Administration (FDA), US law requires that "egg" must clearly appear on the label.[39] Refer to Chapter 9 for more on food allergen labeling and which foods are covered by the FDA regulations.

Some products may have advisory labeling, such as "may contain egg," or "manufactured in a facility that also processes egg." This type of labeling is not regulated, but products so labeled should be avoided because they may cause a reaction in some very sensitive individuals.[40]

Several studies have found that most individuals with egg allergy can tolerate extensively heated or baked egg. Therefore, a small amount in a baked product is usually allowable, as long as the person has eaten the product with impunity in the past.[41]

Important Nutrients in Eggs

Eggs contribute vitamin D, vitamin B-12, pantothenic acid, selenium, folacin, riboflavin, biotin and iron, and in smaller amounts, vitamin A, vitamin E, vitamin B-6, and zinc. These nutrients can easily be supplied in meat, fish, and poultry products; legumes; whole grains; and vegetables (see Chapter 8 for more information); therefore, an egg-free diet should not pose any risk of deficiency of any of these nutrients.

References

1. Rancé F, Kanny G, Dutau G, Moneret-Vautrin D. Food hypersensitivity in children: clinical aspects and distribution of allergens. *Pediatr Allergy Immunol.* 1999;10:33-38.

2. Eggesbo M, Botten G, Halvorsen R, et al. The prevalence of allergy to egg: a population based study in young children. *Allergy.* 2001;56(5):403-411.

3. Martorell Aragonés A, Boné Calvo J, García Ara MC, Nevot Falcó S, Plaza Martín AM; Food Allergy Committee of the Spanish Society of Pediatric Clinical Immunology and Allergy. Allergy to egg proteins. *Allergol Immunopathol* (Madr). 2001;29:72-95.

4. Savage JH, Matsui EC, Skripak JM, Wood R. The natural history of egg allergy. *J Allergy Clin Immunol.* 2007;120(6):1413-1417.

5. Caubet JC, Wang J. Current understanding of egg allergy. *Pediatr Clin North Am.* 2011;58(2):427-443.

6. Clark AT, Skypala I, Leech SC, et al. British Society for Allergy and Clinical Immunology guidelines for the management of egg allergy. *Clin Exper Allergy.* 2010;40:1116-1129.

7. Shek LP, Soderstrom L, Ahlstedt S, Beyer K, Sampson HA. Determination of food specific IgE levels over time can predict the development of tolerance in cow's milk and hen's egg allergy. *J Allergy Clin Immunol.* 2004;114(2):387-391.

8. Boyano-Martinez T, Garcia-Ara C, Diaz-Pena JM, Martin-Esteban M. Prediction of tolerance on the basis of quantification of egg-white specific IgE antibodies in children with egg allergy. *J Allergy Clin Immunol.* 2002;110(2):304-309.

9. Sampson HA, Mendelson L, Rosen JP. Fatal and near-fatal anaphylactic reactions to food in children and adolescents. *N Engl J Med.* 1992;327(6):380-384.

10. Eigenmann PA. Anaphylactic reactions to raw eggs after negative challenges with cooked eggs. *J Allergy Clin Immunol.* 2000;105(3):587-588.

11. Szepfalusi Z, Ebner C, Pandjaltan R, et al. Egg yolk alpha-livetin (chicken serum albumin) is a cross-reactive allergen in the bird-egg syndrome. *J Allergy Clin Immunol.* 1994;93(5):932-942.

12. Tewari A, Du Toit G, Lack G. The difficulties of diagnosing food-dependent exercise-induced anaphylaxis in childhood—a case study and review. *Pediatr Allergy Immunol.* 2006;17(2):157-160.

13. Niggemann B, Slelaff B, Beyer K, et al. Outcome of double-blind, placebo-controlled food challenge tests in 107 children with atopic dermatitis. *Clin Exp Allergy.* 1999; 29(1):91-96.

14. Hill DJ, Hosking CS, de Benedictis FM, et al. Confirmation of the association between high levels of immunoglobulin E food sensitization and eczema in infancy: an international study. *Clin Exp Allergy.* 2008;38(1):161-168.

15. Werfel T, Ballmer-Weber B, Eigenmann PA, et al. Eczematous reactions to food in atopic eczema: position paper of the EAACI and GA2LEN. *Allergy.* 2007;62(7):723-728.

16. Liacouras CA, Spergel JM, Ruchelli E, et al. Eosinophilic esophagitis: a 10-year experience in 381 children. *Clin Gastroenterol Hepatol.* 2005;3(12):1198-1206.

17. Spergel JM, Brown-Whitehorn TF, Beausoleil JL, et al. 14 years of eosinophilic esophagitis: clinical features and prognosis. *J Pediatr Gastroenterol Nutr.* 2009;48(1):30-36.

18. Kondon M, Fukao T, Omoya K, et al. Protein-losing enteropathy associated with egg allergy in a 5-month old boy. *J Investig Allergol Clin Immunol.* 2008;18(1):63-66.

19. Kulig M, Bergmann R, Klettke U, Wahn V, Tacke U, Wahn U. Natural course of sensitization to food and inhalant allergens during the first 6 years of life. *J Allergy Clin Immunol.* 1999;103:1173-1179.

20. Sporik R, Hill DJ, Hosking CS. Specificity of allergen skin testing in predicting positive open food challenges to milk, egg and peanut in children. *Clin Exp Allergy.* 2000 Nov;30(11):1540-1546.

21. Caffarelli C, Cavagni G, Giordano S, et al. Relationship between oral challenges with previously uningested egg and egg-specific IgE antibodies and skin prick tests in infants with food allergy. *J Allergy Clin Immunol.* 1995;95(6):1215-1220.

22. Itoh N, Itagaki Y, Kurihara K. Rush specific oral tolerance induction in school-age children with severe egg allergy: one year follow-up. *Allergol Int.* 2010;59(1):43-51.

23. Lemon-Mule H, Sampson HA, Sicherer SH, et al. Immunologic changes in children with egg allergy ingesting extensively heated egg. *J Allergy Clin Immunol.* 2008;122(5):977-983.

24. Burks AW, Jones SM. Egg oral immunotherapy in non-anaphylactic children with egg allergy: follow-up. *J Allergy Clin Immunol.* 2008;121(1):270-271.

25. Langeland T, Aas K. Allergy to hen's egg white: clinical and immunological aspects. In: Brostoff J, Challacombe SJ, eds. *Food Allergy and Intolerance.* Philadelphia, PA: Bailliere Tindall; 1987:367-374.

26. Cooke SK, Sampson HA. Allergenic properties of ovomucoid in man. *J Immunol.* 1997;159(4):2026-2032.

27. Jarvinen KM, Beyer K, Vila L, et al. Specificity of IgE antibodies to sequential epitopes of hen's egg ovomucoid as a marker for persistence of egg allergy. *Allergy.* 2007;62(7):758-765.

28. Quirce S, Maranon F, Umpierrez A, et al. Chicken serum albumin (Gal d 5) is a partially heat-labile inhalant and food allergen implicated in the bird-egg syndrome. *Allergy.* 2001;56(8):754-762.

29. Heine RG, Laske N, Hill DJ. The diagnosis and management of egg allergy. *Curr Allergy Asthma Rep.* 2006;6(2):145-152.

30. Yamada K, Urisu A, Kakami H, et al. IgE-binding activity to enzyme-digested ovomucoid distinguishes between patients with contact urticaria to egg with and without overt symptoms on ingestion. *Allergy.* 2000;55:565-569.

31. Langeland T. A clinical and immunological study of allergy to hen's egg white, VI: occurrence of proteins cross-reacting with allergens in hen's egg white as studied in egg white from turkey, duck, goose, seagull and in hen egg yolk, and hen and chicken sera and flesh. *Allergy.* 1983;38:399-412.

32. Retailliau HF, Curtis AC, Storr G, et al. Illness after influenza vaccination reported through a nationwide surveillance system. 1976-1977. *Am J Epidemiol.* 1980;111(3):270-278.

33. James JM, Burks AW, Roberson PK, Sampson HA. Safe administration of the measles vaccine to children allergic to eggs. *N Engl J Med.* 1995;332:1262-1266.

34. Baxter DN. Measles immunization in children with history of egg allergy. *Vaccine.* 1996;14:131-134.

35. Peters G, ed. *Red Book: Report of the Committee on Infectious Diseases.* 24th ed. Elk Grove Village, IL: American Academy of Pediatrics Publications; 1997:32-33.

36. Cheloupka I, Schuler A, Marschall M, et al. Comparative analysis of six European influenza vaccines. *Eur J Clin Microbiol Infect Dis.* 1996;15(2):121-127.

37. Greenhawt MJ, Chernin AS, Howe L, Li JT, Sanders G. The safety of the H1N1 influenza A vaccine in egg allergic individuals. *Ann Allergy Asthma Immunol.* 2010;105(5):387-393.

38. Kelso JM, Mootrey GT, Tsai TF. Anaphylaxis from yellow fever vaccine. *J Allergy Clin Immunol.* 1999;103:698-701.

39. US Food and Drug Administration. Food Allergen and Consumer Protection Act of 2004. http://www.fda.gov/Food/LabelingNutrition/FoodAllergensLabeling/GuidanceCompliance RegulatoryInformation/ucm106187.htm. Accessed April 23, 2012.

40. Ford LS, Taylor SL, Pacenza R, et al. Food allergen advisory labeling and product contamination with egg, milk, and peanut. *J Allergy Clin Immunol*. 2010;126(2):384-385.

41. Des Roches A, Nguyen M, Paradis L, et al. Tolerance to cooked egg in an egg allergic population. *Allergy*. 2006;61(7):900-901.

CHAPTER **13**

Wheat Allergy

Wheat is one of the most commonly implicated allergens for food allergy in all Western countries; it is also the most commonly consumed grain in the Western diet. Where legislation regarding labeling of food products exists, wheat is included on lists of foods that must be included as allergens (for more details about labeling of foods, see Chapter 9). Wheat is one of the six most important food allergens for children, especially those with skin reactions, along with milk, soy, egg, peanut, and fish.[1] In the United States, wheat is considered to be a less common cause of food allergy in adults, although recent research is revealing its role as an important cause of food-dependent exercise-induced anaphylaxis in young adults.[2]

The reported incidence of wheat allergy differs between populations; for example, countries in northern Europe report a higher incidence of wheat allergy than those in southern Europe.[3] The incidence of wheat allergy reported in the United States tends to be lower than that in Europe; for instance in a 1990 study in the United States,[4] 2.5% of the subjects were identified as allergic to wheat, whereas in a French study of people with food allergy, 10.9% of the children and 25% of the adults were diagnosed with wheat allergy.[5] However, a study in 2000 in the United States[6] reported an incidence of reactivity to wheat in 20% of the study population (adults and children), suggesting methods of diagnosis and reactivity patterns to wheat (see below) differ between studies. A German multicenter allergy study (MAS)[7] analyzed data from 273 children from ages 2 to 10 years that showed a progressive increase in IgE to wheat from 2% to 10% as the children aged. The investigators in that study speculated that IgE sensitization to wheat occurs primarily in early infancy, whereas wheat allergy is secondary to pollen allergy as a person ages.

In adults, wheat allergy is less frequent than in children. In adults, symptoms of wheat allergy may appear on exertion, as food-dependent exercise-induced anaphylaxis (FDEIA; see below). Adult-onset wheat allergy may occur at any age and tends to persist.[8] An unusual route for sensitization to wheat is through the skin. A 2006 study[9] reported primary sensitization to wheat protein in a cosmetic product that started as contact urticaria and progressed to IgE-mediated hypersensitivity on ingestion of the same proteins, which were identified as albumins and globulins (see below for more details about the allergenic proteins in wheat). Allergy to other grains (eg, oats, rye, barley, corn, or rice) is less common.[10]

Early food allergy is often outgrown as children mature, and wheat is no exception. A 2009 report in the United States indicated that, of the 103 children studied who were allergic to wheat, the majority outgrew their allergy by age 12 years.[11] The rates of resolution were reported to be 29% by 4 years, 56% by 8 years, and 65% by 12 years.

Although the higher wheat IgE levels were generally associated with a reduced probability of the child outgrowing their wheat allergy and the allergy persisting into adolescence, many children with even the highest levels of wheat IgE did outgrow their allergy to wheat.

It is not uncommon for people to react adversely to wheat when they consume it but to test negative in wheat-specific IgE evaluations. This apparent anomaly may be explained by research indicating that not all adverse reactions to wheat are mediated by IgE.[12] Clinical symptoms of allergy toward wheat may cause anything from a mild reaction to anaphylaxis.

Symptoms Associated with Wheat Allergy

The symptoms resulting from wheat allergy or sensitivity can occur in all organ systems and may include:

■ Gastrointestinal (GI) tract symptoms with abdominal pain and loose stools or diarrhea, and occasionally nausea and vomiting, commencing within 12 to 72 hours after eating wheat. GI tract symptoms are the most frequently reported manifestations of wheat allergy. In children, this pattern often accompanies an allergy to cow's milk proteins.[13]

■ Asthma, with bronchospasm, in both adults and children.[14]

■ Skin symptoms, which may include eczema, especially in children;[15] urticaria (hives); and angioedema (tissue swelling), especially of facial areas.[16]

■ Symptoms in the oral cavity and throat, including itching, especially of the roof of the mouth; tongue irritation, swelling, and burning; and throat tightening or constriction.[5]

■ Anaphylactic reactions, especially in children.[17]

■ Exercise-induced anaphylaxis (FDEIA) after eating wheat has been frequently reported[18] (for a discussion of FDEIA, refer to Chapter 4).

■ Eosinophilic esophagitis[19]

Wheat allergy may involve IgE-mediated or non-IgE-mediated reactions. In the former, designated immediate-onset reactions, symptoms typically develop within a few minutes to a few hours after ingesting wheat. Immediate reactions may include skin reactions such as urticaria and/or angioedema; digestive tract complaints such as nausea, vomiting, diarrhea; respiratory signs such as rhinitis or bronchial constriction (bronchospasm); or rarely, anaphylaxis. In non-IgE-mediated reactions, the onset of symptoms is typically delayed from several hours to 1 or 2 days after wheat ingestion. Symptoms of such reactions may include eczema or exacerbation of eczema, loose stools, and diarrhea.[3]

Diagnosis of Wheat Allergy

As with any other food allergy, diagnosis starts with a good medical history. When the history suggests food allergy, tests for food-specific IgE are usually carried out, which may include skin tests and blood tests. To confirm the accuracy of the tests, elimination of the suspect foods, followed by challenge, is frequently implemented (see Chapter 5 for details). However, the diagnostic inaccuracies associated with skin and blood tests for wheat-specific IgE mean that such tests are clinically unsatisfactory, so the diagnosis of wheat allergy depends largely on the results of oral food challenge.[20]

Because several different immunological mechanisms can lead to wheat sensitivity (a term that encompasses both IgE and non-IgE-mediated reactions), tests for food-specific IgE (skin and blood tests) may be negative. However, a food challenge with wheat may induce symptoms, which suggests a reaction mechanism distinct from IgE-mediated allergy. Therefore, tests other than the standard allergy tests are often undertaken in an attempt to diagnose a wheat allergy.

In cases of childhood eczema, some practitioners report good success in the diagnosis of wheat allergy using the atopy patch test (see Chapter 5 for details). A 2001 study reported a 94% correlation between the atopy patch test and wheat oral challenge in children with atopic dermatitis/eczema,[21] and a further study[12] reported a 90% correlation. However, the atopy patch test is not often used in clinical diagnosis in the United States, because it is not yet standardized to the level required for routine diagnosis.

Despite demonstrable immune reactivity (positive skin prick tests or IgE positivity in allergen-specific IgE tests), some people show no clinical evidence of wheat allergy when they consume wheat. On the other hand, many people with demonstrable symptoms after consuming wheat are allergen-specific IgE test negative, especially when the reaction is delayed for an hour or more after the wheat is eaten. These findings further reinforce the importance of elimination and challenge in the identification of a sensitivity to wheat and any other grain before it is excluded from a person's diet for a prolonged period of time.[6]

Mechanisms of Wheat Allergy

Although the carbohydrate content of grains is much higher than the protein content, it is the protein that causes the immune system response in an allergic reaction. Protein makes up about 12% of the dry wheat kernel. Wheat proteins are roughly divided into the following four classes, based on their solubility in a variety of solvents:[22]

- Gliadins (aqueous alcohol)
- Glutenins (dilute acid or alkali)
- Albumins (water soluble)
- Globulins (soluble in dilute salt solutions)

Gliadins and glutenins form the gluten complex. Gliadins contain as many as 40 to 60 distinct components, and glutenins contain at least 15. Many of the proteins in wheat are allergenic.[17]

There are very few studies on the specific allergens responsible for wheat allergy, largely due to the assumed relative unimportance of the allergy compared to the grain's function in celiac disease. Nevertheless, more studies are now looking at allergens responsible for allergy and the symptoms previously mentioned, distinct from those associated with gluten-sensitive enteropathy.

No single protein or class of proteins seems to be responsible for wheat allergy. People allergic to wheat tend to react to several different proteins.[23] Some studies report more reactivity to the albumins and globulins, rather than to the gliadins and glutenins. However, others disagree and believe there is more evidence for immune responses to gliadins and globulins. The dominant allergens tend to differ between populations in which the allergy is reported, possibly indicating a genetic component in the potential for sensitization. In general, it seems that allergy to glutenins is more common, but allergy to gliadins is associated with the most severe cases of the disease.[24]

A 2007 report from Spain compared allergen-specific IgE and the response to the allergen in double-blind food challenges in individuals allergic to wheat. The report indicated the following:[25]

- The major wheat allergens were the alpha-amylase/trypsin inhibitors (enzyme inhibitors), which were present in all of the three protein fractions of raw and cooked wheat tested.
- Another important allergen was a 9-kDa lipid transfer protein (LTP) in the albumin/globulin fraction. LTP was the major allergen only in Italian individuals.
- Several low-molecular-weight (LMW) glutenin proteins in the gluten fraction also showed allergenic activity.
- All of these allergens showed heat resistance and lack of cross-reactivity to grass pollen allergens.

Furthermore, it seems that the allergenic proteins that trigger reactions in children may be different from those affecting adults, and different protein fractions may trigger different symptoms. A 2005 study[26] indicated that α-, β-, γ-gliadins, albumins, and globulins were important allergens in children with atopic dermatitis/eczema, while ω-gliadins were major allergens for adults with food-dependent exercise-induced anaphylaxis (FDEIA) or urticaria. Another study[27] indicated that ω-gliadins may be major allergens in children who are anaphylactic to wheat. (For more information on the structure of food allergens, see Chapter 2.)

Wheat and Celiac Disease

The gluten in wheat, rye, and barley is a cause of celiac disease. Wheat allergy is entirely different and distinct from celiac disease; the only similarity being that in both cases, wheat must be avoided in order to control the condition. It is extremely important that the practitioner be informed about the differences between the two conditions in order to manage the diverse reaction patterns and their outcomes most effectively.

Individuals with gluten-sensitive enteropathy (celiac disease or celiac sprue) react to the alpha-gliadin fraction of gluten. The components of the cereal grains that can cause this immunological response are in the gluten fraction of wheat, rye, and barley. More specifically, the alpha-gliadin component of gluten (in wheat), hordein (in barley), and secalin (in rye).

In celiac disease, the response to gluten is immunologically mediated, but the reaction is quite different and distinct from that of IgE-mediated hypersensitivity (allergy). The antibodies involved in celiac disease are of the IgA class.

Symptoms of celiac disease may include diarrhea, weight loss, malabsorption (especially of fat), iron or folate deficiency, rickets, and indications of other vitamin and mineral deficiencies. Occasionally the condition is accompanied by an itchy rash (dermatitis herpetiformis).

Celiac disease is most definitively diagnosed by a jejunal biopsy that reveals villous atrophy (flattened, short, or absent villi) and other abnormal morphology of the lining of the jejunum. A number of blood tests are available for detecting the presence of a variety of specific antibodies whose presence is indicative of celiac disease (anti-transglutaminase and anti-endomysium antibodies). Treatment is lifelong and consists of the strict avoidance of all grains that contain gluten, namely, wheat, rye, and barley, and in unusual cases oats (celiac disease and the gluten-restricted diet are discussed in Chapter 41).

Management of Wheat Allergy

When wheat has been identified as the trigger for a person's symptoms, regardless of the allergens involved or whether the response is mediated by IgE, the only way to control the reaction is strict avoidance of wheat in any form. This is especially true if there is risk of anaphylaxis. In Western countries, avoiding wheat is one of the more difficult diets to manage because wheat is consumed frequently—often at every meal. Breads, cereals, crackers, cookies, muffins, pasta, snack foods, luncheon meats, sausages, candies, desserts, cakes, pies, pancakes, waffles, and many other wheat-containing products are part of, or accompany, most meals and form the basis of the convenience foods often considered essential in the fast-paced Western lifestyle.

Nowadays, it is easier to avoid wheat than in the past. An increased awareness of the widespread incidence of celiac disease (estimated as greater than 1% of the population in Western countries)[28] has resulted in government-regulated labeling of products containing gluten (and thus wheat) in many countries. A proliferation of gluten-free food products also have appeared in the marketplace. Nevertheless, it is important for individuals with wheat allergy or celiac disease to be aware of all sources of wheat and to recognize products, labeled or not, that are likely to contain wheat.

Wheat-Free Diet

Box 13.1 provides a list of sources likely to contain wheat. The wheat-free diet alone is not suitable for people with celiac disease, because they need to also avoid rye, barley, and sometimes oats. Details about the gluten-free diet are provided in Chapter 41.

Wheat in Manufactured Food Products: Labeling Regulations

In most Western countries, if wheat is included in a manufactured product, it must be listed as an allergen on the label. Sometimes "gluten" may be listed as an ingredient on the label, in which case, individuals allergic to wheat must avoid the product unless it is specifically designated as wheat free. In the United States, manufactured foods regulated by the Food and Drug Administration (FDA) that contain ingredients derived from wheat must list the word "wheat" as an ingredient. For more information on food allergen labeling and which foods are regulated by the FDA, refer to Chapter 9.

BOX 13.1   Foods Likely to Contain Wheat

Gluten	Modified starch
High-gluten flour	Bran
High-protein flour	Vegetable starch
Vital gluten	Wheat bran
Wheat gluten	Gelatinized starch
Wheat starch	Vegetable gum
Enriched flour	Graham flour
Wheat germ	Semolina
Flour	Durum
Starch	Couscous
Farina	Cracker crumbs

Hydrolyzed plant protein (HPP), hydrolyzed vegetable protein (HVP), and monosodium glutamate (MSG) may be made from wheat. However, because the hydrolysis process breaks down the protein to a form that is unlikely to be allergenic, avoiding these products is not always considered necessary on a wheat-free diet. However, these derivatives need to be avoided on an MSG-restricted diet (see Chapter 30).

If rye, oats, barley, corn, and rice are tolerated, baked products, cereals, and pastas using these grains can be used in place of those using wheat. In addition, unusual grains and flours such as millet, quinoa, amaranth, buckwheat, tapioca, sago, arrowroot, soy, lentil, pea, and bean, as well as nuts and seeds, may be used in interesting combinations to make baked products and cereals.

Spelt, kamut, triticale, and flours derived from these are too closely related to wheat to be considered safe on a wheat-free diet, unless specifically demonstrated to be tolerated by elimination and challenge.

Important Nutrients in Wheat

Wheat and wheat products are a significant source of thiamin, riboflavin, niacin, iron, selenium, chromium, and in smaller amounts, magnesium, folate, phosphorus, and molybdenum. Many of these micronutrients are added to wheat cereals and flours as fortifiers.

Alternative choices of foods to replace these include oats, rice, rye, barley, corn, buckwheat, amaranth, and quinoa, some of which are fortified with micronutrients similar to those in wheat products.

Flours that are suitable as replacements for wheat flour include flours and starches from rice, potato, rye, oats, barley, buckwheat, tapioca, millet, corn, quinoa, and amaranth.

References

1. Burks AW, Mallory SB, Williams LW, Shirrel MA. Atopic dermatitis: clinical relevance of food hypersensitivity reactions. *J Pediatr.* 1988;113:447-451.
2. Morita E, Yamamura Y, Mihara S, Kameyoshi Y, Yamamoto S. Food-dependent exercise-induced anaphylaxis: a report of two cases and determination of wheat gamma-gliadin as the presumptive allergen. *Br J Dermatol.* 2000;143:1059-1063.
3. Hischenhuber C, Crevel R, Jarry B, et al. Review article: safe amounts of gluten for patients with wheat allergy or coeliac disease. *Aliment Pharmacol Ther.* 2006;23:559-575.
4. Bock AS, Atkins FM. Patterns of food hypersensitivity during sixteen years of double-blind placebo-controlled food challenges. *J Pediatr.* 1990;117:561-567.
5. Moneret-Vautrin DA, Kanny G, Perrier P, et al. Prospective study 1999-2002 of wheat flour food allergy in children and adults compared to coeliac disease [article in French]. *Alim Inter.* 2003;8:2-8.

6. Sicherer SH. Determinants of systemic manifestations of food allergy. *J Allergy Clin Immunol*. 2000;106(suppl 5):S251-257.

7. Matricardi PM, Bockelbrink A, Beyer K, et al. Primary versus secondary immunoglobulin E sensitization to soy and wheat in the Multicentre Allergy Study cohort. *Clin Exp Allergy*. 2008;38:493-500.

8. Pere-Pimiento AJ, Rodriguez-Cabreros MI, Lombardero M, et al. Late-onset food hypersensitivity to wheat flour. *J Investig Allergol Clin Immunol*. 2007;17:202-203.

9. Lauriere M, Reccardini F, Convento M, et al. Hydrolysed wheat proteins present in cosmetics can induce immediate hypersensitivities. *Contact Dermatitis*. 2006;54:283-289.

10. Rasanen L, Lehto M, Turjanmaa K, Savolainen J, Reunala T. Allergy to ingested cereals in atopic children. *Allergy*. 1994;49:871-876.

11. Keet CA, Matsui EC, Dhillon G, Lenehan P, Paterakis M, Wood RA. The natural history of wheat allergy. *Ann Allergy Asthma Immunol*. 2009;102(5):410-415.

12. Stromberg L. Diagnostic accuracy of the atopy patch test and the skin-prick test for the diagnosis of food allergy in young children with atopic eczema/dermatitis syndrome. *Acta Paediatr*. 2002;91:1044-1049.

13. Bock SA. A critical evaluation of clinical trials in adverse reactions to foods in children. *J Allergy Clin Immunol*. 1986;78:165-174.

14. Atkins FM. A critical evaluation of clinical trials in adverse reactions to foods in adults. *J Allergy Clin Immunol*. 1986;78:174-182.

15. Sampson HA. Immediate hypersensitivity reactions to foods: blinded food challenges in children with atopic dermatitis. *Ann Allergy*. 1986;57:209-212.

16. Scibilia J, Pastorello EA, Zisa G, et al. Wheat allergy: a double-blind, placebo-controlled study in adults. *J Allergy Clin Immunol*. 2006;117(2):433-439.

17. Pastorello EA, Farioli L, Conti A, et al. Wheat IgE-mediated food allergy in European patients: alpha-amylase inhibitors, lipid transfer proteins and low-molecular-weight glutenins. Allergenic molecules recognized by double-blind, placebo-controlled food challenge. *Int Arch Allergy Immunol*. 2007;144(1):10-22.

18. Matsuo H, Morita E, Tatham AS, et al. Identification of the IgE-binding epitope in omega-5 gliadin, a major allergen in wheat-dependent exercise-induced anaphylaxis. *J Biol Chem*. 2004;279(13):12135-12140.

19. Spergel JM, Beausoleil JL, Mascarenhas M, Liacouras CA. The use of skin prick test and patch tests to identify causative foods in eosinophilic esophagitis. *J Allergy Clin Immunol*. 2002;109:363-368.

20. Inomata N. Wheat allergy. *Curr Opin Allergy Clin Immunol*. 2009;9:238-243.

21. Roehr CC, Reibel S, Ziegert M, Sommerfield C, Wahn U, Niggemann B. Atopy patch tests, together with determination of specific IgE levels, reduce the need for oral food challenges in children with atopic dermatitis. *J Allergy Clin Immunol*. 2001;107:548-553.

22. Akagawa M, Handoyo T, Ishii T, Kumazawa S, Morita N, Suyama K. Proteomic analysis of wheat flour allergens. *J Agric Food Chem*. 2007;55(17):6863-6870.

23. Sandiford CP, Tatham AS, Fido R, et al. Identification of the major water/salt insoluble wheat proteins involved in cereal hypersensitivity. *Clin Exp Allergy*. 1997;27(10):1120-1129.

24. Battais F, Pineau F, Popineau Y, et al. Food allergy to wheat: identification of immunoglobulin E and immunoglobulin G-binding proteins with sequential extracts and purified proteins from wheat flour. *Clin Exp Allergy*. 2003;33(7):962-970.

25. Palacin A, Bartra J, Muñoz R, Diaz-Perales A, Valero A, Salcedo G. Anaphylaxis to wheat flour-derived foodstuffs and the lipid transfer protein syndrome: a potential role of wheat lipid transfer protein Tri a 14. *Int Arch Allergy Immunol.* 2010;152(2):178-183.

26. Battais F, Courcoux P, Popineau Y, et al. Food allergy to wheat: differences in immunoglobulin E-binding proteins as a function of age or symptoms. *J Cereal Sci.* 2005;42:109-117.

27. Daengsuwan T, Palusuo K, Phanking-thongkum S, et al. IgE antibodies to ω-gliadin in children with wheat-induced anaphylaxis. *Allergy.* 2005;60:506-509.

28. Leffler DA, Schuppan D. Update on serologic testing in celiac disease. *Am J Gastroenterol.* 2010;105(12):2520-2524.

CHAPTER **14**

Corn Allergy

Although corn is often cited as an allergenic food, cases of allergic reactions after ingestion of corn have rarely been published, and few studies have been devoted to the identification of corn allergens. There is little evidence to suggest that corn is a food that is likely to trigger severe or anaphylactic reactions. In fact, some allergists have questioned whether corn allergy exist at all.[1]

Since 2000, several investigators have been looking more closely at corn allergy, especially in children, and finding evidence that indeed allergy to corn is a valid reaction and may be more prevalent than previously thought.[2] However, most reactions tend to be mild, and not all people sensitized to corn will develop symptoms when they eat it. In one reported study, only 6 out of 16 children who were skin-test positive to corn and who had corn-specific IgE antibodies in their blood actually developed symptoms when they ate corn.[3] The rest of the children were not suffering from food allergy to corn, as revealed both by their clinical history and the negative challenge results.

A 2012 study[4] conducted in Milan suggests that some corn proteins, specifically the prolamins (zeins) in corn, contain amino acid sequences that resemble the proteins in wheat/gluten so closely that eating corn could have a similarly damaging effect on some people with celiac disease as eating wheat. Corn is used as an alternative to wheat in many gluten-free food products. Therefore, these preliminary findings may be of paramount clinical relevance to some individuals with celiac disease, and the use of corn in the formulation and preparation of gluten-free foods may need to be reevaluated in some cases.

A report published in 2006[5] suggested that "maize-related food allergy is more complex than so far anticipated." It is therefore logical to expect that we shall see additional information on corn allergy as more clinicians and scientists become interested in the topic.

Symptoms Related to Corn Allergy

In the 2006 study,[5] nine participants reacted to corn in a double-blind placebo-controlled food challenge (DBPCFC) and reported the following symptoms:

- Erythema (reddening, flushing)
- Pruritus (itching)
- Urticaria (hives)
- Itching, blistering in the oral cavity
- Throat tightening
- Flare of atopic dermatitis (eczema)
- Abdominal pain

In another study, symptoms reported[3] include:

- Asthma
- Angioedema (tissue swelling)
- Rhinoconjunctivitis

A 2008 study[6] reported that 48% of the 27 patients enrolled in the study reacted to corn in DBPCFC. If two or more symptoms occurred, the subject was deemed at risk for anaphylaxis. Exercise-induced anaphylaxis after consumption of corn also has been reported.[7]

In addition to the immediate-onset symptoms described earlier, practitioners in the field of food allergy frequently observe delayed reactions to corn, which become evident when corn is eliminated from the diet and the symptoms resolve. In such individuals, tests for corn-specific IgE (skin and blood tests) are typically negative, and challenge tests that are designed to reveal immediate-onset symptoms show no response. However, when corn is challenged over a 2- to 4-day period, symptoms recur. This pattern of reactivity is very similar to that reported for "cell-mediated" allergy to wheat (see Chapter 13 for details). Because the mechanism of reactivity is currently unknown, some practitioners refer to these delayed responses as corn intolerance rather than allergy.[a] The symptoms reported in this type of delayed response to corn are diverse and include:

- Headaches
- Migraine
- Fatigue
- Mood disturbances
- Joint and muscle pain
- Upper respiratory symptoms

Often such symptoms are considered to be subjective and may be chronic in nature until an exclusion diet reveals the cause of the problem. The possibility of corn being a trigger for these types of symptoms is rarely considered, especially when the diagnosis is so difficult. Hopefully future research will reveal the mechanism responsible

---

[a] Radcliffe M. Consultant in Allergy Medicine and Clinical Research Fellow in Allergy, Royal Free NHS Trust and University of Southampton. "Corn allergy and intolerance—the consultant's view." E-mail communication, June 2011.

and evidence-based research will lead to more individuals with corn allergies being correctly identified and helped in the future.

It is not uncommon for a person who is allergic to wheat and other cereal grains to also be allergic to corn. The common allergen or allergens in these grains remain to be identified. In the meantime, those individuals allergic to cereal grains need to avoid several grains, including gluten-containing grains and corn, to achieve remission of their symptoms.

Mechanism of Corn Allergy

There was virtually no information on the allergenic proteins in corn until about 10 years ago when a research report identified the major corn allergens to be a protein (9 kDa in size) that has the characteristics of a lipid transfer protein (LTP) and a 16-kDa protein that had the potential to induce IgE antibodies.[8] LTPs are proteins in many foods that are often responsible for the most significant allergies. They are generally heat-resistant, and their allergenicity is unaffected by cooking. Furthermore, they can survive stomach acid and digestive enzymes and thus can induce an immunological response when they encounter immune cells in the intestines.

Another group of researchers found a 50-kDa protein that was resistant to both heating and peptic/pancreatic digestion and was thought likely to be an important allergen in triggering corn allergy.[2]

Interestingly, the researchers who reported the existence of the 9-kDa corn allergen found that the corn LTP cross-reacts completely with LTPs in rice and peach, but not with those in wheat or barley.[8] This is further evidence that foods in the same botanic family rarely cross-react, but proteins that are structurally identical in unrelated plants may trigger allergy in a person who is sensitized to only one of them. A 16-kDa protein identified in the same study cross-reacted with similar antigens in grass, wheat, barley, and rice, but the significance of the protein as an allergen was unclear.

Management of Corn Allergy

Elimination of corn does not lead to nutritional deficiencies as long as the usual intake of corn itself is small. However, if the usual diet contains many convenience foods, alternative corn-free products will be needed for adequate nutrition.

In spite of the multitude of foods and products that contain corn in our modern world, it is very rare to encounter anyone who experiences a severe allergic reaction in contact, or after ingestion, of most of them. This is because corn protein is not a highly allergenic allergen, and reactions rarely occur in response to the very small amounts of allergen that are present in most foods. That is the reason why corn is used so extensively—it is considered to be one of the food derivatives that is usually safe and least likely to cause an adverse reaction in the greatest number of consumers.

A study designed to determine a threshold dose of corn likely to elicit an allergic reaction concluded that corn "(maize) is allergenic and can pose a risk for symptomatic food allergy at a dose of 100 mg."[6] However, the dose at which a person reacts to a food is entirely individual, so it would be difficult to predict a level at which all people allergic to corn would be safe.

Because manufactured foods are a reality in our fast-paced lifestyle, and because we demand these products to make our lives easier, we have to accept that a small percentage of the population might react adversely to them. The alternative, of course, is to cook every meal from scratch, using only known, pure ingredients. If individuals allergic to corn are not prepared to do that, then the most important advice is to read all product labels carefully and make your choices judiciously.

The Corn-Free Diet

Avoidance of corn is simple as long as only nonmanufactured foods are eaten. Corn cob, corn niblets, corn in a vegetable mix, and popcorn are usually quite easy to recognize and avoid. When corn is the main ingredient in products such as polenta and baked products such as corn bread, it is not difficult for consumers to find an alternative.

However, when many prepared foods are included in a person's usual diet, it is an entirely different matter. A large number of manufactured foods contain corn in the form of cornmeal, cornstarch, corn syrup, and their derivatives. Corn products are likely to be present in cereals, baked goods, snack foods, syrups, canned fruits, beverages, jams, jellies, cookies, luncheon meats, candies, other convenience foods, and meal replacers, as well as in infant formulas. Even medications may contain cornstarch as a vehicle for the active drug.[9] A person allergic to corn needs to recognize the different forms in which corn can be incorporated into a manufactured product.

Corn oil is not usually allergenic, unless the product contains residual protein from the grain. Because corn protein is an extremely rare cause of anaphylaxis and because the quantity likely to be present is very small, it is usually not necessary to avoid corn oil. However, with the highly sensitive techniques now available for detection, corn proteins in minute quantities can be detected in foods and other materials meant for human consumption. If an individual is highly sensitive to corn, it is wise for them to avoid any derivative of corn such as corn oil, corn syrup, and modified corn products of all types.

Corn is not recognized as a priority allergen, so it is not required to be listed as such on a food label. Anyone who is dealing with a corn allergy, especially in a child, must carefully read all product labels and become familiar with the terms that indicate that an ingredient may be derived from corn (see Box 14.1).

BOX 14.1   Major Foods and Ingredients Derived from Corn

- Caramel
- Caramel corn
- Corn alcohol
- Cornflakes
- Corn flour
- Cornmeal
- Corn oil
- Cornstarch
- Corn sugar
- Corn sweetener
- Corn syrup
- Corn syrup solids
- Dextrate
- Dextrin
- Dextrose (also known as glucose or corn sugar)
- Glucose
- Grits
- High fructose syrup
- Hominy
- Maize
- Maltodextrin
- Maltodextrose
- Modified starch
- Polenta
- Popcorn
- Sorbitol
- Starch
- Vegetable starch
- Vegetable gum
- Vegetable protein
- Vegetable paste

References

1. Moneret-Vautrin DA, Kanny G, Beaudouin E. Food allergy to corn—does it exist? *Allergy Immunol* (Paris). 1998;30(7):230.

2. Pastorello EA, Farioli L, Pravettoni V, et al. Maize food allergy: lipid-transfer proteins. Endochitinases and alpha-zein precursor are relevant maize allergens in double-blind placebo-controlled maize challenge-positive patients. *Anal Bioanal Chem.* 2009;395(1):93-102.

3. Pasini G, Simonatao B, Curioni A, et al. IgE-mediated allergy to corn: a 50 kDa protein, belonging to the reduced soluble proteins, is a major allergen. *Allergy.* 2002;57:98-106.

4. Cabrera-Chávez F, Iametti S, Miriani M, de la Barca AM, Mamone G, Bonomi F. Maize prolamins resistant to peptic-tryptic digestion maintain immune-recognition by IgA from some celiac disease patients. *Plant Foods Hum Nutr.* 2012;67(1):24-30.

5. Weichel M, Vergoossen NJ, Bonomi S, et al. Screening the allergenic repertoires of wheat and maize with sera from double-blind, placebo-controlled food challenge positive patients. *Allergy.* 2006;61(1):128.

6. Scibilia J, Pastorello EA, Zisa G, et al. Maize food allergy: a double-blind placebo-controlled study. *Clin Exp Allergy.* 2008;38(12):1943-1949.

7. Pauls JD, Cross D. Food-dependent exercise-induced anaphylaxis to corn. *J Allergy Clin Immunol.* 1998;101:853-854.

8. Pastorello EA, Farioli L, Pravettoni V, et al. The maize major allergen, which is responsible for food-induced allergic reactions, is a lipid transfer protein. *J Allergy Clin Immunol.* 2000;106(4):744-751.

9. Sims-McCallum RP. Adverse reaction caused by excipients in mercaptopurine tablets. *Ann Pharmacother.* 2007;41(9):1548.

CHAPTER **15**

Peanut Allergy

Peanuts are one of the most frequently cited causes of life-threatening anaphylactic reactions in children and young adults in North America. If an individual has been diagnosed as anaphylactic to peanuts, extreme caution must be exercised in avoiding all sources of peanut. A 2003 review[1] indicates that the first allergic reaction to peanuts usually occurs between 14 and 24 months of age, and commonly occurs at home.

The incidence of peanut allergy tends to vary between countries. The prevalence of peanut allergy in the United States is estimated to be about 0.6% of the population.[2] In Canada, peanut allergy has been estimated to occur in 1% of the population surveyed.[3] Prevalence in the United Kingdom, France, Germany, Israel, and Sweden varies between 0.06% and 5.9% of the population. Definitive numbers are very hard to obtain, as methods of diagnosis, inclusion criteria, and collection of data vary between reports.[4]

In spite of the high incidence of peanut allergy in some Western countries, and the potential for severe anaphylactic reactions to the food, peanut allergy, like many early food allergies, can be outgrown. In 2001, pediatric allergists in the United States reported that about 21.5% of children will eventually outgrow their peanut allergy,[5] and those with a mild peanut allergy, as determined by the level of peanut-specific IgE in their blood, have a 50% chance of outgrowing the allergy.[6] In contrast, only about 9% of people are reported to outgrow their allergy to tree nuts.[7]

Symptoms Associated with Peanut Allergy

As with any food allergy, the organ systems that may be affected include:

- The skin, with symptoms of urticaria (hives); erythema (reddening); angioedema (tissue swelling), especially of the face
- Respiratory tract symptoms, with wheezing, noisy breathing, cough, breathing difficulty, throat tightening, nasal congestion, and asthma in asthmatics

- Gastrointestinal tract symptoms, with vomiting, diarrhea, and abdominal pain
- The cardiovascular system, with drop in blood pressure and irregular heart rate
- Anaphylaxis

In addition, eczema (atopic dermatitis) is often reported as a symptom of peanut allergy in children. But not all individuals allergic to peanuts have all of these symptoms. Like all food allergies, the symptoms experienced are idiosyncratic; some people develop symptoms in one organ system, while others might experience allergy in quite a different way.

Diagnosis of Peanut Allergy

The diagnosis of peanut allergy involves the same procedures as any other food allergy. A good medical history and exam should reveal indications that a person's reactions are likely caused by ingestion of a food and should rule out any other cause for the symptoms. This is typically followed by tests such as skin and blood tests designed to detect food-specific IgE (see Chapter 5 for details).

Because it is possible for sensitization to peanuts to occur through the skin,[8] some authorities question the advisability of skin-testing for peanut allergy at any stage. Pricking the skin through the peanut allergen extract allows the allergen to encounter immune cells below the skin surface; this could cause sensitization of the child who is at risk for allergy.

Most practitioners will not skin-test children who have reacted adversely to peanuts because of the danger of triggering an anaphylactic reaction when the allergen encounters already primed immune cells without the "protective" moderating effect of the gut-associated lymphoid tissue (GALT) that lines the intestines. (For more information on the immune system of the digestive tract, see Chapter 1.)

Mechanism of Peanut Allergies

Peanuts actually contain many different proteins, each with its own distinct structure. Several of these are allergenic and can trigger IgE antibodies—each antibody molecule being specific to its inciting allergen. The term *peanut protein* may thus include some or all of the known peanut allergens.

The major peanut protein allergens have been characterized and named. The "Ara h" in the name of each protein is derived from the Latin name for peanut, *Arachis hypogaea*:

- Ara h 1
- Ara h 2 (5 subtypes)
- Ara h 3
- Ara h 4

- Ara h 5
- Ara h 6
- Ara h 7
- Ara h 8
- Ara h 9
- Ara h agglutinin
- Ara h LTP
- Ara h oleosin
- Ara h TI

The relative quantity of each allergen will affect individuals differently when they are sensitized to one more than another. The assumption that all of the known allergens in a specific food are of equal importance to each subject may not hold true.

Some of these allergens are more frequently detected as triggers of peanut-specific IgE in individuals allergic to peanuts than others. For example, in one study, Ara h 2 was recognized most frequently as the causative allergen in all tests for symptom-triggering allergens and induced a reaction at relatively low concentrations, whereas Ara h 1 and Ara h 3 were recognized less frequently and reacted only at 100-fold higher concentrations than Ara h 2. The authors conclude that for their patient group, Ara h 2 was the most important peanut allergen; a few of the other proteins may be important allergens, but less frequently and at higher concentrations.[9]

In another study, the authors calculated the prevalence of sensitization to every allergen in a population of 40 patients sensitized to peanut. Their results indicated that in addition to Ara h 1 (prevalence 65%) and Ara h 2 (prevalence 85%), Ara h 4 (53%) was also a major allergen, while Ara h 5 (13%), Ara h 6 (38%), and Ara h 7 (43%) were minor allergens. Interestingly, although Ara h 6 was considered a minor allergen, the authors found that sensitization to Ara h 6 was associated with more severe clinical symptoms than most of the other allergens.[10]

Future research will undoubtedly reveal which of the allergenic proteins in peanuts are most important to a specific population and which are affected by various processing methods in the manufacture of foods that include peanuts. This information may then explain why certain populations are at risk for peanut allergy and why others seem to be relatively safe.

Furthermore, improved understanding of the molecular structure of the major peanut allergens and the peanut-specific immune response will eventually lead to effective methods for diagnosis, therapy, and possibly prevention strategies for peanut allergy.[11]

Primary Sensitization to Peanut

In more than 70% of children with peanut allergy, symptoms develop at their first known exposure to peanuts. Because IgE-mediated allergic reactions require an initial exposure to an allergen to induce sensitization, and this primary exposure is characteristically symptom free, it seems logical to assume that children who develop symptoms on the first observed contact with the allergen may have been exposed by an earlier, unknown event.

Although there is evidence for the presence of peanut protein and blood cells (T-cell lymphocytes) that can respond to antigens in amniotic fluid, there is no strong evidence to suggest that peanuts in the maternal diet during pregnancy can sensitize the fetus in utero.[12] In fact, current research indicates that early exposure to food allergens, including peanuts, is likely to promote tolerance to the food.[13] However, a 2010 report indicated that frequent consumption of peanuts by the mother during pregnancy showed a dose-response association with subsequent peanut allergy in the baby.[14] Consequently some authorities recommend that during pregnancy, the mother refrain from consuming *large* quantities of any potentially allergenic food. Small quantities of all foods as part of a balanced diet should promote tolerance rather than sensitization to potential allergens. (For more details about oral tolerance and prevention of food allergy, see Chapter 44.)

Evidence for the passage of peanut protein from mother's diet into her breastmilk during lactation was provided by a study using a very sensitive assay for peanut allergens in breastmilk. In a group of volunteers, samples of breastmilk were tested for the presence of peanut protein at various times after consumption of dry, roasted peanuts. In approximately 50% of the volunteers, the two major peanut allergens associated with anaphylaxis were detected in breastmilk within 1 to 3 hours after ingestion.[15] The authors suggest that exposure to peanut protein during breastfeeding might sensitize at-risk infants to peanuts. However, current research indicates that this may in fact be an important exposure that leads to tolerance of the food within the "safe" environment provided by other components of mother's milk.

Exposure to low doses of food proteins has been shown to tolerize the infant to allergens by "educating" the immune system to recognize the protein as safe. It is this process of immunological tolerization that allows us to consume foods without our immune systems mounting a defense against them. Exposure to peanuts and other food allergens during pregnancy, lactation, and early childhood may be important in the development of immunological tolerance and may prevent allergic sensitization to these foods.

Consequently, the concentration of peanut protein, the timing of the child's exposure to it, and the frequency with which the infant encounters it may lead to either allergic sensitization or to tolerization. Therefore, at this stage in our knowledge, it would not be prudent to suggest that all lactating women avoid peanut products during breastfeeding. While this may protect some children from peanut sensitization, it may predispose other children to acquiring peanut allergy by preventing the process of tolerization.[16]

However, if the baby has already been diagnosed as being allergic to peanut by appropriate tests, it is extremely important that the breastfeeding mother avoid all sources of peanuts in her diet, because peanut protein in her breastmilk will trigger a potentially life-threatening allergic reaction in her baby.

Several studies have suggested that the first exposure to peanuts may be through topically applied peanut oil–containing skin creams used to treat rashes over joints and in skin creases in young babies.[5,8] It is recommended that any skin creams containing peanut oil not be used on babies because of the risk for sensitization to peanut allergens through the skin.

How Much Peanut Will Provoke Allergy?

Several studies have attempted to determine the smallest amount of peanut protein that is likely to trigger an allergic reaction in a person who is allergic to peanuts. However, because there are so many variables associated with peanut allergy, it is difficult to specify a dose of peanut that would elicit symptoms in these people or to define a dose that would be safe for all peanut-sensitive individuals. Each person's *tolerance threshold* or *limit of tolerance* (the dose at which symptoms develop) is different; one person may develop symptoms at a dose of 1 mg of peanut protein, whereas another may not react until he or she consumes at least 500 mg of the protein. Sometimes contact or inhalation of peanut protein may be sufficient to elicit a potentially life-threatening anaphylactic reaction in very sensitive individuals, so usually it is wise for them to avoid even the smallest quantity of peanut in foods or in their environment.[17]

Contact dermatitis and hives from direct peanut contact without ingestion have been reported in the medical literature. A case of contact angioedema in a 9-year-old child who had been allergic to peanuts since the age of 1 year was recently reported in an allergy journal. The child developed angioedema after playing with his Play-Station. This device had been used previously by his uncle, who had eaten peanuts at a family get-together. The authors suggest that this observation illustrates a new way of transmitting food allergies by proxy.[18]

Peanut Allergy and Allergy to Tree Nuts

Peanuts, which are members of the legume family, are unrelated botanically to nuts that grow on trees, which belong to a variety of different botanical families. Most people who are allergic to peanuts can eat tree nuts such as walnuts, pecans, Brazil nuts, almonds, cashews, hazelnuts, macadamia nuts, pine nuts, coconuts, chestnuts, and so on, without difficulty. However, because tree nuts are also highly allergenic foods, they are frequent causes of strong allergic reactions and anaphylaxis.

In the interest of safety, children who are allergic to peanuts should avoid all nuts. Most children and many adults are unable to distinguish between different types of nuts and peanuts and may be unable to determine the presence of peanuts in a nut mixture. Furthermore, sometimes no differentiation is made in the marketing of peanuts and nuts, and the two are often found together in nut mixtures. When sold in bulk, a utensil used to handle nuts has often been previously used with peanuts without cleaning in between. In the manufacture of candies, confectioneries, and ice cream, there is frequent cross-contamination between nuts of different species and peanuts, so anyone with severe peanut allergy is advised to avoid any product containing nuts because of the danger of encountering peanuts inadvertently.

"Mandalona" nut is one of the names given to a manufactured product made from deflavored, decolored peanut meal that is pressed into molds, reflavored and colored, and sold as a cheaper substitute for tree nuts such as almonds, pecans, and walnuts. People with peanut allergy must be cautious when consuming any food that may contain such a product.

Although it is sensible for adults with peanut allergy to determine their sensitivity to nuts of different types to allow more flexibility in their diet, the same is not true for children. Determining a peanut-allergic child's reactivity to nuts should be delayed until he or she is old enough to distinguish one nut from another and to take responsibility for avoiding allergens without supervision. (Tree nut allergy is discussed in Chapter 16.)

Effects of Cooking Methods on Peanut Allergenicity

Roasting of peanuts has been demonstrated to increase their allergenicity, compared to the same variety of peanut processed by other methods.[19] This means that roasted peanuts—which is the form in which most peanuts and peanut butter is consumed in North America because of the improved flavor, taste, and safety from potentially toxic mold—are more likely to trigger a severe anaphylactic reaction than the boiled peanut, which is the form in which people in countries such as China, and in Africa and the South Pacific consume the food.[20] It is a documented fact that the incidence of peanut allergy in China is virtually nonexistent, whereas in the United States, about 3 million people report being allergic to peanuts. Other factors that might affect the allergenicity of peanut proteins are thought to include the type and variety of the peanut (of which there are about 14,000), the conditions under which the peanut has been grown, and the degree of maturation of the peanuts.[21]

Cross-Reactivity Between Peanuts and Other Legumes

A common problem faced by people with peanut allergy is whether they should avoid all legumes (eg, soy, chickpeas, lentils, beans, peas, licorice, carob, and all other members of the *Leguminosae* family, to which peanut belongs).

Although many members of the legume family can be allergenic and trigger allergic symptoms in individuals sensitized to them, there is no evidence to suggest that peanut-allergic individuals should avoid all legumes. In clinical trials, cross-reactivity between different members of the legume family is uncommon; one study reports that only 2 out of 41 peanut-allergic children reacted mildly to other members of the legume family.[22] Furthermore, these reactions may not have been because the foods were related, but because the child had become sensitized to the different foods independently, just as he or she would have been to any other allergenic food.

Allergy to multiple foods is usually due to reactions to botanically unrelated, highly allergenic foods, such as peanut, egg, milk, shellfish, fish, and tree nuts. Highly allergic individuals are most likely to react to the most highly allergenic foods for their age group. Therefore, allergy to specific foods is usually a result of independent sensitization to each individual food allergen.

Allergy to Peanuts and Soy

Previously, the incidence of soy allergy was reported to be low compared to other highly allergenic foods, but recent studies seem to suggest that the prevalence of soy allergy is increasing.[23] It has been suggested that the increase in the incidence of soy allergy in children could be from exposure in early infancy (when the child is at highest risk for allergic sensitization) to the allergenic protein found in soy-based infant formulas. In addition, recent research suggests that an association between peanut and soy allergy could arise from cross-sensitization from soy-based infant formulas. Soy and peanuts contain a similar allergen, and it is thought that exposure to the soy allergen in infant formula could prime the child's immune system to respond to the peanut allergen, even when he or she shows no signs of allergy to soy.[4] As a result, the child could exhibit allergic symptoms on an apparent first exposure to peanuts. (Soy allergy is discussed in Chapter 17.)

Maintaining Tolerance to Peanuts

Research studies indicate that when a child has outgrown an early peanut allergy and there is no longer any evidence of symptoms developing after the child has consumed peanuts, it is preferable for that child to eat peanuts regularly, rather than avoid them, in order to maintain tolerance. Children who outgrow peanut allergy are at risk for recurrence, but the risk has been shown to be significantly higher for those who continue to avoid peanuts after resolution of their symptoms.[24]

The Peanut-Safe Environment

Currently there is strong pressure for public places such as schools, hospitals, and airlines to be peanut free in an attempt to protect vulnerable individuals, especially children and young adults, from accidental exposure to peanuts. However, this could be a mistake, since when people assume that the area is free from contamination, they may relax their guard, and thus be at risk for inadvertent exposure to the allergen. *Peanut-safe* indicates that although people using the facility are requested to avoid bringing peanuts into the area and special precautions are in place to reduce the possibility of exposure of the at-risk population, there must be constant vigilance on everyone's part to maintain the environment in a peanut-safe condition.

Important measures for a peanut-safe environment should include:

▪ Ensuring that all personnel in a peanut-safe facility are well informed about the dangers of accidental contamination to a person with peanut allergy
▪ Having clear strategies for maintaining the facility in a peanut-safe condition, with strict rules about cleaning
▪ Informing everyone entering the facility to avoid introducing peanuts into the area, and the reasons for the restrictions
▪ Educating peanut-allergic individuals about avoiding their own exposure to peanuts, including:

- Avoiding foods likely to contain or be contaminated by peanuts
- Being aware of all terms on food labels that would indicate the possible presence of peanut
- Carrying an EpiPen, Twinject auto-injector, or similar device that contains injectable epinephrine (adrenaline) and being familiar with its use in case of accidental exposure and an allergic reaction
- Wearing a MedicAlert or identification tag or bracelet in case of loss of consciousness during an allergic reaction

■ Informing all staff in the facility about emergency procedures should anyone in the area develop symptoms and require medical treatment. Such information should include:
- Familiarity with the use of the injectable epinephrine (adrenaline) where appropriate
- Contacting key caregivers such as parents and guardians of children, and the child's doctor or other health care provider according to prior instructions, which should be provided to the facility by the parents or guardians
- Instructions for transporting the individual to the nearest hospital in the quickest way possible

Management of Peanut Allergy

Anyone who is allergic to peanuts must avoid peanuts in any and every form as long as he or she develops symptoms after consuming the food. It is important that all sources of peanut be carefully avoided if there is even a moderate risk of an anaphylactic reaction to it.

Because of their nutritive value and their taste, peanuts are widely used in the food industry. Many manufactured foods contain peanuts, resulting in an increased risk for inadvertent ingestion of peanuts by allergic individuals. Additionally, contamination of intended peanut-free products with traces of peanuts during the manufacturing process has sometimes resulted in several fatal and near-fatal allergic reactions.

Many Western countries include peanut as one of the allergens required by law to appear on a product label if peanut is present as an ingredient. In the United States, manufactured foods regulated by the Food and Drug Administration (FDA) must list the word "peanut" on the food label if any of the ingredients are derived from peanuts. However, the FDA does not regulate all foods in the United States; the use of allergen labeling on foods regulated by the U.S. Department of Agriculture (meat products, egg products, and poultry products) is voluntary (see Chapter 9). In addition, patients should be educated that foods purchased in foreign countries and foods without a label may not list *peanut* but may use an alternate term. Sometimes common names (eg, goober peas or goober nuts) are not recognized as being peanuts.

Peanut-allergic individuals and caretakers of peanut-allergic children should be aware of the foods likely to contain peanuts and where peanuts are likely to be encountered, and become familiar with terms on product labels that indicate that peanut is likely to be present.

Important Nutrients in Peanut

Peanuts supply niacin, magnesium, vitamin E, manganese, pantothenic acid, chromium, vitamin B-6, folacin, copper, and biotin. These nutrients are easily replaced by including meat, whole grains, legumes, and vegetable oils in the diet, so a peanut-free diet should not pose any nutritional risk to the average child.

Strict vegans may need to eat tree nuts and seeds in order to obtain adequate quantities of high-grade plant proteins, so this population is strongly advised to undergo a careful investigation of their allergic reactivity to tree nuts and seeds so that they can be assured that these nutritious foods can be consumed in safety.

The Peanut-Free Diet

When a diagnosis of peanut allergy has been determined, it is important that all sources of peanut be avoided. Peanuts are one of the foods most likely to lead to an anaphylactic reaction, which in extreme cases can be fatal.

Allergenicity of Peanut Oil

Most of the oils available to the public for consumption are highly refined. The oil is subjected to physical and chemical methods of purification, such as degumming, refining, bleaching, and deodorization. It is then referred to as *refined oil*, and ingredients other than oil from the plant source are usually undetectable. This is the case with refined peanut oil. Until recently, it was thought that refined peanut oil was completely free from peanut protein, and since an allergic reaction requires the presence of the allergenic protein, pure oil was considered to be incapable of eliciting an allergic response. However, modern extremely sensitive techniques allow detection of much smaller quantities of protein than was previously possible, and it is now recognized that refined oil does indeed contain sufficient peanut allergen to elicit a reaction in highly sensitive individuals.[25] Nevertheless, all but the most highly sensitive individuals can consume the refined oil with impunity. However, if any oil is used to cook peanuts, peanut protein will be detectable in the previously pure oil, which would then be a great hazard to people with peanut allergy. The reuse of oil is common in some homes and in fast-food restaurants, so these sources of contamination with allergenic protein must be avoided by individuals at risk for anaphylaxis.

References

1. Al-Muhsen S, Clarke AE, Kagan R. Peanut allergy: an overview. *CMAJ.* 2003;168:1279-1285.
2. Sicherer SH, Munoz-Furlong A, Burks AW, Sampson HA. Prevalence of peanut and tree nut allergy in the US determined by a random digit dial telephone survey. *J Allergy Clin Immunol.* 1999;103:559-562.
3. Ben-Shoshan M, Harrington DW, Soller L, et al. A population-based study on peanut, tree nut, fish, shellfish, and sesame allergy prevalence in Canada. *J Allergy Clin Immunol.* 2010;125(6):1327-1335.
4. Boyce JA, Assa'ad A, Burks AW, et al. Guidelines for the diagnosis and management of food allergy in the United States: report of the NIAID-sponsored expert panel. *J Allergy Clin Immunol.* 2010;126(6):S1-S58.
5. Skolnick HS, Conover-Walker MK, Koerner CB, Sampson HA, Burks W, Wood RA. The natural history of peanut allergy. *J Allergy Clin Immunol.* 2001;107(2):367-374.
6. Fleischer DM, Conover-Walker MK, Christie L, Burks AW, Wood RA. The natural progression of peanut allergy: resolution and the possibility of recurrence. *J Allergy Clin Immunol.* 2003;112(1):183-189.
7. Fleischer DM, Conover-Walker MK, Matsui EC, Wood RA. The natural history of tree nut allergy. *J Allergy Clin Immunol.* 2005;116(5):1087-1093.
8. Lack G. Epidemiologic risks for food allergy. *J Allergy Clin Immunol.* 2008;121(6):1331-1336.
9. Koppelman SJ, Wensing M, Ertmann M, Knulst AC, Knol EF. Relevance of Ara h1, Ara h2 and Ara h3 in peanut-allergic patients, as determined by immunoglobulin E Western blotting, basophil-histamine release and intracutaneous testing: Ara h2 is the most important peanut allergen. *Clin Exper Allergy.* 2004;34(4):583-590.
10. Becker W-M, Kleber-Janke T, Lepp U. Four novel recombinant peanut allergens: more information, more problems. *Int Arch Allergy Immunol.* 2001;124:100-102.
11. Scurlock AM, Burks AW. Peanut allergenicity. *Ann Allergy Asthma Immunol.* 2004;93(5 suppl 3):S12-18.
12. Hayday K, Shannon S. Are early exposures linked with childhood peanut allergy? *J Fam Pract.* 2003;52(7). http://www.jfponline.com/Pages.asp?AID=1503. Accessed 4/21/2012.
13. Du Toit G, Katz Y, Sasieni P, et al. Early consumption of peanuts in infancy is associated with a low prevalence of peanut allergy. *J Allergy Clin Immunol.* 2008;122(5):984-991.
14. Sicherer SH, Wood RA, Stablein D, et al. Maternal consumption of peanut during pregnancy is associated with peanut sensitization in atopic infants. *J Allergy Clin Immunol.* 2010;126(6):1191-1197.
15. Vadas P, Wai Y, Burks W, Perelman B. Detection of peanut allergens in breast milk of lactating women. *JAMA.* 2001;285(13):1746-1748.
16. Lack G, Fox D, Northstone K, Golding J. Factors associated with the development of peanut allergy in childhood. *New Engl J Med.* 2003;348(11):977-985.
17. Sicherer SH, Furlong TJ, DeSimone J, Sampson HA. Self-reported allergic reactions to peanut on commercial airliners. *J Allergy Clin Immunol.* 1999;104(1):25-27.
18. Pétrus M, Villefranche C, Michaud C, Dutau G. Console de jeu: mode de transmission de l'allergie à l'arachide/PlayStation: a means of transmitting peanut allergy. *Rev Fr Allergol.* 2006;46(4):419-420.
19. Maleki SJ, Hurlburt BK. Structural and functional alterations in major peanut allergens caused by thermal processing. *J AOAC Int.* 2004;87(6):1475-1479.

20. Beyer K, Morrow E, Li X-M, et al. Effects of cooking methods on peanut allergenicity. *J Allergy Clin Immunol.* 2001;107(6):1077-1081.

21. Chung SY, Butts CL, Maleki SJ, Champagne ET. Linking peanut allergenicity to the process of maturation, curing and roasting. *J Agric Food Chem.* 2003;51(15):4273-4277.

22. Bernhisel-Broadbent J, Taylor S, Sampson HA. Cross-allergenicity in the legume botanical family in children with food hypersensitivity. II. Laboratory correlates. *J Allergy Clin Immunol.* 1989;84(5 pt 1):701-709.

23. Sicherer SH, Sampson HA, Burks AW. Peanut and soy allergy: a clinical and therapeutic dilemma. *Allergy.* 2000;55:515-521.

24. Fleischer DM, Conover-Walker MK, Christie L, Burks AW, Wood RA. Peanut allergy: recurrence and its management. *J Allergy Clin Immunol.* 2004;114(5):1195-1201.

25. Olszewski A, Pons L, Moutete F, et al. Isolation and characterization of proteic allergens in refined peanut oil. *Clin Exp Allergy.* 1998;28(7):850-859.

CHAPTER 16

Allergy to Tree Nuts and Edible Seeds

Tree nuts and edible seeds represent a group of foods that tend to be highly allergenic and may trigger an anaphylactic reaction in particularly sensitive individuals. Furthermore, tree nut allergy is especially problematic, because the allergy tends to be persistent and in the majority of cases lasts for a person's lifetime.

Tree Nut Allergy

There is not much information on the prevalence of tree nut allergy in populations, and reports vary in the methods of data collection as well as the ages of the study populations. The few reports available indicate that in the United States, an allergy to tree nuts affects about 0.5% of the population.[1] In Canada, the number is 1.22%;[2] in the United Kingdom, the number varies from 1.4%[3] to 2.2%;[4] France reports an incidence of 0.7%;[5] Germany 8.5%;[6] Sweden 4.1%;[7] and Israel 0.03%.[8]

Previously, it was believed that allergies to tree nuts—including cashews, almonds, Brazil nuts, walnuts, hazelnuts, macadamia nuts, pecans, pistachios, and pine nuts—lasted a lifetime. However, recent research indicates that at least 9% of young children outgrow their nut allergy.[9] Even children who have experienced a severe nut allergy can outgrow it. However, the results of the study indicated that children who are allergic to multiple types of tree nuts are less likely to outgrow their allergy than children who are allergic to only one or at most two types of nuts. Based on their results, the study authors recommend that children with tree nut allergies be reevaluated periodically by an allergist/immunologist. They suggest that oral challenges should be considered in children 4 years of age and older who have less than 5 kilounits per liter of tree nut–specific IgE in their blood.

Allergy to Edible Seeds

Allergy to edible seeds is usually uncommon, although all seeds contain proteins capable of becoming allergenic. Some seeds are eaten as is, some are used as seasoning, and some are pressed for their oil.

Sesame seed is becoming increasingly reported as the trigger for IgE-mediated allergic reactions in all populations. Allergy to sesame seeds has been increasing in incidence in the Western world over the past five decades.[10] The allergy seems to present clinically in two forms:

■ Immediate hypersensitivity, with positive skin prick test or sesame-specific IgE antibody in serum

■ Delayed response to compounds in sesame oil that presents as a contact dermatitis

Symptoms

Symptoms associated with tree nut allergy include:

■ Reactions in the oral cavity and associated tissues, such as tingling of lips; itching of the mouth, ears, and eyes; oral allergy syndrome; contact dermatitis, especially of oral tissues; and throat tightening

■ Reaction in the skin and mucous membranes, including urticaria, angioedema, and conjunctivitis (often from transfer of the allergen to the eye by contaminated hands)

■ Reactions in the respiratory tract, such as asthma (in asthmatics)

■ Reactions in the gastrointestinal tract, including abdominal pain, diarrhea, and vomiting

■ Systemic reactions such as anaphylaxis, which is sometimes life-threatening

Sesame seed allergy is not very different from other food allergies. In a study from three allergy clinics in France[11] that involved 14 children with reported sesame seed allergy and whose median age at the beginning of sesame seed allergy was 5 years (range from 5 months to 16 years old), all of the selected children reacted immediately after sesame seed consumption. The symptoms observed included edema (9 cases, 48%); urticaria (5 cases, 27%); and one report of each of the following symptoms: vomiting, rhinitis, conjunctivitis, asthma, and anaphylactic shock. One patient had recurrent anaphylactic shocks and another had an anaphylactic shock after subsequent sesame seed exposure; these two patients were asthmatic. Three patients outgrew their food allergy. Prior to that study, most of the cases of sesame seed allergy had been reported in adolescents or adults.

Because of the risk for anaphylaxis and the increasing incidence of allergy, sesame seed is considered a "priority allergen" that is required to be listed on food labels in many countries, including Canada and the United Kingdom. Such a requirement is not yet in place in the United States, so people allergic to sesame seeds in the countries that do not require its notation on a label need to be aware of the terms that indicate the presence of sesame seeds in a product.

Diagnosis of Tree Nut and Edible Seed Allergy

The diagnosis of tree nut and edible seed allergies starts with a medical history and exam. Having ruled out any other cause for the symptoms, a physician will typically perform tests for allergen-specific IgE, usually skin prick tests and blood tests. The allergen-specific IgE blood tests should begin with a test for a "nut mix" (which usually includes edible seeds) that, if positive, can be followed by tests for the specific nuts and seeds within the mix.

However, many reports indicate a low level of correlation between the tests and the development of symptoms on challenge with the individual nuts and seeds. Based on the study of 96 children investigated for nut allergy using skin prick tests, allergen-specific IgE in blood serum, and oral challenge over a 27-month period, one report concludes that "skin prick testing and IgE measured by radioallergosorbent testing [ImmunoCAP-RAST] are inadequate tests for nut allergy. The definitive diagnostic test for nut allergy in the hospital setting is direct oral challenge."[12] A 2003 study[13] supports this conclusion, reporting that 46% of their study population of 1,000 adults and children who tolerated a nut on consumption, tested positive on skin prick tests. There was poor concordance between these tests and allergen-specific IgE in blood serum. Of patients with a clear history of nut allergy, only 0.5% had negative skin prick tests, but 22% had negative ImmunoCAP. The authors further determined that the severity of the reaction on oral consumption cannot be predicted by the size of the skin prick wheal or the level of allergen-specific IgE in serum.

In contrast, a 2008 study[14] of 324 atopic adults and children allergic to peanuts, tree nuts, and sesame seeds in the United States found a good correlation between the results of their tests, stating that, "quantification of food-specific IgE is a valuable tool that will aid in the diagnosis of symptomatic food allergy and might decrease the need for double-blind, placebo-controlled food challenges."

The apparent discrepancies in these studies can be partly explained by the methods employed in evaluating the results, such as prospective or retrospective trials, selection of subject populations, and the parameters used in quantifying the data. It remains for future research to clarify the value of the various testing modalities in clinical practice.

Mechanisms of Tree Nut and Edible Seed Allergy

Nuts and seeds represent the reproductive part of the plant. In the majority of cases, the most highly allergenic molecules of plants are associated with the storage proteins in the seed. Nuts, grains, legumes (eg, peas, beans, lentils), and seeds all contain similar types of storage albumins, which may be highly allergenic. The seed storage albumins are used by the growing plant during germination. They possibly have a defensive role against pathogens, since many of these types of albumins have been shown to have antifungal properties.

It is possible that many of the huge number of *dicot seeds* (seeds that have two parts) contain cross-reacting albumins. However, the degree of clinical cross-reactivity, in which a person allergic to one nut, seed, grain, or legume is allergic to another from a different plant species, has not been determined with any degree of confidence. It appears that each storage albumin is unique to the species of plant that produces it.

In addition to the storage proteins, nuts and seeds contain other proteins that are often allergenic. These include the profilins and pathogenesis-related proteins.[15] Profilins are active in cellular activities, including regeneration; pathogenesis-related proteins are produced in a plant "under stress" and act as defensive chemicals. These two classes of proteins are considered to be *panallergens*, which means that they are similar in a wide range of plants and may be responsible for cross-reactivity in which allergy to one leads to allergy to many (see Chapter 2 for more details).

A person's allergic profile (the range of foods to which he or she is allergic) depends on exactly which types of proteins trigger their hypersensitivity reactions. In practice, it is not possible to identify the individual allergens within a specific food to which a person is sensitized; it is sufficient to know that symptoms develop when a person eats that food.

In theory, it is only necessary to avoid the specific species of nut that has been identified as the culprit allergen. But, because allergy to certain tree nuts is often associated with anaphylactic reactions, in the interest of safety, a person who is known to be allergic to one or more species of nut should avoid all nuts, since many people find it very difficult to identify individual nuts in nut mixtures (see Box 16.1). Additionally, the risk of cross-contamination of one type of nut with another is high.

BOX 16.1   Botanic Families of Nuts

Nuts belong to a wide array of different biological families. For example:

- Walnuts and pecans belong to the *Judanglacea* family, which also includes the hickory nut.
- Almond is of the *Drupacea* family, which includes peaches, apricots, plums, nectarines, and cherries.
- Cashews and pistachios belong to the *Anacardiaceae* family group, which also includes mango.
- Hazelnut (filbert) is part of the *Betulaceae* family, to which birch trees belong.
- Chestnuts belong to the *Fagaceae* family, which includes beech trees.
- Coconut belongs to the *Arecaceae* family group, which also includes date and palm trees.
- Brazil nuts belong to the *Lecythidaceae*, a family of tropical trees that includes the anchovy pear (*Grias cauliflora*; a West Indian species with edible fruit used for pickles) and several lumber trees of South America.
- Macadamia nuts belong to a tropical plant family called the *Proteaceae*, which includes the coneflower and pincushion tree.

Some edible seeds are also highly allergenic, and it is important that the specific seed responsible for a person's allergic reaction be correctly identified. However, like nuts, if an anaphylactic reaction has been experienced after consuming seeds, it is usually advisable for the allergic person to avoid all seeds in the interest of safety.

Note on Coconut and Nutmeg

Coconut and nutmeg are not usually included on lists of tree nuts. Most people allergic to tree nuts can eat coconut and nutmeg without difficulty. Occasionally a person will be sensitized independently to coconut or nutmeg, apart from any tree nut allergy. In these cases, the allergic person must recognize the presence of their allergens in manufactured and prepared foods and avoid them. If a person is allergic to a specific seed, all sources of the seed should be investigated and avoided.

Management of Allergies to Tree Nut and Edible Seeds

Diet Free from Tree Nuts

Tree nuts are not a common constituent of foods and are included in recipes and manufactured foods selectively. It is very important to recognize the sources where nuts are likely to be found and to recognize terms that would indicate the presence of nuts on manufacturers' labels or in recipes

Diet Free from Edible Seeds

Some seeds are eaten as is, some are used as seasoning, and some are pressed for their oil. If a person is allergic to a specific seed, all sources of the seed should be recognized and avoided. Refer to Box 16.2 for a list of edible seeds with allergenic potential.

BOX 16.2 Selected Potentially Allergenic Seeds

- Celery seed
- Cottonseed
- Flax seed (linseed)
- Melon seeds
- Mustard seeds
- Pomegranate seed
- Poppy seed
- Psyllium
- Pumpkin seed
- Rape seed
- Safflower seed
- Sesame seed
- Squash seeds
- Sunflower seed

References

1. Sicherer SH, Munoz-Furlong A, Burks AW, Sampson HA. Prevalence of peanut and tree nut allergy in the US determined by a random digit dial telephone survey. *J Allergy Clin Immunol.* 1999;103:559-562.
2. Ben-Shoshan M, Harrington DW, Soller L, et al. A population-based study on peanut, tree nut, fish, shellfish, and sesame allergy prevalence in Canada. *J Allergy Clin Immunol.* 2010;125(6):1327-1335.
3. Venter C, Pereira B, Grundy J, Clayton CB, Arshad SH, Dean T. Prevalence of sensitization reported and objectively assessed food hypersensitivity amongst six-year old children: a population-based study. *Pediatr Allergy Immunol.* 2006;17(5):356-363.
4. Pereira B, Venter C, Grundy J, Clayton CB, Arshad SH, Dean T. Prevalence of sensitization to food allergens, reported adverse reactions to foods, food avoidance and food hypersensitivity among teenagers. *J Allergy Clin Immunol.* 2005;116(4):884-892.
5. Rance F, Grandmottet X, Garndjean H. Prevalence and main characteristics of schoolchildren diagnosed with food allergies in France. *Clin Exp Allergy.* 2005;35(2):167-172.
6. Schafer T, Bohler E, Ruhdorfer S, et al. Epidemiology of food allergy/food intolerance in adults: association with other manifestations of atopy. *Allergy.* 2001;56(12):1172-1179.
7. Marklund B, Ahlstedt S, Nordstrom G. Health-related quality of life among adolescents with allergy-like conditions—with emphasis on food hypersensitivity. *Health Qual Life Outcomes.* 2004;2:65-77.
8. Dalal I, Binson I, Reifen R, et al. Food allergy is a matter of geography after all: sesame as a major cause of severe IgE-mediated food allergic reactions among infants and young children in Israel. *Allergy.* 2002;57(4):362-365.
9. Fleischer DM, Conover-Walker MK, Matsui EC, Wood RA. The natural history of tree nut allergy. *J Allergy Clin Immunol.* 2005;116(5):1087-1093.
10. Gangur V, Kelly C, Navaluni L. Sesame allergy: a growing food allergy of global proportions? *Ann Allergy Asthma Immunol.* 2005;95(1):4-11.
11. Agne PS, Bidat E, Rance F, Paty E. Sesame seed allergy in children. *Allergie et Immunologie* (Paris). 2004;36(8):300-305.
12. Armstrong D, Rylance G. Definitive diagnosis of nut allergy. *Arch Dis Child.* 1999;80:175-177.
13. Clark AT, Ewan PW. Interpretation of tests for nut allergy in one thousand patients, in relation to allergy or tolerance. *Clin Exper Allergy.* 2003;33(8):1041-1045.
14. Maloney JM, Rudengren M, Ahlstedt S, Bock SA, Sampson HA. The use of serum-specific IgE measurements for the diagnosis of peanut, tree nut, and seed allergy. *J Allergy Clin Immunol.* 2008;122(1):145-151.
15. Crespo JF, James JM, Fernandez-Rodriguez C, Rodriguez J. Food allergy: nuts and tree nuts. *Br J Nutr.* 2006;96(suppl 2):S95-S102.

CHAPTER 17

Soy Allergy

Allergy to soy has apparently been increasing in incidence since soy allergy was first reported in 1934.[1,2] The prevalence of soy allergy has not been specifically studied to any great extent. Estimates suggest that soy allergy may affect about 0.4% of children in the United States.[3] A population-based study of food allergy in the United Kingdom indicated that soy was the least frequent cause (0.3%) of allergy among 16 foods and food ingredients reported.[4] In a multicenter study in Italy,[5] only 6 out of 505 (1.2%) children with a history of food allergy reacted to soy.

Many studies of the incidence of soy allergy use selected populations and look at the effect of soy allergy in specific conditions. Therefore, they do not reflect the incidence of soy allergy in the population as a whole. For example, among children with atopic dermatitis examined for food hypersensitivity, 5 out of 113 (4.4%)[6] reacted to soy. In another such study, 3 out of 168 (1.8%)[7] reacted to soy. It is difficult to obtain a good idea about the actual incidence of soy allergy, because the calculations are based on different criteria for subject inclusion, as well as different methods of determining the presence of the allergy; for example, skin tests, evidence of allergen-specific IgE, or oral food challenge.

It is estimated that 10% to 14% of babies who are allergic to cow's milk develop an allergy to soy when given soy-based infant formulas.[8] This does not mean there is any cross-reactivity between allergens of milk and soy; rather it indicates that an allergic (atopic) baby is likely to develop allergy to any food, especially those deemed highly allergenic, such as milk and soy.

The incidence of soy allergy in adults is presently unknown, although soy is included in the list of the most important ("priority") food allergens affecting populations in the United States and other Western countries. The Food and Agriculture Organization of the United Nations includes soy in its list of the eight most significant food allergens. In the United States, the Food and Drug Administration (FDA) includes soy as one of the eight major foods or food groups that are responsible for 90% of food allergies (milk, eggs, fish, crustacean shellfish, tree nuts, peanuts, and wheat are the others). In an effort to make manufactured foods safe for people with food allergies, the Food Allergen Labeling and Consumer Protection Act (FALCPA) took effect on January 1, 2006.[9] FALCPA requires that the major food allergens be properly labeled on foods regulated by the FDA (see Chapter 9 for more detailed information on food labeling and which foods are covered by FALCPA). Similar regulations on declaring the presence of "priority allergens" are in place in many Western countries, including Canada. These actions on the part of governments emphasize that allergy to soy has assumed a greater prominence in incidence and severity and is now a significant health concern.

Soy allergy is usually considered to be a transient allergy of infancy and childhood, which is frequently outgrown. In one study,[10] all of the 480 infants with food allergies became tolerant of their allergenic foods, including soy, by the age of 3 years. In another study, two-thirds of the 113 children studied lost their soy allergy 2 years after a positive oral challenge.[6] In a study of Danish children with cow's milk allergy, 5.1% demonstrated soy allergy in infancy, but all the cases had resolved by the age of 3 years.[11]

In a prospective study of 133 people with soy allergy, the predicted age of resolution of the allergy was 25% by age 4 years; 45% by age 6 years; and 69% by age 10 years. In this study, 50% of children with soy allergy had outgrown it by the age of 7 years.[3]

Symptoms of Soy Allergy

Allergy to soy protein has many features similar to those of cow's milk protein allergy. Like cow's milk, soy is a frequent contributor to atopic dermatitis (eczema) in atopic children. In infants, soy allergy can cause loose stool and diarrhea, vomiting, abdominal discomfort, irritability, crying, intestinal blood loss, anemia, and slow or no weight gain (failure to thrive). Respiratory tract symptoms include cough, wheeze, asthma, and rhinitis. Symptoms in the skin include hives, angioedema, and atopic dermatitis (eczema). Unlike peanut allergy, anaphylactic reactions to soy are extremely rare and were virtually unknown until a report from Sweden in 1999.[12]

Soy protein is sometimes a cause of a digestive condition of childhood known as *food-protein-induced enterocolitis syndrome*.[3] Symptoms of this condition include vomiting and diarrhea that may have their onset several hours after the child has consumed soy. In extreme cases, severe dehydration, failure to thrive (little or no weight gain, or weight loss), and shock may occur. The same symptoms may be triggered by cow's milk protein, in which case the condition is known as *cow's milk protein-induced enterocolitis*. Approximately 50% of infants with this condition who react to cow's milk also react to soy.[13] Additional information on these conditions can be found in Chapter 39.

Diagnosis of Soy Allergy

As in all cases of food allergy, the diagnosis of soy allergy begins with a medical history and exam. Although most practitioners do carry out allergy tests, the often wide discrepancies between skin tests, allergen-specific IgE, and oral challenge make the diagnosis difficult.[14] Many of the apparent discrepancies frequently reported between the results of allergy tests for soy and oral challenge with soy, in which the former are negative but the latter positive, may be explained by conditions such as soy protein enteropathies in which IgE is not involved, but symptoms develop when soy is consumed.

Mechanism of Soy Allergy

Soybeans are legumes. Soy and peanut (which belongs in the same botanic family as soy) are the most allergenic of the *Leguminosae* family, which has over 30 species, including peas, beans, all types of lentils, carob, and licorice.

Symptomatic reactivity to more than one member of the legume family is rare. Because an individual is allergic to peanut and/or soy, it does not follow that they also will be allergic to other members of the family. Each type of legume must be investigated individually to determine a person's sensitivity to it; avoiding all legumes when only one causes allergy will place unnecessary restrictions on a person's diet. This can be especially detrimental to nutritional health if the individual is vegetarian, and even more so if they are vegan.

Soy Protein Allergens

Investigations of soy proteins have identified numerous protein fractions, but the allergenicity of most of them is unknown.[4] Some studies identified no particular allergenic protein,[15] while others[16,17] identified as many as ten fractions with significant allergenicity (ie, potential to trigger allergic sensitization). It remains for future research to definitively identify the allergenic protein fractions responsible for soy protein allergy.

Soy-Based Infant Formulas and Allergy

In the United States, soy-based infant formulas were first used to feed babies with cow's milk allergy in 1929. Since then, soy protein formulas (SPFs) containing purified soy proteins, a mixture of vegetable oils, and purified carbohydrate have been developed. SPFs have been used for managing various conditions in babies and children, including cow's milk allergy, lactose and galactose intolerance, and severe gastroenteritis.

However, not all authorities recommend soy protein–based formulas for babies allergic to cow's milk. Among the 2008 recommendations of the Committee on Nutrition of the American Academy of Pediatrics on the use of soy protein–based infant formulas are the following:[18]

▪ In term infants, although isolated soy-protein based formulas may be used to provide nutrition for normal growth and development, there are few indications for their use in place of cow's milk-based formula. These indications include:
  • For infants with galactosemia and hereditary lactase deficiency (rare)
  • In situations in which a vegetarian diet is preferred
▪ For infants with documented cow milk protein allergy, extensively hydrolyzed (cow's milk) protein formula should be considered, because 10% to 14% of these infants will also have a soy protein allergy.
▪ Infants with documented cow milk protein-induced enteropathy or enterocolitis frequently are as sensitive to soy protein and should not be given isolated soy protein-based formula. They should be provided formula derived from hydrolyzed protein or synthetic amino acids.

Management of Soy Allergy

In recent years, soybeans and soy products have become an increasingly important part of the average diet in North America. As well as their inclusion in Asian foods as tofu and fermented soy products such as soy sauce and miso, soy is frequently included as an additional source of protein in many processed foods, infant formulas, breakfast cereals, baked goods, crackers, soups, packaged meals, and sauces.

The Soy-Free Diet

The soy-free diet omits soybeans and all soy products. All sources of soy must be avoided when soy protein allergy has been diagnosed. Although anaphylactic reactions to soy are extremely rare, soy allergy can contribute to many types of allergies, such as eczema, asthma, hives, digestive tract disorders, and respiratory allergies, making the symptoms significantly more severe.

In the United States, most manufactured foods that contain soy will indicate its presence on the label. Because soy is one of the eight major allergens identified in FALCPA, FDA-regulated foods that contain soy must list it in the ingredients list or in a "contains" statement. However, the word *soy* may not appear on foods regulated by the USDA or foods purchased abroad. Therefore, people who are allergic to soy are advised to become familiar with terms that indicate the likely presence of soy.

On a food label, soy may be indicated by terms such as *textured vegetable protein* (TVP) or *hydrolyzed plant protein* (HPP). Lecithin is often derived from soy, and Asian foods such as tempeh, tofu, miso, and bean curd are made from soy, which may not be obvious to the consumer who is unfamiliar with Asian cuisines.

Unlabeled products such as bulk foods and unwrapped breads and baked goods may contain soy, especially if flour is an ingredient. People who are allergic to soy are advised not to purchase these products unless the specific ingredients can be ascertained.

Pure soy oil is not considered to be allergenic, unless soy protein residues remain in its manufacture. However, modern, highly sensitive techniques may detect minute quantities of soy protein even in highly refined oils. People who are very allergic to soy are advised to avoid soy oil, although most will tolerate a small amount of the oil without any difficulty. When a child is highly sensitive to soy, it is recommended that all products containing soy oil, especially where it is listed as the main ingredient (eg, soy oil, soy-based margarines, cooking sprays), should be avoided because of the possibility that soy protein may also be present. Cold-pressed oils (also referred to as *pure-pressed*, *expeller-pressed*, or *unrefined*) are very likely to contain soy proteins and should not be used.

Important Nutrients in Soy Beans

Soybeans contribute thiamin, riboflavin, vitamin B-6, phosphorus, magnesium, iron, folacin, calcium, and zinc to the diet. However, soy is typically used in commercial products in amounts that are too small to be considered a significant source for these nutrients. Therefore, elimination of soy from the diet does not compromise the nutritional quality of most diets.

References

1. Duke WW. Soybean as a possible important source of allergy. *J Allergy*. 1934;5:300-302.
2. Cordle CT. Soy protein allergy: incidence and relative severity. *J Nutr*. 2004;134(5 suppl): 1213S-1219S.
3. Savage JH, Kaeding AJ, Matsui EC, Wood RA. The natural history of soy allergy. *J Allergy Clin Immunol*. 2010;125(3):683-686.
4. Young E, Stoneham MD, Petruckevitch A, Barton J, Rona R. A population study of food intolerance. *Lancet*. 1994;343:1127-1130.
5. Bruno G, Giampietro PG, Del Guercio MJ, et al. Soy allergy is not common in atopic children: a multicenter study. *Peditr Allergy Immunol*. 1997;8:190-193.
6. Sampson HA, McCaskill CC. Food hypersensitivity and atopic dermatitis: evaluation of 113 patients. *J Pediatr*. 1985;107:669-675.
7. Burks AW, James JM, Hiegel A, et al. Atopic dermatitis and food hypersensitivity reactions. *J Pediatr*. 1998;132-136.
8. Klemola T, Vanto T, Juntunene-Backman K, Kalimo K, Korpela R, Varjonene E. Allergy to soy formula and to extensively hydrolyzed whey formula in infants with cow's milk allergy: a prospective, randomized study with a follow-up to age 2 years. *J Pediatr*. 2002;140(2):219-224.
9. US Food and Drug Administration, Department of Health and Human Services. Public Law 108-282, Food Allergen Labeling and Consumer Protection Act of 2004. http://www.fda.gov/Food/LabelingNutrition/default.htm. Accessed April 24, 2012.
10. Bock SA. Prospective appraisal of complaints of adverse reactions to foods in children during the first 3 years of life. *Pediatrics*. 1987;79:683-688.

11. Høst A, Halken S. A prospective study of cow milk allergy in Danish infants during the first 3 years of life. *Allergy.* 1990;45:587-596.

12. Foucard T, Malmhedan Yman I. A study on severe food reactions in Sweden—is soy protein an underestimated cause of food anaphylaxis? *Allergy.* 1999;54(3):261-265.

13. Sicherer SH, Eigenmann PA, Sampson HA. Clinical features of food protein-induced enterocolitis syndrome. *J Pediatr.* 1998;133:214-219.

14. Sicherer SH, Sampson HA, Burks AW. Peanut and soy allergy: a clinical and therapeutic dilemma. *Allergy.* 2000;55:515-521.

15. Burks AW, Brollks JR, Sampson HA. Allergenicity of major component proteins of soybean determined by ELISA and immunoblotting in children with atopic dermatitis and positive soy challenges. *J Allergy Clin Immunol.* 1988;81:1135-1142.

16. Shibasaki M, Suzuki S, Tajma S, et al. Allergenicity of major component proteins of soybean. *Int Arch Appl Immunol.* 1980;61:441-448.

17. Houston NL, Lee DG, Stevenson SE, et al. Quantitation of soybean allergens using tandem mass spectrometry. *J Proteome Res.* 2011;10(2):763-773.

18. Bhatia J, Greer F, Committee on Nutrition of the AAP. Use of soy protein-based formulas in infant feeding. *Pediatrics.* 2008;121(5):1062-1068.

CHAPTER **18**

Seafood Allergy

Seafood (free-swimming fish and shellfish) is among the most common causes of food allergy and is a trigger for anaphylaxis, especially in adults. Most developed countries include seafood as one of the "priority allergens" that must be listed on food labels to indicate the presence of allergens.

Edible seafood is abundant and is consumed in most countries of the world. It comprises three major divisions:

- Chordata (fin fish): free-swimming fish such as tuna, salmon, trout, cod, sole, catfish, halibut, mackerel, pollock, sea bass, and so on
- Mollusca (mollusks): bivalves such as mussels, oysters, scallops, clams; gastropods such as snails and abalone; and cephalopods such as squid and octopus
- Arthropoda (shellfish): crustaceans such as shrimp, crab, lobster, crawfish (crayfish), prawns, and scampi

The incidence of fish allergy varies among populations. A 2004 telephone census of U.S. households that encompassed 14,948 individuals[1] reported that fish or shellfish allergy occurred in 5.9% of households. Individuals allergic to seafood reported their specific allergy as follows: 2.3% for any seafood, 2% for shellfish, 0.4% for fish, and 0.2% for both types of seafood. Seafood allergy was more common in adults compared with children (2.8% and 0.6%, respectively) and occurred more in women than in men (3.6% and 2%, respectively).

Shellfish constitutes the number one cause of food allergy in American adults.[2] In a 2011 study[3] of 167 children with a clinical reaction to seafood, with one-fifth reporting a history of seafood anaphylaxis, prawn and shrimp were the most common seafood allergens implicated in their allergy. Over 50% of the children allergic to crustaceans could tolerate noncrustacean fish. One-third of the children reacted to two or more species of fish. Sixteen percent developed reactions to seafood vapors. (For more details on the amount of an allergen required to elicit a response, see Chapter 2.)

Symptoms of Seafood Allergy

The symptoms of allergy to seafood are the same as allergy to any food and differ among individuals.[4] Gastrointestinal tract symptoms include diarrhea, nausea, and vomiting. The respiratory tract also may be involved, resulting in asthma and rhinitis. Skin and mucous membrane symptoms include urticaria (hives), angioedema (tissue swelling), and itching. Swelling of the oral tissues, including the lips and tongue, may occur. Anaphylaxis can also occur and can be fatal.

Certain nonallergic conditions also can cause adverse reactions to fish. Food protein–induced enterocolitis syndrome (FPIES) is an uncommon condition that occasionally occurs in infants. Typical symptoms include profuse vomiting and/or diarrhea several hours after ingestion of a given food. The disorder is a non-IgE-mediated food hypersensitivity, so skin tests and blood tests that look for food-specific IgE will be negative. The most frequently involved foods are milk and soy, but some cases of FPIES induced by other foods have been described. The syndrome has also been reported in response to fish protein in children aged from 9 to 12 months.[5] As with food allergies, the diagnosis is confirmed by elimination and challenge (see Chapters 6 and 7). In many cases, the child outgrows the condition by about 7 years of age after a usually prolonged period of avoiding the food (see Chapter 40 for more details).

Diagnosis of Seafood Allergy

Diagnosis of seafood allergy follows the same pattern as in any allergic condition (see Chapters 6 and 7). A medical history is typically followed by tests for allergen-specific IgE, which may be skin or blood tests. Allergen-specific IgE blood tests for seafood are most conveniently carried out by starting with a "seafood mix" containing a variety of fish and shellfish allergens. If the seafood mix is positive, individual fish and shellfish within the mix are then tested separately. This is a far better method for determining a person's reactions to individual fish species than basing the choice of types of fish to be tested on the patient's reports of their reactions to consumed fish.

An intriguing observation from a study on testing for allergy to shellfish[6] indicated that allergen extracts from boiled shrimp and American and spiny lobsters showed statistically significant larger wheals in skin tests than raw extracts. This result was confirmed by measuring allergen-specific IgE in the extracts. In addition, more individuals with these seafood allergies were identified using boiled extracts of the shrimp and lobster than with raw extracts. These results emphasize the fact that the results of skin and blood tests for allergen-specific IgE vary, depending on the state of the allergen extracts used in the tests. Even more significantly, it further supports the observation that the allergenicity of food can change during food preparation. Whereas many foods decrease in allergenicity after heating, especially those associated with conditions such as oral allergy syndrome (see Chapter 2 for more information), others actually become more allergenic. Peanut is another food that becomes more highly allergenic after being exposed to high heat (for details, see Chapter 15).

Mechanism of Allergy

The question as to whether antigens in different types and species of fish cross-react, making it necessary for an individual allergic to fish to avoid all species of fish if they are allergic to one, has not yet been answered satisfactorily. Traditionally it was thought that it is usually only necessary for the allergic person to avoid the specific type of fish to which they are allergic, as evidenced by their response to elimination and challenge. However, there is increasing evidence that certain fish allergens may be common to several, or even most, species.

Not a great deal is known about individual fish allergens except for the antigen in cod (*Gadus callarias*), named Gad c 1, which was one of the first food allergens of any type to be studied.[7] The antigen is a protein called a *parvalbumin* that can be found in a variety of fish species unrelated to cod (eg, carp, tuna, and salmon). In some studies using a double-blind, placebo-controlled food challenge, individuals allergic to cod reacted to other fish species, such as herring, plaice, and mackerel.[8]

Research in 2010 indicates that the parvalbumin content of most commonly consumed fish species varies considerably. Differences range from severalfold to a hundredfold.[9] It is thought that the variability in a person's reactivity to different species is a function of the level of parvalbumin in the fish rather than a result of unrelated allergens in different species. This must be taken into account when designing food challenge tests and advising individuals allergic to fish.

It is unclear whether a person allergic to one species should avoid all fish. At the present time, in order to avoid unnecessary dietary restrictions, people are advised to avoid only the fish species that have demonstrated clinical reactivity—unless there is a risk of an anaphylactic reaction. However, because it is often impossible to determine when a person who is allergic to fish may be at risk for anaphylaxis, many clinicians advise these patients to avoid all species of fish in the interests of safety.

Sometimes it is difficult to determine the type of fish being consumed. In addition to the obvious forms of fish and shellfish, seafood meat is often used as the basis of a variety of food products. For example, surimi, protein derived from Alaskan pollock, is used in making imitation crabmeat, imitation shrimp, sausages, sauces, and flavorings.[10]

The allergenic part of the fish is usually in the meat (muscle), but there is evidence that fish gelatin made from skin and bones may also be allergenic. Fish gelatin contains a high level of collagens, so there is concern that certain collagens made from fish might cause allergy.[11] This subject needs to be investigated further.

Fish and shellfish are quite distinct antigenically, so a person who is allergic to shellfish rarely needs to avoid free-swimming fish. In shrimp, the major allergenic protein (Pen a 1) has been identified as *tropomyosin*, a 36-kDa protein that also occurs in lobster, crab, squid, oyster, snail, mussels, clams, and scallops.[12] The protein is present in the shrimp meat and can also be detected in the water in which the shrimp has been boiled.[12] Because of the ubiquity of tropomyosin, anyone allergic to one species of shellfish is advised to avoid them all.

Sensitization to Fish

Fish consumption during infancy has traditionally been regarded as a risk factor for allergic disease; in fact, some authorities recommend not introducing fish until after 1 or even 2 years of age. However, recent evidence is suggesting otherwise. A study of 4,089 newborn infants followed for 4 years found that regular fish consumption during the first year of life was associated with a reduced risk for allergic disease by age 4 years.[13]

Another study[14] found that frequent intake of fish during pregnancy reduced the incidence of skin-test positivity to foods in the offspring of mothers who did not have allergies. In the whole study population—that is, mothers with and without allergies—there was a similar trend between increased consumption of fish (two to three times per week or more) and decreased prevalence of skin-test positivity for foods. In fact, babies of the mothers who consumed fish regularly had over one-third less food sensitization compared to infants of mothers who did not consume fish.

In light of the conflicting information, it is difficult to make any clear recommendations regarding the best time to introduce fish to a potentially allergic child. It is probably safe to try fish in the later quarter of the first year until further well-conducted research indicates otherwise (see the section in Chapter 44 on the introduction of solid foods).

Shellfish Allergy

A person who is allergic to shellfish is usually advised to avoid shellfish of all types, because even unrelated species tend to cause an adverse reaction when eaten by a sensitized individual. Therefore, a shellfish-restricted diet eliminates all species of crustaceans, such as crab, lobster, shrimp, and prawn, as well as mollusks (bivalves) such as clams, mussels, and scallops.

Fish Oils

Although pure oils are nonallergenic, it is very likely that any fish oil is contaminated with protein of the fish from which it was extracted. A person allergic to fish is usually advised to avoid oil from the species of fish to which they are sensitive. If the fish species is not specified, then all fish oil should be avoided, especially if there is a risk of anaphylaxis.

Fish Proteins in Wine or Beer

Isinglass, a type of gelatin that is derived from the air bladders of certain fish and is mostly collagen, may be commercially used to fine (clarify) wine or beer.[15] Fish-allergic individuals, especially those with a risk of anaphylaxis, should avoid wines and beers clarified with isinglass.

Important Nutrients in Fish

Fish is a significant source of niacin, vitamin B-6, vitamin B-12, vitamin E, phosphorus, selenium, and, in smaller amounts, vitamin A, magnesium, iron, and zinc. These nutrients are also present in meats, grains, legumes, and oils, so foods with equivalent nutrients can be readily obtained when fish and shellfish are removed from the diet.

It is usually easy to avoid fish, because its presence in a recipe tends to be obvious. In the United States, fish and crustacean shellfish are identified as major food allergens by the Food and Drug Administration (FDA) under the Food Allergen Labeling and Consumer Protection Act (FALCPA). If a manufactured food regulated by the FDA contains fish or crustacean shellfish as ingredients, the label must clearly identify these ingredients. (See Chapter 9 for more information on food allergen labeling and which foods are covered by FALCPA.)

References

1. Sicherer SH, Muñoz-Furlong A, Sampson HA. Prevalence of seafood allergy in the United States determined by a random telephone survey. *J Allergy Clin Immunol.* 2004;114(1):159-165.
2. Wild LG, Lehrer SB. Fish and shellfish allergy. *Curr Allergy Asthma Rep.* 2005;5(1):74-79.
3. Turner P, Ng I, Kemp A, Campbell D. Seafood allergy in children: a descriptive study. *Ann Allergy Asthma Immunol.* 2011;106(6):494-501.
4. O'Neil C, Heilbling AA, Lehrer SB. Allergic reactions to fish. *Clin Rev Allergy.* 1993;11(2):183-200.
5. Zapatero Remon L, Alonso Lebrero E, Martin Fernandez E, Martinez Molero MI. Food-protein-induced enterocolitis syndrome caused by fish. *Allergol Immunopathol* (Madr). 2005;33(6):312-316.
6. Carnés J, Ferrer A, Huertas AJ, Andreu C, Larramendi CH, Fernández-Caldas E. The use of raw or boiled crustacean extracts for the diagnosis of seafood allergic individuals. *Ann Allergy Asthma Immunol.* 2007;98(4):349-354.
7. Elsayed S, Aas K, Sletten K, Johansson SG. Tryptic cleavage of a homogeneous cod fish allergen and isolation of two active polypeptide fragments. *Immunochemistry.* 1972;9(6):647-661.
8. Poulsen LK, Hansen TK, Norgaard A, Vetsergaard H, Skov PS, Bindslev-Jensen C. Allergens from egg and fish. *Allergy.* 2001;56:39.

9. Kuehn A, Scheuermann T, Hilger C, Hentges F. Important variations in parvalbumin content in common fish species: a factor possibly contributing to variable allergenicity. *Int Arch Allergy Immunol.* 2010;153(4):359-366.

10. Lehrer SB, Ayuso R, Reese G. Seafood allergy and allergens: a review. *Marine Biotechnol.* 2003;5:339-348.

11. Hamada Y, Nagashima Y, Shiomi K. Identification of collagen as a new fish allergen. *Biosci Biotech Biochem.* 2001;65(2):285-291.

12. Daul CB, Slattery M, Reese G, Lehrer SB. Identification of the major brown shrimp (*Penaeus aztecus*) allergen as the muscle protein tropomyosin. *Int Arch Allergy Clin Immunol.* 1994;105:49-55.

13. Kull I, Bergstrom A, Lilja G, Pershagen G, Wickman M. Fish consumption during the first year of life and development of allergic diseases during childhood. *Allergy.* 2006;61(8):1009-1015.

14. Calvani M, Alessandri C, Sopo SM, et al. Consumption of fish, butter and margarine during pregnancy and development of allergic sensitizations in the offspring: role of maternal atopy. *Pediatr Allergy Immunol.* 2006;17(2):94-102.

15. Hickman D, Sims TJ, Miles CA, Bailey AJ, de Mari M, Koopmans M. Isinglass/collagen: denaturation and functionality. *J Biotechnol.* 2000;79:245-257.

CHAPTER **19**

Allergy to Multiple Foods: The Top Ten Allergens (Milk, Egg, Wheat, Corn, Peanuts, Soy, Tree Nuts, Seeds, Shellfish, and Fish)

It is common for a person with food allergies to react to more than one food. Chapters 10 through 18 provide information on individual food allergies, but it is a complex task to combine each of the directives together to provide healthy, balanced meals.

Milk and milk products, egg, wheat, corn, soy, peanut, tree nuts, edible seeds, fish, and shellfish are the most common causes of food allergy. The more foods that need to be avoided, the greater the risk for nutritional deficiency. When these foods are removed from the diet at the same time, it is important to find substitutes that will replace the important nutrients that are restricted. Table 19.1 provides examples of foods allowed on a diet that avoids the top ten allergens. If additional foods need to be avoided, care must be taken to provide substitutes that supply the missing nutrients.

Including Tolerated Foods

If a person does not need to avoid all the allergenic foods on this list, it is a fairly easy matter to include those that cause no problems. Information on the foods allowed can be incorporated from the individual chapters.

A very restricted diet should not be followed for any longer than 4 weeks, after which time each food should be "challenged' (see Chapter 7) to confirm that it really needs to be avoided. If any of the excluded foods is not a problem, it can be included in the diet, which will then become more nutritionally complete and easier to manage.

TABLE 19.1

Avoidance of the Top Ten Allergens: Diet Free From Milk, Egg, Wheat, Corn, Soy, Peanut, Tree Nuts, Seeds, Fish, and Shellfish

Type of Food	Foods Allowed
Milk and milk products	• Milk-free, nut-free, and soy-free products, such as rice beverages (made from brown rice and safflower oil, usually fortified with calcium), potato-based beverages (made from potato starch) • In recipes that call for milk, substitute fruit or vegetable juice, homemade soup stock, water used to cook vegetables or potatoes
Grains and flours	• Amaranth and amaranth flour • Barley and barley flour • Buckwheat and buckwheat flour • Chickpea or garbanzo bean flour (besan) • Millet and millet flour (bajri) • Teff • Oats and oat flour • Potato starch and flour • Quinoa and quinoa flour • Rice and rice flour • Wild rice and wild rice flour • Rye and rye flour • Sago and sago flour • Tapioca, and tapioca starch, and flour • Cassava flour and starch
Breads and baked goods	• Baked goods and specialty baking mixes containing allowed ingredients, such as Ener-G rice, brown rice, or tapioca bread; Celimix rice or flax meal bread • Homemade baked goods made with allowed flours and grains
Crackers and snacks	• Potato chips made without corn oil, soy oil, peanut oil, or oils from restricted sources • Pure rye crisp crackers • Rice cakes without wheat, corn, sesame seed, or other restricted ingredients • Rice crackers without wheat, corn, sesame seed, or other restricted ingredients
Cereals	• Cream of rice • Puffed rice • Rice flakes • Oatmeal • Rolled oats • Oat bran • Rye flakes • Granola made with only allowed ingredients • Puffed amaranth • Puffed millet • Quinoa flakes • Other cereals made with only allowed ingredients
Pasta	• Brown rice pasta • Wild rice pasta • Mung bean pasta • Green bean pasta • Buckwheat pasta (soba noodles; confirm they are wheat-free) • Rice pasta • Rice noodles • Potato pasta • Quinoa pasta • Other pastas made with allowed ingredients only

Continues

TABLE 19.1

Avoidance of the Top Ten Allergens: Diet Free From Milk, Egg, Wheat, Corn, Soy, Peanut, Tree Nuts, Seeds, Fish, and Shellfish (*Continued*)

Type of Food	Foods Allowed
Vegetables	• All plain fresh and frozen vegetables and their juices *except* corn, soybeans, soy bean sprouts, sprouted wheat, mixed sprouts
Fruit	• All plain fresh and frozen fruits and their juices
Meat and poultry	• All fresh or frozen pure meat or poultry; *avoid* any meat mixed with additional ingredients, such as processed meats, sausages, and all deli meats
Fish and shellfish	• None
Eggs	• None; use egg-free egg replacer products
Legumes	• All plain legumes (peas, beans, lentils) and legume dishes prepared with allowed foods; *avoid* soy and peanut
Nuts and seeds	• None
Fats and oils	• Vegetable oils such as olive, canola, sunflower, safflower, flaxseed, grapeseed • Meat drippings • Lard • Poultry fat • Whey-free, soy-free, corn-free margarine (eg, canola or safflower oil-based); olive oil • Homemade dressings on vegetables and salads made with only allowed ingredients (eg, olive oil with herbs) • Homemade gravy with allowed ingredients only
Spices, herbs, and sweeteners	• All pure fresh or dried herbs (leaves and flowers of the plant) • Note: Many spices are derived from seeds, but these are usually tolerated. However, if seed allergy is a severe problem, avoid all spices except for the nonseed spices that are derived from the root or bark of the plant. The following *are* allowed: cinnamon, nutmeg (this is not a nut), mace, ginger, turmeric, and clove. • Pure jelly, jam, and honey

Notes on the Diet

Each of the foods restricted on this diet can be found in many products and has many derivatives. It would require extensive lists of foods and their products to cover all possible dietary sources. This can become a very unwieldy project. Reading food labels is essential to detect the allergen as an ingredient in processed and prepared foods. The allergic person should be provided with lists of terms indicating the presence of their allergenic foods as appropriate.

Because so many foods are restricted, information is provided only for the foods allowed (see Table 19.1). Most of the information for individual restrictions has already been included in Chapters 10 through 18.

Nutritional Adequacy of the Diet

If sufficient substitute foods from Table 19.1 are consumed, and the diet is limited to 4 weeks, nutritional deficiency should not be a concern. Possibly the only supplements required are calcium and vitamin D. In addition, it is usually a good idea for the allergic person to consume an appropriate (additive free, and free from the listed allergenic foods) multivitamin and mineral daily to ensure adequacy of micronutrients. Anyone, especially a child, who needs this diet for longer than 4 weeks must be provided with adequate information and supervision to ensure that all macro- and micronutrients are provided in the substitute foods or appropriate supplements.

CHAPTER 20

Yeast and Mold Allergy

Yeasts and molds are minute, single-celled fungi. They belong to the same biological group as mushrooms but are much smaller. Fungi are organisms that depend on external nutrients and therefore live as saprophytes,[a] parasites,[b] or symbionts[c] of animals and plants under nearly all environmental conditions. Out of over 100,000 known fungal species, about 100 are known to cause infections (mycoses) in humans and animals.

Many species of mold fungi have been implicated in inhalant allergy; about 150 individual fungal allergens from approximately 80 mold genera have been identified in the last 20 years.[1] Asthma is the most common allergic disease triggered by molds and mold spores. Other allergy symptoms triggered by molds include rhinitis (hay fever symptoms), atopic dermatitis (eczema), urticaria (hives), and very rarely anaphylaxis.[2] However, the primary causative role of fungal species in rhinitis, atopic dermatitis, and urticaria remains to be definitively established.[3]

A person sensitized to fungi and fungal spores produces IgE against the fungal allergenic proteins. These IgE antibodies can be detected in blood tests such as allergen-specific IgE. In addition, skin tests for the fungal allergen are usually positive. This indicates that IgE is present in the body and could presumably trigger inflammatory mediator release from mast cells whenever the allergen enters. The allergen is usually in the inhaled form but could be ingested in foods containing the specific allergen to which sensitization has occurred.

---

[a] A saprophyte is an organism that obtains its nutrients from, and usually lives on, dead or decaying matter.

[b] A parasite is an organism that lives upon another living organism from whom it obtains an advantage, in this case nutrients.

[c] A symbiont is an organism living in symbiosis with another in which both derive an advantage, or in which the symbiont does no harm to the other.

People sensitive to inhaled fungi and fungal spores must avoid inhalation of all sources of the fungi, such as in the moist soil of houseplants and damp rooms, especially basements where molds grow. Because mold spores are released from damp ground softened by the first thaw of spring, mold-sensitive people with asthma may need to limit their time outdoors to avoid inhaling the spores in the air at this time of year.

A small percentage of asthmatic people sensitive to inhaled fungal spores, and some nonasthmatic people, develop eczema or urticaria (hives) when they come into contact with their specific allergen or if they eat or drink substances containing yeast or molds. Extremely sensitive people can suffer an anaphylactic reaction, with breathing difficulty; hives; angioedema (tissue swelling), especially in the throat; and cardiac symptoms.[4] These people must be particularly careful to avoid all sources of fungi in their diet.

Allergy to yeast is often associated with inhalant allergy to *Saccharomyces cerevisiae* in conditions such as baker's asthma[5] and some cases of atopic dermatitis (eczema).[6]

The yeast *Pityrosporum ovale* is sometimes associated with atopic dermatitis, and studies indicate the presence of allergen-specific IgE to the yeast in sensitized individuals with eczema.[7]

Occurrence of Yeast and Mold in Foods

Mold

Mold colonies are often seen growing on the surface of moist foods such as bread, jam, and cheese. Molds range from a unicellular to a filamentous form on these media.

Some mold-restricted diets advocate avoiding wheat flour because in the past, stored wheat was often contaminated by mold. However, because modern flour milling does not permit the use of moldy wheat, flour need not be avoided.

Fresh fruit may also be a source of mold. Fresh fruits are prone to fungal contamination in the field; during harvest, transport, marketing; and in the home.[8]

Molds are used in the production of certain types of cheese, such as the soft white cheeses Brie and Camembert (which are inoculated with *Penicillium camemberti*), blue cheeses (which are inoculated with *Penicillium roqueforti* or *Penicillium glaucum*), and goat milk cheeses (which may be treated with white or blue molds).

Some lists of foods to avoid in mold sensitivity cite milk, because it could be a source of penicillin, an antibiotic derived from the mold belonging to the genus *Penicillium*. In the past, dairy cows were treated with penicillin to protect them from infection. However, this practice has been discontinued because of the danger to penicillin-sensitive people, so milk need not be avoided.

Yeast

Yeasts (*Saccharomyces* species) are used in food production to ferment the nutrient source on which they grow. In baking, fermentation of the substrate (starch) leads to the generation of gases (mainly carbon dioxide), which is the process that makes the dough rise in breads and other leavened baked products. Another by-product of yeast fermentation of a substrate (sugar) is alcohol. This is the basis of production of alcoholic beverages. Both baker's and brewer's yeast are strains of *Saccharomyces cerevisiae*.

Savory spreads made from yeast extract, a by-product of beer brewing, are popular in many parts of the world. In Britain, the product is marketed as Marmite; in Australia, it is marketed as Vegemite; and in Switzerland, there is a similar product called Cenovis. Meat extract products and some gravy brownings usually contain yeast extract: The label will indicate if yeast is present in the product. All these products contain *Saccharomyces cerevisiae*.

Saccharomyces exiguus (also known as *S. minor*) is a wild yeast found on plants, fruits, and grains that is occasionally used for baking; however, it is not generally used in a pure form but comes from being propagated in a sourdough starter in which lactobacilli are also included.

Yeast is a source of B vitamins and is present in many multivitamin preparations containing B vitamins. The B vitamins thiamin, riboflavin, folic acid, and niacin are usually derived from the yeast *Saccharomyces cerevisiae*.

Milk and milk products may also contain yeasts. A 1987 study reported that yeasts were isolated, identified, and enumerated from 161 samples of retail dairy products. Highest yeast populations (up to 10^6 to 10^7 cells/g) were found in yogurt and cheese, while lower counts occurred in pasteurized milk, cream, butter, and ice cream.[9] While not all of these products are restricted on a yeast- and mold-free diet, it is wise to keep in mind these possible sources of yeast if symptoms do not resolve on a restricted diet. If symptoms resolve when these foods are restricted, a reaction to these sources of the fungi might be indicated.

Dietary Management of Yeast and Mold Sensitivity

Dietary management of yeast and/or mold sensitivity requires the elimination of all foods that might contain yeast or mold. Foods excluded as probable sources of yeasts or molds are baked products leavened with yeast, many cheeses, certain fruits and vegetables, certain beverages, and moldy foods. Also, because enriched flours contain vitamins that may be derived from yeast, vitamin-enriched flours must also be avoided.

Even if a cheese does not have mold in its production (eg, cheddar), cheese and other milk products provide a rich substrate that is ideal for mold growth. Therefore, cheese, even when stored in the fridge, should be carefully examined for the presence of a mold on its surface and avoided. It is not sufficient to cut out the moldy bits, as mold filaments can invade the cheese below the surface and products of mold growth can be present even when the mold itself seems to have been cut out.

Foods containing sugar are particularly vulnerable to colonization by molds; therefore, jams, jellies, and other sugar-based products should be avoided if mold is visible on their surface. Some molds will even grow on frozen food. Examine any food that has been stored for a prolonged period of time for the presence of mold and discard it if mold is present.

Leftover foods and leftover tea and coffee are potential media for the growth of molds; therefore, only fresh foods and freshly brewed tea and coffee should be consumed. All raw fruits and vegetables should be carefully examined for the presence of mold and must be avoided if mold is present. It is not sufficient to merely wash the food.

Candidiasis

Candida albicans is a dimorphic fungus, which means that it grows as a yeast form in a carbohydrate medium and forms hyphae (strands) when the medium is low in nutrients. Thus, it is commonly referred to as a *pseudoyeast.*

Candida species are common members of the body's resident microflora. Usually they are innocuous, as they are kept in check by other resident microorganisms such as bacteria. However, this balance can be upset when, for example, antibiotics eliminate several species of bacteria or the immune system is not functioning efficiently. In these instances, *Candida* multiply unchecked and soon cause infections such as oral thrush, vaginal moniliasis, and skin eruptions.

The role of *Candida* as a cause of allergy has been much disputed. Positive skin reactions often occur in people without clinical evidence of *Candida* infection or allergic disease. Some practitioners believe that repeated imbalances in *Candida* in the body can lead to chronic *Candida* sensitivity, which in turn can lead to numerous food and chemical sensitivities.[10] A "*Candida* diet" is prescribed to treat this condition, usually excluding foods that contain sugars and more complex carbohydrates. In addition, the *Candida*-sensitive individual is advised to avoid dietary forms of other fungi, which are believed to cross-react with *Candida* and produce similar reactions.

Although *Candida* infection or sensitivity may contribute to mold and yeast sensitivity, this connection has not been proven.[11] The instructions in this chapter are for a yeast and mold allergy (usually IgE-mediated hypersensitivity) and should not be used to manage a suspected *Candida* sensitivity.

References

1. Simon-Nobbe B, Denk U, Pöll V, Rid R, Breitenbach M. The spectrum of fungal allergy. *Int Arch Allergy Immunol.* 2008;145:58-86.
2. Bennett AT, Collins KA. An unusual case of anaphylaxis: mold in pancake mix. *Am J Forensic Med Pathol.* 2001;22(3):292-295.
3. Bush RK, Portnoy JM, Saxon A, Terr AI, Wood RA. Position paper: the medical effects of mold exposure. *Envir Occup Respir Disorders.* 2006;117(2):326-333.

4. Airola K, Petman L, Mäkinen-Kiljunen S. Clustered sensitivity to fungi: anaphylactic reactions caused by ingestive allergy to yeasts. *Ann Allergy Asthma Immunol.* 2006;97(3):294-297.

5. Baldo BA, Baker RS. Inhalant allergies to fungi: reactions to bakers' yeast (*Saccharomyces cerevisiae*) and identification of bakers' yeast enolase as an important allergen. *Int Arch Allergy Immunol.* 1988;86:201-208.

6. Kortekangas-Savolafnen O, Kalimo K, Lammintausta K, Savolainen J. IgE-binding components of baker's yeast (*Saccharomyces cerevisiae*) recognized by immunoblotting analysis. Simultaneous IgE binding to mannan and 46–48 Kd allergens of *Saccharomyces cerevisiae* and *Candida albicans. Clin Exp Allergy.* 1992;23(3):179-184.

7. Wessels MW, Dolkes G, Van Ieperen-Van Dijk A, Gkoers WJ, Young E. IgE antibodies to *Pityrosporum ovale* in atopic dermatitis. *Br J Dermatol.* 1992;125(3):227-232.

8. Tournas VH, Katsoudas E. Mould and yeast flora in fresh berries, grapes and citrus fruits. *Int J Food Microbiol.* 2005;105(1):11-17.

9. Fleet GH, Mian MA. The occurrence and growth of yeasts in dairy products. *Int J Food Microbiol.* 1987;4(2):145-155.

10. Crook WG. *The Yeast Connection: A Medical Breakthrough.* Jackson, TN: Professional Books; 1984.

11. Position statement: Executive Committee of the American Academy of Allergy and Immunology. Candidiasis sensitivity syndrome. *J Allergy Clin Immunol.* 1986;78(2):271-273.

CHAPTER **21**

Sulfite Sensitivity

Sensitivity to sulfites is most common in people with asthma. Of these people, individuals who are steroid dependent are considered most at risk for sulfite sensitivity. Although the incidence of adverse reactions to sulfites is estimated to be as high as 1% of the U.S. population, sulfite sensitivity in people without asthma is considered rare.[1] Most studies report a 3% to 10% prevalence of sulfite sensitivity among asthmatic subjects following ingestion of sulfite-containing additives.[2] Reported symptoms have occurred in most organ systems, including the lungs, gastrointestinal tract, skin, and mucous membranes. Reports of life-threatening anaphylactic reactions to sulfites in asthmatics have been reported but are very rare.[3]

Symptoms

Symptoms reported to be due to sulfite sensitivity include:

- Asthma in asthmatics
- Severe respiratory reactions, including bronchospasm, wheezing, and a feeling of tightness in the chest
- Flushing, feeling of temperature change
- Onset of hypotension (low blood pressure)
- Gastrointestinal symptoms (abdominal pain, diarrhea, nausea, vomiting)
- Swallowing difficulty
- Dizziness, loss of consciousness
- Urticaria (hives), angioedema (swelling, especially of the mouth and face)
- Contact dermatitis
- Anaphylaxis (in people with asthma); anaphylactoid reaction (in people without asthma)

People with impaired kidney and liver function are advised to avoid sulfites because the enzymes in the kidney and liver that are required to break down sulfites will be inadequate, resulting in sulfite excess and development of symptoms of sulfite intolerance just listed.[4]

There is no evidence that avoiding all dietary sources of sulfites improves asthma. For people who are not sensitive to sulfites, exposure to sulfiting agents poses very little risk. Toxicity studies in volunteers showed that ingestion of 400 mg of sulfites daily for 25 days produced no adverse effects.[5]

Diagnosis of Sulfite Sensitivity

Because the exact mechanism involved in sulfite sensitivity is presently unknown (see the next topic, "Mechanism of Action of Sulfites," in this chapter), there are no laboratory tests available for diagnosis of the condition. Sensitivity to sulfites rarely involves allergen-specific IgE, so in general skin tests and blood tests are of very little value. Typically, the diagnosis is suggested by a history of adverse reactions after consuming sulfite-containing foods or medications.

In order for the diagnosis to be confirmed, an allergist may perform an oral metabisulfite challenge for a patient suspected of having sulfite allergy. This procedure involves giving a person increasing amounts of metabisulfite to swallow, usually enclosed in gelatin capsules. Lung function and vital signs are carefully measured with each increasing dosage of the sulfite. The typical response to sulfite is bronchospasm in an asthmatic; a significant drop in lung function confirms sensitivity to sulfites. This test should only be performed under direct supervision of a physician who has been trained and is experienced with such a procedure. Any other signs of a reaction to sulfite (as detailed in the "Symptoms" section earlier) will be assessed at the same time.

Mechanism of Action of Sulfites

The precise mechanism responsible for sulfite sensitivity remains to be determined. However, research suggests several possible mechanisms that might be responsible for triggering symptoms in sulfite-sensitive individuals. One or all of these processes may play a role in sulfite intolerance.

Sulfur Dioxide Acts as a Respiratory Irritant

Respiratory symptoms caused by sulfites are thought to be caused by sulfur dioxide, which acts as a direct irritant on hypersensitive airways. Sulfur dioxide is released from sulfurous acid, which forms when sulfites dissolve in water. This effect is enhanced when the sulfite is present in an acidic food. People with asthma can experience significant bronchospasm after inhaling as little as one part per million of sulfur dioxide.[6] Wheezing, flushing, and other symptoms of asthma have been induced by the inhalation of the vapors from a bag of dried apricots.

Sulfite-Specific IgE

In a few studies, sulfite-sensitive individuals have exhibited a positive skin test to sulfite. Consequently, an IgE-mediated reaction has been suggested. Because the sulfite molecule is nonprotein and is too small to elicit an immunologically mediated reaction on its own, it has been proposed that sulfite acts as a hapten, combining with a protein in food to form a neoantigen that elicits antigen-specific IgE.[7] In the process, some reports indicate that histamine and other inflammatory mediators associated with IgE-mediated allergy may be released. This provides additional weight to the idea of a possible IgE-mediated response and the potential involvement of mast cells and basophils in the process.[8] However, IgE-mediated reactions are considered to be unlikely or very rare, and no evidence of sulfite-specific IgE has been demonstrated in research studies.[7]

Sulfite Oxidase Deficiency

A deficiency in the enzyme sulfite oxidase, which normally rapidly converts sulfite to sulfate, has been suggested as a possible cause of abnormally high levels of sulfites in some sensitive individuals.[2,4] Sulfates do not trigger the adverse responses associated with sulfites. However, this hypothesis has not yet been substantiated.

Use of Sulfites in Foods and Medications

Sulfites are used as preservatives in beverages, fruits, vegetables, prepared and presliced foods, and packaged snack foods. The active component is sulfur dioxide, which has been used as a preservative since Roman times, especially for wine. Today it is the most versatile food additive in use in the food manufacturing industry. Its uses include:

- Preventing food spoilage by (a) inhibiting the growth of microorganisms, especially enterobacteria such as *Salmonella*; (b) inhibition of enzymatic and nonenzymatic browning in food plants; (c) antioxidant effects; (d) preservation of the red color of meat by preventing oxidation of myoglobin to metmyoglobin; and (e) prevention of discoloration of shrimp and lobster by inhibiting the enzyme tyrosinase.
- Bleaching of flour, maraschino cherries, citrus peel before recoloring
- Improving agent
- Physically modifying dough by sulfitolysis of disulfite bonds in the gluten of the flour. This reduces the elasticity of the dough and reduces the time required for mixing and standing of the dough in making batches of baked goods.
- Stabilizing vitamin C
- Inhibiting nitrosamine formation (eg, in kilning of barley to make malt)

Sulfites are also used as preservatives in some medications, including inhalable and injectable drugs, where they act as antioxidants and prevent browning. Some forms of epinephrine (adrenaline) contain sulfite as a preservative. However, the action of epinephrine appears to overcome any adverse effects of sulfite, and administration of epinephrine in anaphylactic emergencies is the recommended treatment.

Cooking foods does not cause sulfites to lose their effect. In addition, because sulfites bind to several substances in foods, such as protein, starch, and sugar, washing foods, even if a detergent is used, will not remove all traces of sulfites.

Sulfates in foods do not cause the same adverse reactions as sulfites and need not be avoided by people who are sensitive to sulfites. Table 21.1 provides examples of sources and uses of sulfites.

TABLE 21.1

Examples of Sources and Uses of Sulfites, and European E Numbers[a]

Additive (European E Number)	Function	Foods Likely to Contain Sulfite
Sulfur dioxide (E220)	Occurs naturally	Fruit juices
	May be produced chemically	Fruit pulp
	Prevents browning by destroying plant enzymes	Fruit syrup
		Fruit salad
		Fruit spreads
		Packet soups
		Glacé cherries
		Dried bananas and apricots
		Jams and jellies
		Desiccated coconut
		Beer
		Wine
		Cider
		Cider vinegar
		Candied peel
		Canned crabmeat
		Fruit-based milk and cream desserts
		Flavorings
		Fruit fillings
		Powdered garlic
		Gelatin
		Dry ginger root
		Glucose
		Soft drinks
		Frozen mushrooms
		Dehydrated vegetables and fruits
		Sausage meat

Continues

TABLE 21.1

Examples of Sources and Uses of Sulfites, and European E Numbers[a] (*Continued*)

Additive (European E Number)	Function	Foods Likely to Contain Sulfite
Sodium sulfite (E221)	Used in food manufacture to:	Preserved egg yolk
	Sterilize fermentation equipment	Quick-frozen shrimps, prawns, lobster
	Sterilize food containers	Beer
	As a preservative to prevent browning especially of prepeeled and sliced apples and potatoes	Wine
		Concentrated pineapple juice
	In some countries used to control microorganisms such as enterobacteria, especially salmonella	Caramel
	Preservation of the red color of meat and shellfish	
Sodium hydrogen sulfite (E222)	Preservative for alcoholic beverages	Beer
	Bleaching agent	Wine
	Antimicrobial preservative	Cider
	Antioxidant	Bleaching of cod
	Antibrowning agent	Bleaching of sugar
		Quick-frozen shrimp, prawn, lobster
		Quick-frozen French fries
		Dehydrated instant mashed potatoes
		Fruit juices
		Vegetable juices
		Relishes and some condiments
		Gelatin-containing puddings
Sodium metabisulfite (E223)	Antimicrobial preservative	Soft drinks
	Antioxidant	Pickled onions
	Bleaching agent	Pickled red cabbage
		Packet mashed potatoes
		Quick-frozen shrimp, prawns, lobster
		Quick-frozen French fries
		Gelatin puddings
		Alcoholic beverages
		Dried fruits and nuts
Potassium metabisulfite (E224)	Antimicrobial preservative	Quick-frozen French fries
	Especially for preserving fruit and homemade wine	Quick-frozen shrimp, prawns, lobster
		Wine
	Used to halt fermentation process in commercial breweries	Wine-making tablets (Campden tablets)
	Antibrowning agent	

Continues

TABLE 21.1

Examples of Sources and Uses of Sulfites, and European E Numbers[a] (*Continued*)

Additive (European E Number)	Function	Foods Likely to Contain Sulfite
Calcium sulfite (E226)	Preservative	Cider
	Firming agent in canned fruits and vegetables	Fruit juices
		Canned fruits and vegetables
	Disinfectant in brewing vats	
Calcium bisulfate (E227)	Preservative	Beer
	Prevents secondary fermentation in brewing	Jams
		Jellies
	Used in washing beer casks to prevent the beer becoming cloudy or sour	Canned fruits and vegetables
	Firming agent in canned fruit and vegetables	

[a] *E numbers* are used in the European Union to identify food additives on food labels.

Detection of Sulfites in Foods

Chemically treated strips have been developed to test foods for the presence of sulfites. However, because of the high number of false-positive and false-negative results obtained with these test strips, their use is not recommended.[9]

Government Regulations on the Use of Sulfites

Sulfiting agents or sulfites, traditionally used as food preservatives, are causing concern among consumers in all countries, and many government health departments have regulations regarding their use.

Labeling regulations in the United States require that food products indicate the presence of sulfites if the amount of sulfite in the product is equal to or exceeds 10 parts per million (ppm).[10] A Food and Drug Administration (FDA) regulation banned the use of sulfites on fresh fruit and vegetables, except sliced potatoes and raw grapes, in the United States in 1986; a similar ban in Canada came into effect in 1987. Canadian regulations state that "no person shall sell any fresh fruit or vegetable that is intended to be consumed raw, except grapes, if sulfurous acid or any salt thereof has been added thereto."[11] The FDA prohibits the use of sulfites in foods that are important sources of thiamin (vitamin B-1), such as enriched flour, because sulfites destroy the nutrient. In many countries, including Canada,[12] the European Union, Australia, and New Zealand, sulfites are required to be listed on food and beverage labels if the level is or exceeds 10 ppm.

Permitted Forms of Sulfites

In the United States, sulfites are permitted for use in the form of:

- Sodium metabisulfite
- Potassium metabisulfite
- Sodium bisulfite
- Potassium bisulfite
- Sodium sulfite
- Sodium dithionite
- Sulfurous acid
- Sulfur dioxide

Foods That May Have Sulfites Added to Them

Under U.S. regulations, a specified level of sulfites (calculated in parts per million) may be added to the following foods and beverages, because no suitable alternatives are currently available (not all manufacturers of these products use sulfites).

- Fruits and vegetables:
  - Dried fruits and vegetables
  - Fruit juices (except frozen concentrated orange juice)
  - Frozen sliced apples
  - Frozen sliced mushrooms
  - Grapes
  - Sliced potatoes
- Beverages:
  - Alcoholic
  - Dealcoholized wines and beers
- Sweeteners:
  - Glucose solids and syrup
  - Dextrose (used in making confectionery)
  - Molasses
- Fish: crustaceans (shellfish)
- Others:
  - Jams, jellies, marmalades (sulfite is in the pectin)
  - Mincemeat
  - Pickles and relishes
  - Tomato paste, pulp, ketchup, purée
  - Gelatin
  - Pectin

- Snack foods
- Candies and confectioneries
- Frozen pizza dough
- Frozen pastry shells

As noted previously, U.S. government regulations state that if any food contains 10 ppm or more, the sulfite must be identified in the ingredient list on the label.

Sulfites in Unlabeled Foods

Some foods do not require labels. The presence of sulfites in the following may not be listed:

▪ Some bulk foods
▪ Individually sold candies
▪ Individually portioned foods such as those sold in vending machines, mobile canteens, and delis
▪ Manufactured foods that contain sulfite as a secondary ingredient (eg, if one of the ingredients in a prepared cake is jam that contains sulfites, the jam must be listed but not the sulfite contained in it; this is because the final level of sulfite in the finished product is below the amount required by law to be disclosed.)

When eating in restaurants, people who are sensitive to sulfites should ask whether sulfite agents are present in the foods.

Alcoholic Beverages

Labeling regulations of sulfites in alcoholic beverages differ among countries; for example:

▪ In the United States, if sulfite levels are 10 ppm or more in wine bottled after mid-1987, distilled spirits, and malt beverages, sulfites must be listed on the labels.
▪ In the European Union, an equivalent regulation came into effect in November 2005.
▪ In Canada, at the present time, ingredients of alcoholic beverages, including sulfites, need not be listed on the label.

Sulfites in Medications

Sulfites are used in a wide range of medications and pharmaceuticals. The Compendium of Pharmaceuticals and Specialties (CPS) provides a list of sulfite-containing products. A pharmacist should be consulted about the possible sulfite in any medications; formulations change frequently.

Other Sources of Sulfites

Food-processing equipment and food packaging materials (eg, plastic bags) may be sanitized with sulfites. These sources of sulfites will not be listed on any labels. Sulfite-sensitive individuals should avoid opening any packages likely to contain sulfites, especially sealed plastic bags containing dried fruits and vegetables.

Note: Some food manufacturers publish extensive lists of their products in which they specify ingredients to which food-allergic and food-additive sensitive consumers might react. People with sulfite sensitivity are advised to obtain these publications if they wish to purchase manufactured foods such as cookies, breakfast cereals, boxed entrées, and so on. However, the ingredients in manufactured foods and pharmaceuticals change frequently. People with sulfite sensitivity are advised to obtain updated information at regular intervals.

Sulfites and Thiamin (Vitamin B-1)

When sulfur dioxide dissolves, the disulfide chemical bonds that result break up certain protein molecules in food. Enzymes are proteins, and this ability of sulfites confers its property of preserving and inhibiting browning of foods. However, it also has a negative effect on the food: It destroys thiamin,[13] which is essential to the nutrient value of the food. Therefore, U.S. government regulations require that sulfites not be used in high-protein foods that are a significant source of thiamin, especially meat of all types, cereal grains, and milk products. (Meats may be "washed" with a sulfite solution to prevent browning, but sulfites cannot be used as an additive.)

Management of Sulfite Sensitivity

Avoiding foods containing sulfites is the only way to prevent an adverse reaction to sulfite.

References

1. Lester MR. Sulfite sensitivity: significance in human health. *J Am Coll Nutr*. 1995;14(3): 229-232.
2. Vally H, Misso NL, Madan V. Clinical effects of sulphite additives. *Clin Exp Allergy*. 2009;39(11):1643-1651.
3. Tsevat J, Gross GN, Dowling GP. Fatal asthma after ingestion of sulfite-containing wine (letter). *Ann Intern Med*. 1987;107:263.
4. Kajiyama H, Nojima Y, Mitsuhashi H, et al. Elevated levels of serum sulfite in patients with chronic renal failure. *J Amer Soc Nephrol*. 2000;11(5):923-927.
5. Simon RA. Sulfite sensitivity. *Ann Allergy*. 1987;57:100-105.

6. Fine JM, Gordon T, Sheppard D. The roles of pH and ionic species in sulphur dioxide- and sulfite-induced bronchoconstriction. *Am Rev Respir Dis.* 1987;136:1122-1126.

7. Boxer MB, Bush RK, Harris KE, Patterson R, Pruzansky JJ, Yang WH. The laboratory evaluation of IgE antibody to metabisulfites in patients skin test positive to metabisulfite. *J Allergy Clin Immunol.* 1988;82:622-626.

8. Sokol WN, Hydick IB. Nasal congestion, urticaria and angioedema caused by an IgE-mediated reaction to sodium metabisulfite. *Ann Allergy.* 1990;65:233-237.

9. Nordlee JA, Naidu SG, Taylor SL. False positive and false negative reactions encountered in the use of sulfite test strips for the detection of sulfite-treated foods. *J Allergy Clin Immunol.* 1988;81:537-541.

10. US Food and Drug Administration. Sulfites in standardized food. 21 CFR § 130.9 Revised April 1, 2011. http://www.accessdata.fda.gov/scripts/cdrh/cfdocs/cfcfr/CFRSearch.cfm?fr=130.9. Accessed April 24, 2012.

11. Department of Justice, Canada. Food and Drugs Act. Regulation B.11.001.1 amended on June 16, 2008. Act current to August 29, 2011.

12. Regulations amending the Food and Drug Regulations (1220—enhanced labeling for food allergen and gluten sources and added sulphites). *Canada Gazette.* 2011 (Feb 16);145(4). http://gazette.gc.ca/rp-pr/p2/2011/2011-02-16/html/sor-dors28-eng.html. Accessed June 26, 2012.

13. Jaroensanti J, Panijpan B. Kinetics of bisulphate cleavage of the three biological phosphorylated derivatives of thiamine. *Int J Vit Res.* 1981;51(1):34-38.

22

Nickel Allergy

Nickel is a well-known cause of contact dermatitis in nickel-sensitive people, inducing a reaction wherever it is in close contact with the skin or mucous membrane for a period of time.[1] This response is known as a *cell-mediated delayed* (type IV) *hypersensitivity reaction*. The nickel induces local T-cell lymphocytes to produce cytotoxic cytokines that cause the itching, reddening, and scaling of contact dermatitis.[2]

Food allergy caused by nickel was first suspected when dermatologists noticed that some people exhibited symptoms of dermatitis on skin surfaces that were not in contact with any known allergen. These dermatologists suspected that the allergenic source might be in something ingested and looked for sources of known contact allergens, such as nickel, in commonly eaten foods.[3] Nickel occurs naturally in many foods and may be introduced during food processing—for example, from metal containers or cooking utensils.

Symptoms of Nickel Allergy

Nickel-contact dermatitis develops in areas in direct contact with nickel-containing objects such as jewelry, metal studs, and watchbands and in occupations where metal contact is frequent. Ingested dietary nickel may trigger reactions in the skin in individuals who react systemically to nickel.[4]

Eczema, especially on the hands, may develop as a secondary response to nickel sensitization. The eczematous rash may later spread to other body surfaces. This may be a reaction to nickel in foods in individuals primarily sensitized by direct nickel contact.[5] Occasionally, cases of *erythema multiforme*[6] and vasculitis[7] after ingestion of nickel in food have been reported.

Diagnosis of Nickel Allergy

Contact allergy to nickel is diagnosed by a patch test. The nickel allergen (usually in the form of nickel sulfate) within the patch is placed on the skin and left in place for up to 72 hours. The area under the skin is usually observed after 48 hours. Because type IV hypersensitivity is a delayed response, the reaction takes 2 or 3 days to become visible. In a positive reaction, the area of skin under the patch will turn red and possibly itch and blister if the reaction is severe. A similar dermatological patch test is used for any suspected contact allergy.

Dermatitis due to ingested nickel is usually suspected when a chronic dermatitis persists without obvious contact with nickel-containing objects. Elimination and challenge is at present the only method to identify this cause of a chronic dermatitis. A low-nickel diet is followed for a period of 4 weeks. If the rash subsides, a challenge with foods with high nickel content will usually indicate that ingested nickel is a trigger for the reaction.

Because all foods contain some level of nickel, a nickel-free diet is not possible. However, some foods are much higher in their nickel content than others. Table 22.1 provides a comparative list of nickel levels from a variety of studies.[8–11]

TABLE 22.1
Level of Nickel in Common Foods

	Nickel, µg/g	Serving Size	Nickel, µg/ serving
Dairy Products			
Cheese	0.1	½ cup (28 g)	2.8
Fat-free milk	0.02	½ cup (123 g)	2.46
Whole milk	0.02	½ cup (123g)	2.46
Dried milk	< 0.09	½ cup (15 g)	< 1.35
Yogurt	0.01	½ cup (114 g)	1.14
Cream	0.03	½ cup (15 (g)	0.45
Butter	0.1	1 tsp (5 g)	0.5
Fruit			
Canned fruit	0.69	½ cup (125 g)	86.25
Pears	0.26	1 med (166 g)	43.16
Bananas	0.32	1 med (114 g)	36.48
Fruit juice, canned	< 0.15	½ cup (125 g)	< 18.75
Plums	0.12	2 med (132 g)	15.84
Fruit juice, bottled	< 0.11	½ cup (125 g)	< 13.75
Cloudberries	0.18	½ cup (73 g)	13.14
Raspberries	0.21	½ cup (61 g)	12.81
Pears	0.068	1 med (166 g)	11.29

Continues

TABLE 22.1
Level of Nickel in Common Foods (*Continued*)

	Nickel, µg/g	Serving Size	Nickel, µg/ serving
Apples	0.07	1 med (138 g)	9.66
Black currants	0.16	½ cup (56 g)	8.96
Rhubarb	0.13	½ cup (68 g)	8.84
Strawberries	0.05	½ cup (125 g)	6.25
Blueberries	0.065	½ cup (73 g)	4.745
Currants	0.06	½ cup (72 g)	4.32
Citrus fruit	0.03	1 med orange (140 g)	4.2
Lingonberries	0.044	½ cup (73 g)	3.212
Bananas	0.02	1 med (114 g)	2.28
Raisins	0.03	½ cup (76 g)	2.28
Apples	0.009	1 med (138 g)	1.242
Grapes	0.02	½ cup (46 g)	0.92
Grains			
Oatmeal	1.76	½ cup (117 g)	205.92
Oats	2.3	½ cup (56 g)	128.8
Buckwheat	2.2	½ cup (56 g)	123.2
Wheat germ	1	¼ cup (28 g)	28
Wheat flour extracted	0.35	½ cup (56 g)	19.6
Wheat bran	0.53	½ cup (28 g)	14.84
Wheat grain	< 0.19	½ cup (56 g)	< 10.64
Flour—whole grain	0.165	½ cup (56 g)	9.24
Rice	0.07	½ cup (94 g)	6.58
Rye flour	0.096	½ cup (56 g)	5.376
Flour—white, self-rising	< 0.09	½ cup (56 g)	< 5.04
Bread—whole grain	0.19	1 slice (25 g)	4.75
Flour—white plain	< 0.06	½ cup (56 g)	< 3.36
Bread—white	< 0.06	1 slice (56 g)	< 3.36
Various Foods			
Cocoa	9.8	1 Tbsp (22 g)	215.6
Soy proteins	4.3	50 g	215
Walnuts	3.6	12 halves (30 g)	108
Peanuts	2.8	1 oz (28 g)	78.4
Dark chocolate	2.2	1 oz (28 g)	61.6
Dried soup powder	1.1	1 package (39 g)	42.9
Tea—instant	15.5	2 tsp (2 g)	31
Milk chocolate	0.34	1 oz (28 g)	9.52

Continues

TABLE 22.1
Level of Nickel in Common Foods (*Continued*)

	Nickel, µg/g	Serving Size	Nickel, µg/serving
Soft drink, concentrated bottles	0.05	½ cup (125 g)	6.25
Curry powders	1.7	1 tsp (2 g)	3.4
Sugar—brown	< 0.23	1 Tbsp (14 g)	< 3.22
Stock cubes	0.6	1 cube (5 g)	3
Herbs	< 2.9	1 tsp (1 g)	< 2.9
Spices	1.4	1 tsp (2 g)	2.8
Coffee—instant	1.2	2 tsp (2 g)	2.4
Margarine	0.34	1 tsp (5 g)	1.7
Coffee—ground	0.8	2 tsp (2 g)	1.6
Sugar—white	< 0.13	1 Tbsp (12 g)	< 1.56
Mustard	< 0.5	1 tsp (2 g)	1
Meat, Fish, and Other Protein Foods			
Fish	0.7	4 oz (113 g) cooked; 5.25 oz (150 g) raw	105
Fish pastes	0.53	4 oz (113 g) cooked; 5.25 oz (150 g) raw	79.5
Kidney (ox, lamb)	< 0.25	4 oz (113 g) cooked; 5.25 oz (150 g) raw	< 37.5
Chicken	0.11	4 oz (113 g) cooked; 5.25 oz (150 g) raw	16.5
Liver (ox, lamb, pig)	< 0.1	4 oz (113 g) cooked; 5.25 oz (150 g) raw	< 15
Lamb	< 0.09	4 oz (113 g) cooked; 5.25 oz (150 g) raw	< 13.5
Pork	< 0.06	4 oz (113 g) cooked; 5.25 oz (150 g) raw	< 9
Egg	0.05	4 oz (113 g) cooked; 5.25 oz (150 g) raw	7.5
Baltic herring	0.036	4 oz (113 g) cooked; 5.25 oz (150 g) raw	5.4
Cod	0.021	4 oz (113 g) cooked; 5.25 oz (150 g) raw	3.15
Beef	0.02	4 oz (113 g) cooked; 5.25 oz (150 g) raw	3
Trout	0.017	4 oz (113 g) cooked; 5.25 oz (150 g) raw	2.55
Cattle kidney[1]	0.015	4 oz (113 g) cooked; 5.25 oz (150 g) raw	2.25
Pike	0.013	4 oz (113 g) cooked; 5.25 oz (150 g) raw	1.95
Perch	0.012	4 oz (113 g) cooked; 5.25 oz (150 g) raw	1.8
Pig kidney	0.012	4 oz (113 g) cooked; 5.25 oz (150 g) raw	1.8
Pig liver	0.011	4 oz (113 g) cooked; 5.25 oz (150 g) raw	1.65
Beef	0.011	4 oz (113 g) cooked; 5.25 oz (150 g) raw	1.65
Whitefish	< 0.010	4 oz (113 g) cooked; 5.25 oz (150 g) raw	< 1.5
Pike/perch	< 0.010	4 oz (113 g) cooked; 5.25 oz (150 g) raw	< 1.5
Cattle liver	< 0.010	4 oz (113 g) cooked; 5.25 oz (150 g) raw	< 1.5
Kingklip red	< 0.010	4 oz (113 g) cooked; 5.25 oz (150 g) raw	< 1.5
Chilean hake	< 0.010	4 oz (113 g) cooked; 5.25 oz (150 g) raw	< 1.5

Continues

TABLE 22.1
Level of Nickel in Common Foods (*Continued*)

	Nickel, µg/g	Serving Size	Nickel, µg/ serving
Pork	< 0.010	4 oz (113 g) cooked; 5.25 oz (150 g) raw	< 1.5
Arctic char	< 0.008	4 oz (113 g) cooked; 5.25 oz (150 g) raw	< 1.2
Atlantic mackerel	< 0.005	4 oz (113 g) cooked; 5.25 oz (150 g) raw	< 0.75
Vegetables and Legumes			
Green lentils	3	½ cup (125 g)	375
Soy beans	2.9	½ cup (125 g)	362.5
Dried legumes	1.7	½ cup (125 g)	212.5
Brown beans	1.7	½ cup (125 g)	212.5
Chickpeas	1.6	½ cup (125 g)	200
Alfalfa seeds	4	50 g	200
Linseeds	1.9	½ cup (100 g)	190
Yellow peas, dried	0.93	½ cup (125 g)	116.25
Beans (frozen and fresh)	0.4	½ cup (125 g)	50
Spinach	0.52	½ cup packed (90 g)	46.8
Asparagus	0.42	½ cup (83 g)	34.86
Broccoli	0.28	1 stalk (100 g)	28
Canned vegetables	< 0.31	½ cup (83 g)	< 25.73
Canned peas	0.28	½ cup (76 g)	21.28
Kale	0.2	½ cup (100 g)	20
Poppy seeds, blue	1.3	1 Tbsp (15 g)	19.5
Poppy seeds, white	1.2	1 Tbsp (15 g)	18
Mushrooms	0.16	10 small (100 g)	16
Endive	0.31	10 long leaves (50 g)	15.5
Cauliflower	0.3	½ cup, pieces (50 g)	15
Potatoes	0.14	1 med (100 g)	14
Leeks	0.11	3 to 4 med (100 g)	11
Cabbage	0.17	½ cup shredded (50 g)	8.5
Brussels sprouts	0.16	5 small (50 g)	8
Tomatoes	0.07	1 small (100 g)	7
Carrots	0.054	1 large (100 g)	5.4
Green peas	0.076	½ cup (67 g)	5.092
Potatoes	0.048	1 med (100 g)	4.8
Carrots	0.04	1 large (100 g)	4
Celery	0.06	½ cup (50 g)	3
Chinese cabbage	0.046	½ cup shredded (50 g)	2.3

Continues

TABLE 22.1
Level of Nickel in Common Foods (*Continued*)

	Nickel, µg/g	Serving Size	Nickel, µg/ serving
Cucumber	0.04	½ med (50 g)	2
Onions	0.08	1 Tbsp diced (10 g)	0.8
Lettuce	0.027	0.7 oz (20 g)	0.54

Listed from highest to lowest levels of nickel per serving in each food category. *Note:* The stated level of nickel in food such as apples is the mean for several varieties. All fruit is raw, unless otherwise stated. Where the same food appears with different nickel levels, it indicates different independent analysis reports. When the amount of nickel is reported as *less than* (<) a certain level, this indicates that the authors who provided the data found that levels varied among reports and samples but no reported levels exceeded the stated amount.

Source: Data compiled from Booth J. Nickel in the diet and its role in allergic dermatitis. *J Hum Nutr Diet*. 1990;3:233-243; Han HJ, Lee BH, Park CW, Lee CH, Kang YS. A study of nickel content in Korean foods. *Korean J Dermatol*. 2005;43:593-598; Jorhem I, Sundström B. Levels of lead, cadmium, zinc, copper, nickel, chromium, manganese, and cobalt in foods on the Swedish market, 1983–1990. *J Food Compost Anal*. 1993;6:233-241; Ysart G, Miller P, Crews H, et al. Dietary exposure estimates of 30 elements from the UK Total Diet Study. *Food Addit Contam*. 1999;16(9):391-403.

Level of Nickel in Food

The level of nickel in foods varies with the variety of the plant species and with the nickel content of the soil in which the plant was grown or, in the case of seafood, of the aquatic environment. In addition, different laboratories employ a variety of tests to detect nickel in food, so frequently data from one source can disagree markedly with that from another. In most studies, the richest sources of dietary nickel are found in nuts, dried peas and beans, whole grains, and chocolate (see Table 22.1).

In addition, processing a food can increase its nickel content. For example, minute traces of nickel from metal grinders used in milling flour can increase the nickel in flour considerably, and stainless-steel cookware will increase the level of nickel in the food cooked in it.

The Relationship Between Nickel and Iron

Most ingested nickel remains unabsorbed and is excreted in the feces. Usually less than 10% of the nickel in food is absorbed[6] but this amount increases in people with iron-deficiencies and lactating mothers. Nickel and iron use the same transport system to cross the intestinal mucosa, so if iron is being transported, nickel is excluded. Accordingly, individuals who are sensitive to nickel should include iron-rich foods in their diet.

Nickel Contact Dermatitis and Oral Tolerance

The most common cause of nickel dermatitis is direct contact with nickel-containing objects. People who have tested positive for nickel using a patch test (on the skin of the forearm or back) should avoid contact with all objects containing the metal.

An increasing number of studies are indicating that reducing the severity of contact dermatitis related to nickel or preventing symptoms can be achieved by oral exposure to nickel.[12,13] According to other studies, oral exposure to nickel can worsen established nickel contact dermatitis initially, but prolonged exposure can reduce the clinical symptoms.[14]

The subject of nickel-contact dermatitis, nickel allergy, and achievement of tolerance is confusing from a practical point of view because of the extremely complex series of events that occur in the immune system. Nickel contact dermatitis is part of a cell-mediated (type IV) hypersensitivity reaction; nickel allergy is possibly an IgE-mediated (type I) hypersensitivity,[15] and the precise mechanism that allows the immune system to achieve tolerance, especially to foods, is unclear at present.

Management Allergy to Ingested Nickel

Clinical studies suggest that some nickel-sensitive people benefit from avoiding foods with high amounts of nickel. However, opinions differ on what constitutes a nickel-restricted diet. In one research study, an oral dose of nickel (as nickel sulfate) as low as 0.6 mg produced a positive reaction in some nickel-sensitive people.[16] Another report indicated that 2.5 mg was required to induce a flare-up.[17] Because the levels of nickel required to induce a reaction have varied widely in different studies, it is difficult to determine a "safe level" of dietary nickel for nickel-sensitive people.

However, dietary nickel often is not the sole cause of the dermatitis. In these cases, avoiding nickel in the diet may improve the situation but does not entirely eradicate the symptoms. If symptoms have resolved on the diet, challenge with foods with high nickel content should lead to a flare-up of skin reactions if a person is indeed allergic to dietary nickel.

References

1. Schram SE, Warshaw EM, Laumann A. Nickel hypersensitivity: a clinical review and call to action. *Int J Dermatol.* 2010;49(2):115-125.
2. Walsh ML, Smith VH, King CM. Type 1 and type IV hypersensitivity to nickel. *Australas J Dermatol.* 2010;51(4):285-286.
3. Veien N. Dietary treatment of nickel dermatitis. *Acta Dermatol Venereol.* 1985;65: 138-142.
4. Nijhawan RI, Molenda M, Zirwas MJ, Jacob SE. Systemic contact dermatitis. *Dermatol Clin.* 2009;27(3):355-364, vii.
5. Christensen OB, Moller H. External and internal exposure to the antigen in the hand eczema of nickel allergy. *Contact Dermatitis.* 1975;1:136-141.
6. Friedman SJ, Perry HO. Erythema multiforme associated with contact dermatitis. *Contact Dermatitis.* 1985;12:21-23.
7. Hjorth N. Nickel dermatitis. *Contact Dermatitis.* 1976;2:356-357.
8. Booth J. Nickel in the diet and its role in allergic dermatitis. *J Hum Nutr Diet.* 1990; 3:233-243.

9. Han HJ, Lee BH, Park CW, Lee CH, Kang YS. A study of nickel content in Korean foods. *Korean J Dermatol.* 2005;43:593-598.

10. Jorhem l, Sundström B. Levels of lead, cadmium, zinc, copper, nickel, chromium, manganese, and cobalt in foods on the Swedish market, 1983–1990. *J Food Compost Anal.* 1993;6:233-241.

11. Ysart G, Miller P, Crews H, et al. Dietary exposure estimates of 30 elements from the UK Total Diet Study. *Food Addit Contam.* 1999;16(9):391-403.

12. Morris DL. Intradermal testing and sublingual desensitization for nickel. *Cutis.* 1998;61(3):129-132.

13. Panzani RC, Schiavino D, Nucera E, et al. Oral hyposensitization to nickel allergy: preliminary clinical results. *Int Arch Allergy Immunol.* 1995;107(1-3):251-254.

14. Santucci B, Cristaudo A, Canmistraci C, Picardo M. Nickel sensitivity: effects of prolonged oral intake of the element. *Contact Dermatitis.* 1988;19:202-205.

15. Estlander T, Kanerva L, Tupsela O, Keskinen H, Jolanski R. Immediate and delayed allergy to nickel with contact urticaria, rhinitis, asthma and contact dermatitis. *Clin Exper Allergy.* 1993;23:306-310.

16. Cronin E, de Michiel A, Brown SS. Oral nickel challenge in nickel-sensitive women with hand eczema. *Ann Clin Lab Sci.* 1981;11:91.

17. Veiein NK, Menne T. Nickel contact allergy and a nickel-restricted diet. *Semin Dermatol.* 1990;9(3):197-205.

CHAPTER **23**

Disaccharide Intolerance

Disaccharide intolerance is due to impaired digestion and/or absorption of sugars. Complex carbohydrates (polysaccharides and oligosaccharides) are broken down by digestive enzymes to disaccharides. Disaccharides are then split into their monosaccharide components by disaccharidase enzymes in the brush border cells lining the small intestine. The monosaccharides are then absorbed into circulation after crossing the intestinal epithelium by a variety of absorption mechanisms (ie, active and passive transport or diffusion). Monosaccharide sugars are normally efficiently absorbed in the small intestine. However, if there is a deficiency in the brush border enzyme production, disaccharides remain undigested and move into the large bowel intact. Symptoms result from the presence of the disaccharide in the colon and its fermentation by the resident microorganisms.

The Problem Disaccharides

The carbohydrate composition of the normal diet is about 60% starch, 30% sucrose, and 10% lactose. Each carbohydrate is treated slightly differently in the process of digestion.[1]

Lactose

Lactose is the sugar in milk. It occurs mostly in the whey (liquid) fraction of milk, although foods made mainly of casein (such as cheeses) may still contain a small amount of lactose, especially in the softer cheeses with a higher content of whey. Lactase, the enzyme that breaks down lactose, splits lactose into two monosaccharides: glucose and galactose. A person whose intestinal cells are producing very little lactase cannot break down much lactose. Undigested lactose moves into the colon, where it causes osmotic imbalance and provides a substrate for microbial fermentation. Lactose intolerance is quite different from milk allergy, in which a person's immune system reacts to the protein in milk. (See Chapter 11 for more details.)

Sucrose

Table sugar and syrups are examples of sucrose. It is usually derived from sugar beet or sugarcane but is also present in many plants, especially fruits, grains, and vegetables. The enzyme that breaks down sucrose, *sucrose alpha-glucosidase*, commonly known as *sucrase*, splits sucrose into the two monosaccharides: glucose and fructose. The monosaccharides are transported across the digestive epithelium into circulation. Deficiency in sucrase results in intact sucrose moving into the large bowel, causing osmotic imbalance and providing a substrate for microbial fermentation.

Maltose

Maltose is the disaccharide resulting from digestion of the starches in grains and starchy vegetables. Starch is gradually split into smaller and smaller chains of glucose molecules by amylase enzymes, ultimately resulting in maltose. Further breakdown by the disaccharidase enzymes maltase and isomaltase in the brush border cells results in individual glucose molecules.

Starches

Starches are composed of long chains of glucose molecules. The linkages between the glucose molecules all have to be split to release the free glucose before it can be absorbed. The enzymes (amylases) that begin starch breakdown are present in saliva and in pancreatic secretions in the small intestine. When the starch is reduced to the disaccharide (two joined glucose molecules) as maltose or maltotriose (depending on the structure of the starch), it is then broken down into its constituent monosaccharides by alpha-dextrinase and glucoamylase (sometimes referred to as *maltase* and *isomaltase*); they split maltose into single molecules of glucose, which are moved by active transport across the digestive epithelium into circulation. If there is a deficiency in the enzymes that split these linkages, free glucose molecules will not be released, and the remaining undigested starch or sugar will be passed to the large bowel where bacteria will ferment it. Digestion of polysaccharides into their constituent monosaccharides is depicted in Figure 23.1.

Symptoms

Diarrhea, abdominal distention, pain, and flatulence characterize disaccharide intolerance.[2] Fluid is drawn into the large intestine to normalize the increased osmotic pressure produced by excess sugar. Watery diarrhea or loose stool results from the increase in fluid in the bowel.[3] Gases are produced as a result of an increase in microbial growth and fermentation in the bowel. This results in abdominal bloating, pain, and flatulence. Organic acids are produced by microbial fermentation in the bowel, which tend to increase motility in the digestive tract, which may promote diarrhea, and increase osmotic imbalance, leading to a net influx of fluid into the bowel.

FIGURE 23.1

Carbohydrate digestion in the mouth and small intestine. Digestion of carbohydrates in the form of polysaccharides, sugars, and starches begins with breakdown by amylase enzymes within the intestinal lumen in the mouth and small intestine. When the breakdown reaches the disaccharide stage, the individual disaccharides (sucrose, lactose, maltose) are further broken down by disaccharidase enzymes produced by cells in the brush border of the small intestine. The disaccharidase enzymes release individual monosaccharides, which are transported across the intestinal barrier into circulation. The percentages in parentheses indicate the relative amounts in the normal North American diet.

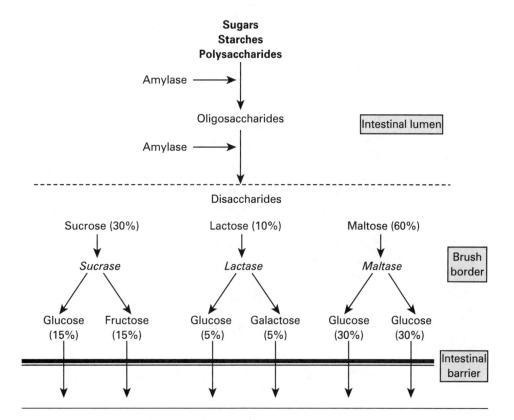

Maldigested disaccharide leads to symptoms in a cyclical pattern:[4] The initial diarrhea caused by fermentation products and osmotic imbalance in the colon leads to speeding up of intestinal transit (decreased transit time) of food. As contact with intestinal enzymes (pancreatic and brush-border derived) is reduced because of inadequate churning and mixing, more undigested starches and sugars move into the colon. This increases the amount of fermentation products and osmotic imbalance in the colon, which perpetuates the cycle. Once it starts, removal of all maldigested carbohydrate is required to interrupt the cycle.

In most cases, a disaccharide intolerance is dose-related. Usually the brush-border cells are producing a limited amount of enzyme, and small doses of foods containing disaccharides can be processed. Problems occur when the amount of disaccharide in the food exceeds the capacity of the enzymes to digest it. The important thing is to determine a person's capacity to handle the sugar. As long as the amount consumed remains within an individual's limits, they should remain symptom free.

Conditions That May Result in Disaccharide Intolerance

Disaccharide intolerance may occur in a variety of conditions that result in the lack of, or decrease in activity of, the disaccharidase enzymes:[5]

- Inherited (congenital) enzyme deficiency, which is a rare condition that is present from birth
- Inherited (congenital) deficiency in components of transport systems needed to assimilate sugars
- Protein enteropathy, such as cow's milk, soy, fish protein enteropathy that leads to inflammation in the small intestine and damage to the enzyme-producing cells
- Gluten-sensitive enteropathy (celiac disease)
- Infections in the digestive tract with parasites such as amoebas, helminths, nematodes, and microorganisms such as *Giardia lamblia* and viruses such as the rotavirus group
- Food allergy affecting the digestive tract
- Strong drugs and antibiotics
- In infants, additional causes may include immaturity of enzymes and transport components

In all cases of disaccharidase deficiency, symptoms are confined to the digestive tract.

Congenital Lactase Deficiency

In cases of congenital lactase deficiency (CLD),[6] symptoms are obvious from birth. Usually the mother reports watery diarrhea, generally after the first feeding of breastmilk but at the latest by age 10 days.[7] If the condition is not recognized, dehydration and malnutrition can lead to death. Implementation of a lactose-free diet with lactose-free formula or lactase-treated breastmilk leads to rapid recovery. The condition is very rare, with 42 cases of CLD reported between 1966 and 1998 in Finland.[8] The condition was first recognized in 1958.

Congenital Sucrase-Isomaltase Deficiency

Congenital sucrase-isomaltase deficiency usually becomes apparent after an infant is weaned and starts to consume fruits, juices, and grains. After ingestion of sucrose or maltose, an affected child will typically experience stomach cramps, bloating, gassiness, and diarrhea. These digestive problems can lead to failure to gain weight and grow at the expected rate (failure to thrive) and malnutrition.[9] Most affected children are better able to tolerate sucrose and maltose as they get older.

The prevalence of congenital sucrase-isomaltase deficiency is estimated to be 1 in 5,000 people of European descent. This condition is much more prevalent in the native populations of Greenland,[10] Alaska, and Canada, where as many as 1 in 20 people may be affected. This condition is inherited in an autosomal recessive pattern, which means both copies of the gene in each cell have mutations. The parents of an individual with an autosomal recessive condition each carry one copy of the mutated gene, but they typically do not show signs and symptoms of the condition.

Duration of the Condition

If the deficiency is a result of damage to the intestinal cells, caused by infection, food allergy, food protein enteropathy, or strong drugs, it is called a *secondary deficiency* and is usually temporary. When the primary cause is removed, the cells will start to heal and gradually resume production of the enzymes. Over time, foods to which an affected individual was intolerant will be processed adequately and tolerated.

If the deficiency is a result of an inherited tendency, it is likely that the intolerance will be lifelong. This is called a *primary deficiency*. The foods that cause the problem must always be avoided.

In some cases, the deficient enzyme can be provided as medication to be consumed with the food or as drops to be added to foods (eg, lactase in the form of Lactaid or Lacteeze). A certain amount of the treated food will be tolerated.

Identifying the Disaccharide That Is Deficient

Except in the case of a lactase deficiency, which improves dramatically when lactose is removed from the diet, it is often difficult to separate specific disaccharide intolerances from each other. If the deficiency is due to extensive damage to intestinal cells, reduction in the activity of all the disaccharidases may result.

The most definitive method of diagnosing deficiency in any of the brush-border cell disaccharidases is by measuring the activity of the enzyme in the epithelial cells of the small intestine.[11] This technique involves taking an endoscopic biopsy of the epithelium and homogenizing the tissue. A sample of the homogenate is then mixed with each of the substrates: sucrose, lactose, and maltose. The activity of the enzyme is then calculated by measuring the amount of glucose released from each substrate, since all of the disaccharides contain glucose.

Because the test is invasive, many people prefer to try to control the symptoms by dietary methods. If the deficiency is due to a temporary deficiency, dietary exclusion of all the disaccharides, followed by reintroducing each one individually in increasing doses, may be feasible.

If the deficiency is permanent, it is often due to loss, or lack, of the ability to produce one specific disaccharidase; in this case, the specific deficiency must be identified, especially in babies and young children in whom nutritional deficiency and failure to thrive can lead to serious consequences for health and survival.

Requirements for Nutritional Supplements

In general, if an individual is consuming a wide range of the allowed foods and the condition is a secondary (temporary) deficiency, nutritional supplements should not be necessary. The amount of supplement that may be required will depend on individual tolerances to the disaccharide-containing food; some people will be able to tolerate a small amount of the food and so any deficiencies will be minimal.

For people with primary (permanent) deficiencies, or those who need to follow the diet for an extended period of time, the following supplements should be considered:

▪ Lactose restricted: calcium and vitamin D
▪ Sucrose restricted: vitamin C
▪ Maltose restricted: vitamin B complex

Feeding the Disaccharide-Intolerant Baby

A breastfed baby will ingest significant quantities of lactose in the mother's milk. The lactose composition of her milk will remain constant, regardless of whether the mother consumes milk and dairy products. Human milk contains 6% (weight in volume [w/v]) lactose compared to 4% (w/v) in cow's milk. Human milk does not contain sucrose, maltose, or starch, so intolerance of other disaccharides is not a problem for the baby during breastfeeding.

If the baby's lactose intolerance is secondary to a gastrointestinal tract infection or other transient condition, some authorities advise continuing breastfeeding and expect the diarrhea to gradually diminish as the underlying inflammation disappears.

Alternatively, the mother can pump her breastmilk and treat the milk with lactase drops (4 drops per 250 mL milk), and allow the enzyme to act for 24 hours in the fridge. The baby will be fed the lactose-free milk the next day. This is continued until the diarrhea abates, when the baby can be gradually put back to the breast. (For more information on feeding the lactose-intolerant breastfed baby, see Chapter 11.)

Infant formulas that are lactose free and sucrose free can be given to a disaccharidase-deficient infant. If the baby is not allergic to milk, a milk-based formula that is free from lactose and sucrose is suitable. If the infant is allergic to cow's milk proteins but tolerates soy, a sucrose-free soy-based formula may be suitable, although an extensively hydrolyzed sucrose-free casein formula is preferable for feeding infants with milk allergies (see Chapter 10 for details). If the infant is allergic to both cow's milk and soy proteins, a casein hydrolysate formula that is free from lactose and sucrose—such as Enfamil Nutramigen (Mead Johnson) and Enfamil Pregestimil (Mead-Johnson)—should be tolerated.

The Disaccharide-Restricted Diet

A convenient way to manage disaccharide intolerances is to conduct the diet in three phases:[3]

■ Phase 1 (restriction of all disaccharides) should be followed until symptoms resolve.
■ Phase 2 (reintroduction) should identify which disaccharides are not tolerated.
■ Phase 3 introduces each individual food in a step-wise dose to determine a person's limit of tolerance.

Phase 1 restricts all disaccharides. The disaccharide-restricted diet (Consumer factsheet) should be followed for a minimum of 4 weeks to determine if disaccharidase deficiency is the cause of the gastrointestinal symptoms, specifically diarrhea.

Phase 2 should determine exactly which disaccharide is not tolerated. It involves challenge with foods containing the suspect disaccharide and monitoring for the recurrence of abdominal symptoms. A serving size or more of each of the following food types should be consumed. Development of symptoms (particularly diarrhea) over the following 24 hours should indicate the culprit disaccharide.

■ *Maltose* tolerance is determined by consuming starch in the form of "white" grains and flours.
■ *Sucrose* tolerance is determined by consuming table sugar.
■ *Lactose* tolerance is determined by consuming complete milk.

Phase 3 involves introducing one food from the restricted list of the specific disaccharide every other day until diarrhea recurs. Because the intolerance to disaccharide is dose-related, it is a good idea to introduce each food in increasing doses, as described in Chapter 7.

The foods used to test for tolerance of each disaccharide are as follows:

■ *Maltose* tolerance is determined by introducing grain products—for example, white bread, white rice.
■ *Sucrose* tolerance is determined by introducing vegetables, fruits, nuts, seeds, and refined sugars and syrups.
■ *Lactose* tolerance is determined by introducing dairy products and milk. Specific details for determining a person's degree of lactose intolerance are provided in Chapter 11.

References

1. Gray G. Intestinal disaccharidase deficiencies and glucose-galactose malabsorption. In: Stanbury JB, Wybgaarden JB, Fredrickson DS, Goldstein JS, Brown MS, eds. *The Metabolic Basis of Inherited Disease.* 5th ed. New York, NY: McGraw-Hill; 1983:1729-1742.

2. Sibley E. Carbohydrate intolerance. *Curr Opin Gatroenterol.* 2004;20(2):162-167.

3. Lloyd-Still JD, Listernick R, Buentello G. Complex carbohydrate intolerance: diagnostic pitfalls and approach to management. *J Pediatr.* 1988;112(5):709-713.

4. Joneja JMV. Maldigestion of carbohydrates. In: Joneja JMV. *Digestion, Diet and Disease. Irritable Bowel Syndrome and Gastrointestinal Function.* New Brunswick, NJ: Rutgers University Press; 2004:116-134.

5. Perman JA. Carbohydrate malabsorption. In: Lifshitz F, ed. *Nutrition for Special Needs in Infancy.* New York, NY: Marcel Dekker; 1985:145-157.

6. Torniainen S, Savilahti E, Järvelä I. Congenital lactase deficiency—a more common disease than previously thought? *Duodecim.* 2009;125(7):766-770.

7. Savilahti E, Launiala K, Kuitunen P. Congenital lactase deficiency: a clinical study on 16 patients. *Arch Dis Child.* 1983;58:246-252.

8. Jarvela I, Enattah NS, Kokkonen J, Varilo T, Savilahti E, Peltonen L. Assignment of the locus for congenital lactase deficiency to 2q21, in the vicinity of but separate from the lactase-phlorizin hydrolase gene. *Am J Hum Genet.* 1998;63:1078-1085.

9. Belmont JW, Reid B, Taylor W, et al. Congenital sucrase-isomaltase deficiency presenting with failure to thrive, hypercalcemia, and nephrocalcinosis. *BMC Pediatr.* 2002;2:2-4.

10. Gudmand-Hoyer E, Fenger HJ, Kern-Hansen P, Madsen PR. Sucrase deficiency in Greenland. Incidence and genetic aspects. *Scand J Gastroenterol.* 1987;22:24-28.

11. Lu J, Grenache DG. High-throughput tissue homogenization method and tissue-based quality control materials for a clinical assay of the intestinal disaccharidases. *Clin Chim Acta.* 2010;411(9-10):754-757.

CHAPTER 24

Fructose Intolerance

Intolerance of fructose, especially in childhood, probably occurs more frequently than diagnostic figures currently suggest.[1] The condition typically presents as loose stools or diarrhea after consumption of fruits such as apples and pears or the juice of these fruits.

Fructose intolerance is usually caused by impaired absorption of fructose. However, there are rare cases in which intolerance of fructose is due to a deficiency in one of the enzymes responsible for the digestion of fructose (see "Inherited Conditions Causing Fructose Intolerance" [page 234]).

Fructose is consumed in three forms:

- As the pure monosaccharide, fructose
- In the disaccharide, sucrose, where fructose is complexed with glucose in a 1:1 ratio of glucose to fructose
- In carbohydrates in a polymerized form as oligosaccharides and polysaccharides. These include inulins, fructans, and fructooligosaccharides. These are considered to be dietary fiber and are not readily broken down by human digestive enzymes. They are often used as prebiotics,[a] as they provide a substrate for microbial metabolism in the colon.

FODMAP and the Inability to Digest Fructose Polymers

An inability to digest and absorb fructose polymers is not intolerance in the context of food sensitivity, because all humans lack the hydrolase enzymes necessary to split the bonds between the fructose molecules in the polymer chain. Hence, molecules

---

[a] Prebiotic: a nondigestible food ingredient that stimulates the activity and growth of microorganisms in the colon that are beneficial to the body's health.

of fructose are not free to be transported across the digestive epithelium and instead remain within the digestive lumen. The term *fermentable oligosaccharides, disaccharides, monosaccharides, and polyols* (FODMAP)[2] has been introduced to define a previously seemingly unrelated group of poorly absorbed short-chain carbohydrates and sugar alcohols that move into the distal small bowel and colon, where they are fermented by the resident microflora, producing symptoms of excessive gas, abdominal bloating, pain, and diarrhea. Strictly speaking, these symptoms do not indicate intolerance, because anyone consuming large quantities of FODMAPs will develop them; this is not an idiosyncratic response limited only to sensitive people.

However, intake of FODMAPs has been identified as a possible cause of gastrointestinal (GI) symptoms, especially in individuals who have been diagnosed with irritable bowel syndrome (IBS). As a result, the FODMAP diet,[3] which eliminates excess fructose, fructose polymers, and sugar alcohols, is often followed in an attempt to reduce GI symptoms. The following section provides information explicitly for the management of diagnosed fructose intolerance.

The Mechanism of Fructose Malabsorption

Intestinal fructose absorption depends on the low-affinity transporter molecule GLUT2, which will carry the monosaccharides glucose, fructose, and galactose across the small intestine epithelium. GLUT2 transports the hexose sugars down a concentration gradient. This carrier mechanism is facilitated by glucose, which permits lower concentrations of glucose to be taken up by the cell by an active process.[4] The process is not entirely understood, but because glucose is preferentially absorbed, an excess of fructose will result in its inefficient absorption. The resultant unabsorbed fructose moves into the large bowel, where it causes an increase in osmotic pressure and a net influx or reduced outflow of water, resulting in loose stool or frank diarrhea. It also acts as a substrate for microbial fermentation with production of gas (especially hydrogen) and organic acids. These activities are responsible for the symptoms of fructose intolerance.

Sucrose contains both glucose and fructose in a 1:1 ratio. Consumption of sucrose does not result in malabsorption of fructose, because when sucrose is split into its constituent monosaccharide sugars by sucrase, the fructose level does not exceed that of the glucose. However, some sucrose-containing fruits contain a higher fructose-to-glucose ratio than most other fruits (Table 24.1). Diarrhea after eating apples, pears, watermelon, blackcurrant, cherries—or juices from these fruits—and honey and high fructose corn syrup, when no other cause for the loose stool is evident, is a sign that fructose malabsorption may be the problem.[5,6]

TABLE 24.1
Fructose and Glucose Content of Fruits and Other Foods
Foods with a high fructose-to-glucose ratio are highlighted.

Food Type	Fructose, g/100 g Edible Portion	Glucose, g/100 g Edible Portion
Fruits		
Apple	5	1.7
Banana	3.5	4.5
Blackberry	2.9	3.2
Black currant	3.7	2.4
Cherry	7.2	4.7
Date	23.9	24.9
Fig	8.2	9.6
Gooseberry	4.1	4.4
Grape	7.3	8.2
Grapefruit	1.2	2
Greengage plum	4	5.5
Lemon	1.4	1.4
Loganberry	1.3	1.9
Melon	1.5	2.1
Mulberry	3.6	4.4
Orange	1.8	2.5
Peach	1.6	1.5
Pear	6.5	2.6
Pineapple	1.4	2.3
Plum	3.4	5.2
Prune	15.9	30
Raisin	29.7	27.8
Raspberry	2.4	2.3
Red currant	1.9	2.3
Strawberry	2.3	2.6
Tomato	1.2	1.6
Watermelon	3.4	1.6
White currant	2.6	3
Other Foods		
Sucrose (for reference)	50	50
Potato	0.1	0.1
Honey	40.5	34.2
Royal jelly	11.3	9.8
Molasses	8.0	8.8
High fructose corn syrup	55–90	45–58

Source: Data are from David TJ. *Food and Food Additive Intolerance in Childhood.* Blackwell Scientific Publications; 1993:164; and US Department of Agriculture. National Nutrient Database Release 20. September 2007. http://www.ars.usda.gov/SP2UserFiles/Place/12354500/Data/SR20/SR20_doc.pdf. Accessed April 25, 2012.

Absorption of Fructose

Free fructose has limited absorption in the small intestine, with up to one-half of the population unable to completely absorb a dose of 25 g of fructose.[7] Average daily intake of fructose is estimated to vary from 11 g to 54 g around the world, depending on the dietary habits of the population sampled.

When used as a sweetener in soft drinks as consumed in North America, fructose can quickly approach levels at which malabsorption is seen in healthy adults. Evidence suggests that when solutions containing 25 g to 50 g of fructose (equivalent to more than 500 mL of sweetened soft drink) are consumed, more than 50% of healthy subjects demonstrate malabsorption of fructose and consequently experience symptoms of abdominal pain, gas, and loose bowels.[8] The high fructose content in sports drinks has also been implicated in impeded athletic performance and abdominal symptoms.[9]

Diagnosis

Diagnosis of fructose intolerance can be confirmed by a hydrogen breath test. The patient consumes a drink made of water containing a known amount of fructose powder dissolved in it. For the next 2 hours, the amount of hydrogen in the person's breath is measured every 15 minutes by having him or her breathe into a tube attached to a measuring device.

If the fructose is not carried across the digestive tract lining and transported into circulation (which is what happens in people without fructose malabsorption), it moves into the large bowel, where it is fermented by the resident microorganisms. A major product of fermentation is hydrogen. The hydrogen produced by fructose fermentation passes from the bowel into circulation, is removed in the lungs, and finally excreted in the breath. This method of testing is often used to diagnose lactose intolerance, but malabsorption of any sugar can be tested in the same way.

However, the problem with this method of testing for fructose intolerance is that if an excessive quantity of fructose is consumed, everyone will experience some degree of malabsorption and will develop loose stool and an increase in breath hydrogen. Usually the quantity of fructose used in the test is 2 mg/kg body weight (that means a child of 15 kg would be tested with a dose of 30 mg of fructose in water). This is the amount of fructose that is usually tolerated by most people who do not have clinical fructose malabsorption.

Inherited Conditions Causing Fructose Intolerance

Although many people, especially children, develop loose stool and diarrhea after consuming a high dose of fructose, there are inherited conditions in which metabolism of fructose is impaired and that require more careful avoidance of all sources of fructose. This may include avoidance of sucrose, sorbitol, and the polymerized forms of fructose listed above, depending on the mechanism of the deficiency. These diseases are more accurately described as inborn errors of metabolism, and are relatively rare.[10] Diagnosis and treatment typically takes place in a specialized clinic staffed by specially trained doctors, registered dietitians, nurses, and other health care practitioners. The most well-known conditions include fructose-1,6-bisphosphatase deficiency, hereditary fructose intolerance, and essential fructosuria.

Fructose-1, 6-Bisphosphatase Deficiency

Inheritance is through an autosomal recessive gene,[11] and the worldwide incidence of the condition is unknown. The enzyme deficiency leads to the accumulation of certain amino acids, lactic acid, and ketoacids. Symptoms include fasting hypoglycemia, ketosis, and acidosis. It can be fatal to newborns. Infections and other fever-inducing illnesses can trigger episodes throughout life.

Hereditary Fructose Intolerance

The inheritance of hereditary fructose intolerance is through an autosomal recessive gene.[12] The condition is due to a deficiency in the enzyme aldolase B. The disease was first recognized in Switzerland, where the incidence has been estimated to be 1 in 20,000 births. The incidence in adults is unknown.[13]

The condition is first noticed in infancy, usually after the first feeding of fruit juice or fruit. Symptoms include hypoglycemia, sweating, tremor, confusion, nausea, vomiting, abdominal cramping pain, and in extreme cases, convulsions and coma. Prolonged consumption of fructose can lead to degeneration of renal function, resulting in cirrhosis and mental deterioration. Ingestion of more than a very small amount of fructose or sucrose results in symptoms.

Diagnosis can be confirmed by a fall in blood glucose 5 to 40 minutes after giving 250 mg/kg body weight of fructose by intravenous delivery. Liver biopsy shows the absence of the enzyme. Treatment involves the strict avoidance of dietary fructose, sucrose, and sorbitol.

Essential Fructosuria

This condition is characterized by a deficiency in an enzyme called *fructokinase*, which results in excretion of fructose in the urine.[14] It is inherited as an autosomal recessive gene, and the incidence has been estimated to be 1 in 130,000. Since the fructose is excreted in blood and urine, there is no effect of excess fructose in the digestive tract, and the condition is usually asymptomatic. Treatment is typically not required, but a false diagnosis of diabetes mellitus might occur due to the high level of fructose in the blood.

Management of Fructose Intolerance

Management of fructose intolerance involves reducing the intake of foods that contain fructose.[15] A fructose-restricted diet inevitably means limiting the consumption of fruit, especially those with a high fructose-to-glucose ratio. Table 24.1 provides information on the levels of natural fructose and glucose in common foods. It is usually only necessary to avoid the fruits and foods that contain considerably more fructose than glucose. The worst culprits are:

■ Apple
■ Pear
■ Cherry
■ Black currant
■ Watermelon
■ Honey
■ High fructose corn syrup

Grapes and the raisins derived from them are sometimes listed as a "high fructose fruit," but levels of fructose vary between varieties of grapes and methods of measuring fructose. Furthermore, where there is a difference between glucose and fructose content, it is relatively small (see Table 24.1).

Fruits with approximately the same levels of glucose and fructose may be tolerated when they are eaten in *small to moderate quantities*. However, if a large amount of fruit is consumed, the amount of fructose released from sucrose may exceed the overall ability of the system to transport it efficiently across the digestive lining. Unabsorbed fructose then moves into the large bowel and causes the symptoms previously described. In addition, the sugar content of a fruit will change with the degree of ripeness; the riper the fruit, the more likely a person will react to it.

Some practitioners suggest a limit of fructose consumption to reduce the possibility of symptom development in GI disorders such as IBS (see FODMAPS diet earlier). A 2010 review[3] suggests the following should be avoided:

■ Foods and beverages containing greater than 0.5 g fructose in excess of glucose per 100 g
■ Greater than 3 g fructose in an average serving quantity regardless of glucose intake
■ Greater than 0.2 g of fructans per serving

Following these expanded guidelines, the foods listed in Box 24.1 are likely to be problematic. Fruit juices are more of a problem than the whole fruit, because the sugar tends to be concentrated in the juice, which will then have a higher level of fructose than the whole fruit. It is always wise to dilute all fruit juices in a 1:1 ratio for children younger than 7 years.

Fructose malabsorption is an individual characteristic. The level of fruit or juice that each person can tolerate will probably require some experimentation with different fruits and different quantities of each.

A practical approach to determining the foods involved in individual cases is to start by limiting the foods with a high fructose-to-glucose ratio (Table 24.1). If the symptoms do not resolve, increase the restrictions to include foods in Box 24.1.

> **BOX 24.1 Foods Likely to Be Problematic in Fructose Intolerance**[a]
>
> Apple
> Black currant
> Cherry
> Pear
> Raisins
> Watermelon
> Royal jelly
> Honey
> High fructose corn syrup

[a]The foods listed in this box have a high fructose-to-glucose ratio and should be avoided by people on a fructose-restricted diet. Foods with a low fructose-to-glucose ratio (ie, those with a ratio that is close to 1:1) need not be avoided.

Since fruit is an important source of vitamin C, supplementary vitamin C may be necessary for individuals following a low-fructose diet. This is especially important for children, who have the most frequent problem with fructose intolerance. Consult the Dietary Reference Intakes to identify daily requirements for healthy individuals.

Additional Sources of Fructose

Fructose is sweeter than sucrose and much sweeter than glucose. Hence, fructose is sometimes added to reduced-calorie foods to increase the sweet taste, without the extra calories of sucrose that would be required to give the same amount of sweetness.

Fructose is often used in foods recommended for diabetics to provide sweetness, while avoiding the insulin-dependent mechanisms required for metabolism of glucose. These additional sources of fructose need to be avoided by people who have a problem with the absorption of fructose.

Fructose on Product Labels

There are no government regulations requiring fructose to be identified on a product label in the way an allergen is listed. If fructose is included in a product, it may appear on a food label as:

■ Fructose
■ Fruit sugar
■ Levulose

References

1. Gaby AR. Adverse effects of dietary fructose. *Altern Med Rev.* 2005;10:294-306.

2. Gibson PR, Shepherd SJ. Personal view: food for thought—Western lifestyle and susceptibility to Crohn's disease. The FODMAP hypothesis. *Aliment Pharmacol Ther.* 2005;21:1399-1409.

3. Gibson PR, Shepherd SJ. Evidence-based dietary management of functional gastrointestinal symptoms: the FODMAP approach. *J Gastroenterol Hepatol.* 2010;25(2):252-258.

4. Helliwell PA, Richardson M, Affleck J, Kellett GL. Stimulation of fructose transport across the intestinal brush-border membrane by PMA is mediated by GLUT2 and dynamically regulated by protein kinase C. *Biochem J.* 2000;350:149-154.

5. David TJ. *Food and Food Additive Intolerance in Childhood.* Boston, MA: Blackwell Scientific Publications; 1993:164.

6. US Department of Agriculture. National Nutrient Database Release 20. September 2007. http://www.ars.usda.gov/SP2UserFiles/Place/12354500/Data/SR20/SR20_doc.pdf. Accessed April 25, 2012.

7. Gibson PR, Newnham E, Barrett JS, Shepherd SJ, Muir JG. Review article: fructose malabsorption and the bigger picture. *Aliment Pharmacol Ther.* 2006;25:349-363.

8. Beyer PL, Caviar EM, McCallum RW. Fructose intake at current levels in the United States may cause gastrointestinal distress in normal adults. *J Am Diet Assoc.* 2005;105:1559-1566.

9. van Nieuwenhoven MA, Brouns F, Kovacs EMR. The effect of two sports drinks and water on GI complaints and performance during an 18-km run. *Int J Sports Med.* 2005;26:281-285.

10. Mayatepek E, Hoffmann B, Meissner T. Inborn errors of carbohydrate metabolism. *Best Pract Res Clin Gastroenterol.* 2010;24(5):607-618.

11. Asberg C, Hjalmarson O, Alm J, Martinsson T, Waldenström J, Hellerud C. Fructose 1,6-bisphosphatase deficiency: enzyme and mutation analysis performed on calcitriol-stimulated monocytes with a note on long-term prognosis. *J Inherit Metab Dis.* 2010. [Epub ahead of print.]

12. Boutelda N, Timson DJ. The biochemical basis of hereditary fructose intolerance. *J Inherit Metab Dis.* 2010;33:105-112.

13. Yasawy MI, Folsch UR, Schmidt WE, Schwend M. Adult hereditary fructose intolerance. *World J Gastroenterol.* 2009;15:2412-2413.

14. Asipu A, Hayward BE, O'Reilly J, Bonthron DT. Properties of normal and mutant recombinant human ketohexokinases and implications for the pathogenesis of essential fructosuria. *Diabetes.* 2003;52(9):2426-2432.

15. Shepherd SJ, Gibson PR. Fructose malabsorption and symptoms of irritable bowel syndrome: guidelines for effective dietary management. *J Am Diet Assoc.* 2006;106(10):1631-1639.

CHAPTER **25**

Benzoate Intolerance

Benzoic acid, sodium, potassium, calcium benzoate, and various forms of these chemicals are used in many different manufactured food products. They have a wide range of uses, such as keeping food free from contaminating microorganisms, preserving food color, and preventing separation of oils and water (emulsifying). In addition, benzoates occur naturally in some foods, such as berries, prunes, tea, and cinnamon.

For most people, benzoates pose no threat and cause no adverse symptoms even when eaten in relatively high doses.[1] The International Programme on Chemical Safety found no adverse effects in humans at doses of 647 to 825 mg per kg of body weight per day in processed foods.[2]

Acceptable daily intakes were established by the World Health Organization to be 5 mg/kg for benzyl alcohol, benzoic acid, and sodium benzoate.[1] However, a small group of people do react adversely to benzoates and develop a range of symptoms that sometimes mimic allergy. Recently, benzoates have been implicated, together with certain food-coloring agents, as triggers of hyperactivity in children.[3] This is discussed in more detail in Chapter 45.

Adverse Reactions to Benzoates

Although benzoate sensitivity is not an allergy and is not triggered by a response of the immune system, reactions to benzoates are often allergy-like in character. They often cannot be distinguished clinically from an IgE-mediated response. The following symptoms have been reported by people sensitive to benzoates:[4,5]

- Asthma
- Urticaria (hives)
- Angioedema (tissue swelling)
- Rhinitis (nasal congestion such as hay fever)

- ▩   Atopic dermatitis (eczema)
- ▩   Contact dermatitis
- ▩   Cutaneous vasculitis
- ▩   Headaches

The chronic inflammatory disorder *orofacial granulomatosis* (OFG), with symptoms of lip swelling and involvement of other areas of the oral cavity, has been reported in several studies to respond positively to a diet that excludes all sources of cinnamon and benzoates.[6] Subjects exhibited positive patch tests to cinnamon and benzoate. The authors recommend a benzoate-restricted diet as a first line treatment for the condition.

People who have immediate-onset IgE-mediated hypersensitivity reactions (allergy) such as respiratory tract symptoms, including asthma, or skin reactions such as hives and eczema may be particularly vulnerable to benzoate sensitivity. Benzoate does not trigger allergy but may exacerbate an existing allergy.

Benzoic acid can act as a mild irritant to the skin, eyes, and mucous membranes. Its adverse effects often increase when combined with other additives.[7]

Mechanism of Action

The mechanism of adverse reactions to benzoate is unknown, but evidence suggests that the cyclooxygenase pathway of arachidonic acid metabolism may be affected (see Chapter 1 for details of this pathway). People sensitive to acetylsalicylic acid (aspirin) are particularly vulnerable to benzoate sensitivity.[8]

Diagnosis and Laboratory Tests

There is no definitive diagnostic test for benzoate intolerance. The following process is helpful in diagnosing benzoate intolerance as a cause for a person's symptoms:

- ▩   A clear and detailed clinical history of the patient is essential.
- ▩   A detailed food and symptom record that indicates symptoms typical of benzoate intolerance when the patient consumes benzoate-rich foods.
     A reaction following intake of cinnamon is highly suggestive of benzoate sensitivity, as cinnamon contains a high level of natural benzoate.
- ▩   Elimination of benzoates from the diet for a period of 4 weeks, followed by challenge with benzoate-rich foods will determine benzoate sensitivity.
- ▩   Patch testing with benzoate when contact dermatitis to benzoate is suspected.

Information on Specific Benzoates in Foods

Benzoic Acid and Sodium Benzoate

Both benzoic acid and sodium benzoate are used to prevent spoilage by microorganisms in a wide variety of processed foods, beverages, and pharmaceuticals, thus extending their shelf life.

Benzoic acid is a common ingredient in flavorings (specifically, chocolate, lemon, orange, cherry, fruit, nut, and tobacco) that are used in carbonated and noncarbonated beverages, ice cream, ices, candies, baked goods, pie and pastry fillings, icings, and chewing gum. It may also be used in pickles and margarines. Concentration as a preservative is limited by the U.S. Food and Drug Administration to 0.1% by weight.[1]

Benzoic acid occurs naturally in foods at varying levels (Table 25.1). High levels occur in:

■ Most berries, especially strawberries and raspberries
■ Prunes
■ Tea
■ Spices and herbs such as cinnamon, cloves, nutmeg, and thyme
■ Cherry bark and cassia bark

TABLE 25.1
Benzoates: Examples of Their Sources and Use as Additives

Food Label Term (E-number)[a]	Natural Food Sources[b]	Foods That May Contain Benzoate as an Additive
Benzoic acid (E210)	Edible berries, especially cranberries, raspberries, strawberries	Jam
		Dessert sauces
	Stone fruits, especially apricots, cherries, nectarines, papaya, peaches, plums, prunes	Flavored syrups
		Fruit pulp and puree
	Citrus fruits, especially oranges, grapefruit	Fruit juice
		Concentrated fruit juice
	Vegetables: avocado, red beans, pumpkin, soy beans, spinach	Soft drinks (soda pop)
		Yogurt
	Other foods, spices, herbs, and beverages, such as honey, cinnamon, nutmeg, clove, pimento, thyme, tea (black and green)	Margarine
		Table olives
		Marinated fish (herring, mackerel)
		Pickles
		Salad dressing
		Flavored coffee
		Beer

Continues

TABLE 25.1

Benzoates: Examples of Their Sources and Use as Additives (*Continued*)

Food Label Term (E-number)[a]	Natural Food Sources[b]	Foods That May Contain Benzoate as an Additive
Sodium benzoate (E211)	No natural source	Caviar
		Cod
		Prawns
		Margarine
		Concentrated pineapple juice
		Fruit pies
		Cheesecake mix
		Jams and jellies
		Candies
		Soft drinks
		Oyster sauce
		Soy sauce
		Salad dressing
		Barbecue sauce
		Taco sauce
		Dill pickles
		Table olives
Potassium benzoate (E212)	No natural source	Margarine
		Table olives
		Dill pickles
		Concentrated pineapple juice
Calcium benzoate (E213)	No natural source	Concentrated pineapple juice
Ethyl 4-hydroxybenzoate (E214)	No natural source	Beer
		Cooked, packaged beet
		Coffee and chicory essence
Propyl 4-hydroxybenzoate (E216)	No natural source	Coloring dyes in solution
		Dessert sauces
		Flavored syrups
Methyl 4-hydroxybenzoate (E218)	No natural source	Frozen drink concentrates
		Fruit-based pie fillings
		Fruit pulp or puree
		Glucose
		Marinated fish (herring and mackerel)
		Pickles
		Salad dressing

[a] E-numbers are used on food labels in the European Union to indicate the type of food additive.
[b] For a more comprehensive list of foods containing natural benzoates, see Table 25.2.

Sodium benzoate may be used as a preservative in margarine, codfish, bottled soft drinks, maraschino cherries, mincemeat, fruit juices, pickles, fruit jelly preserves, and jams. In addition, it may be added to the ice used for cooling fish and may be an ingredient in eye creams, vanishing creams, and toothpastes.

When ingested, benzoic acid and sodium benzoate are rapidly absorbed. On reaching the liver, they combine with the amino acid glycine and are excreted. The metabolization process proceeds as follows:[9]

■ Benzoic acid and sodium benzoate are rapidly absorbed through the intestine and transported to the liver.

■ Benzoate is converted to a thioester with coenzyme A (CoA) to form benzoyl-CoA in the mitochondria and other sites within the liver:

$$\text{Benzoic acid} + \text{CoA} \rightarrow \text{benzoyl-CoA} + \text{water}$$

■ Benzoyl-CoA then reacts with glycine to form hippuric acid, which is excreted in urine:

$$\text{Benzoyl-CoA} + \text{glycine} \rightarrow \text{hippuric acid} + \text{CoA}$$

The success of this process depends on a healthy functioning liver and a sufficient nutritional supply of glycine.

Benzoyl Peroxide

Benzoyl peroxide is used primarily as a bleaching agent in the manufacture of white flour, some cheeses (especially blue cheeses, such as Gorgonzola), and lecithin. Lecithin is derived from soy, safflower, or corn oil by solvent extraction. The lecithin is then bleached by hydrogen peroxide and benzoyl peroxide and dried by heating. It is used as an emulsifier in manufactured foods containing fats and oils. Its action is improved when benzoyl peroxide, hydrogen peroxide, acetic or lactic acid, or sodium hydroxide is added to produce hydroxylated lecithin, which disperses more readily in water and acts as a better emulsifier than pure lecithin.

Certain vitamins can be destroyed by adding benzoyl peroxide to food. Where the loss could be significant, such as in the destruction of beta carotene in milk, U.S. government regulations require that the vitamin be replaced, such as in the addition of vitamin A to cheese made from bleached milk.

Most benzoyl peroxide added to food has been converted to benzoic acid by the time the food is eaten. Only a small fraction of the bleach is ingested, most of which is converted in the intestine to benzoic acid or a similar product that is metabolized as described previously and readily excreted in the urine.

Benzyl and Benzoyl Compounds

A large number of benzyl and benzoyl compounds are allowed in foods—for example, benzyl acetate, benzyl alcohol, benzyl ether, benzyl butyrate, benzyl cinnamate, benzyl formate, benzyl propionate, and benzyl salicylate.[10] On food labels, this ingredient will include the word *benzyl* or *benzoyl*. Most of these compounds are used as synthetic flavorings in a wide variety of processed and manufactured foods, beverages, and chewing gum, and are also used to provide scents for soaps, hair spray, hair dye, skin cream, sunscreen, perfume, and cosmetics.

Some of these compounds are skin irritants and can cause hives and contact dermatitis. Others are digestive tract irritants and can cause intestinal upset, vomiting, and diarrhea, and in very high concentrations can have a narcotic effect. A few irritate the eyes and cause respiratory symptoms when inhaled.

Parabens

Parabens, a class of derivatives of benzoic acid, are sometimes used as preservatives in foods. People who are sensitive to benzoates may also react to parabens because parabens metabolism mimics that of benzoates in the later stages. There are no naturally occurring parabens. On food labels, parabens will be indicated by the term *methyl p-hydroxybenzoate* or *propyl p-hydroxybenzoate*.

Parabens are used in processed fruits and vegetables, baked goods, fats, oils, and seasonings. They may be present in foods such as cakes, pies, pastries, icings, fillings, fruit products (eg, sauces, juices, fruit salads, syrups, preserves, jellies), syrups, olives, pickles, beer, cider, and carbonated beverages.

Management of Benzoate Sensitivity

People differ in their sensitivity to chemicals like benzoates. Consequently, it is impossible to define a limit of benzoate intake that applies to all people intolerant of benzoate. The general recommendation is to reduce benzoate intake by avoiding foods known to contain natural and added benzoates. Therefore, people sensitive to benzoate should avoid:

▪ Natural sources of benzoic acid (see Table 25.1)
▪ Any processed foods containing benzoic acid or sodium benzoate (read labels carefully) (see Table 25.1)
▪ Bleached flour
▪ Products containing hydrolyzed lecithin such as margarine, salad and cooking oils, frozen desserts, chocolate, and baked goods

Table 25.2 lists the levels of benzoates in a variety of natural food sources.[11,12] Not all foods have been analyzed for levels of benzoates. This table should be used to:

- Select foods suitable for a food challenge to confirm benzoate intolerance
- Determine a person's limit of tolerance by dosage
- Develop a benzoate-restricted diet based on individual needs and preferences

TABLE 25.2
Level of Benzoates in Selected Natural Foods[a]

Food	Benzoates, mg/kg	Serving Size	Benzoates, mg/serving
Fruits			
Strawberry	13.9	½ cup	1.04
Navel orange	2.3	1 medium	0.32
Peach	2.7	1 medium	0.24
Papayas	1.5	½ medium	0.23
Nectarine	1.3	1 medium	0.18
Avocado	1.7	½ medium	0.15
Grapefruit	0.7	½ medium	0.09
Cherry	1.1	10 cherries	0.08
Valencia orange	0.6	1 medium	0.07
Quince	0.7	1 medium	0.06
Mandarin orange	0.5	½ cup	0.06
Pomegranate	0.3	1 medium	0.05
Plum	0.4	1 medium	0.03
Watermelon	0.3	½ cup	0.02
Banana	0.2	1 medium	0.02
Lemon	0.7	½ medium	0.02
Fig	0.2	5 figs	0.02
Lime	0.4	½ medium	0.01
Pineapple	0.1	½ cup	0.007
Kumquat	0.4	1 medium	0.007
Kiwi	0	1 medium	0
Grape	0	½ cup	0
Japanese pear	0	1 small	0
Persimmon	0	2 medium	0
Apple	0	1 medium	0

Continues

TABLE 25.2

Level of Benzoates in Selected Natural Foods (*Continued*)

Food	Benzoates, mg/kg	Serving Size	Benzoates, mg/serving
Beans and Grains			
Soy bean	1.9	½ cup	0.19
Red bean	1.8	½ cup	0.18
Rice	0.4	½ cup	0.05
Barley	0.3	½ cup	0.03
Corn	0.2	½ cup	0.02
Wheat	0.3	½ cup	0.02
Nuts and Seeds			
Walnut	1.2	8 to 10 halves	0.02
Pistachio	0.5	30 nuts	0.01
Almond	0.4	12 to 15 nuts	0.01
Sesame seed	0.6	1 Tbsp	0.005
Hazelnut	0.3	10 to 12 nuts	0.005
Cashew	0.3	6 to 8 nuts	0.005
Spices, Herbs, and Condiments			
Cinnamon	336	1 tsp	0.67
Soy sauce	8.9	1 Tbsp	0.16
Nutmeg	44.1	1 tsp	0.09
Worcestershire sauce	4.9	1 Tbsp	0.07
Clove	28.1	1 tsp	0.06
Pimento	14.1	1 tsp	0.03
Light soy sauce	1.4	1 Tbsp	0.03
Celery seed	8.9	1 tsp	0.02
Tomato ketchup	1.1	1 Tbsp	0.02
Thyme	15.9	1 tsp	0.02
Cayenne pepper	7.0	1 tsp	0.01
Black pepper	4.7	1 tsp	0.01
Mustard seed	5.0	1 tsp	0.01
Coriander	3.2	1 tsp	0.01
Cumin	3.2	1 tsp	0.01
White pepper	2.6	1 tsp	0.01
Paprika	2.3	1 tsp	0.01
Parsley	0.6	1 Tbsp	0.01
Bay leaf	4.3	1 tsp	0.004
Garlic	0.8	1 tsp	0.002

Continues

TABLE 25.2
Level of Benzoates in Selected Natural Foods (*Continued*)

Food	Benzoates, mg/kg	Serving Size	Benzoates, mg/serving
Vegetables			
Pumpkin	1.4	½ cup	0.14
Spinach	1	3½ oz	0.1
Chinese cabbage	0.7	1 cup	0.04
Carrots	0.3	1 large	0.03
Tomato	0.2	1 small	0.02
Radish	0.1	5 small	0.01
Broccoli	0	½ cup	0
Potato	0	1 medium	0
Cabbage	0	1 cup	0
Lettuce	0	3½ oz	0
Celery	0	½ cup or 1 stalk	0
Cauliflower	0	½ cup	0
Onion	0	1 Tbsp	0

[a] In each food category, benzoate levels are listed from highest to lowest per serving size.

Source: Data are from Heimhuber B, Herrmann K. Benzoe-, Phenylessig-, 3-Phenylpropan- und Zimtsäure sowie Benzoylglucosen in einigen Obst- und Fruchtgemüsearten. *Deutsche Lebensmittel-Rundschau* 1990;86: Jahrg. Heft 7 [article in German]; and Ishiwata H, Nishijima M, Fukasawa, Ito Y, Yamada T. Evaluation of preservatives contents in foods and the daily intake deduced from the results of the official inspection in Japan in F.Y. 1994. *J Food Hyg Soc Jpn*. 1997;38:145-154.

References

1. Nair B. Final report on the safety assessment of benzyl alcohol, benzoic acid, and sodium benzoate. *Int J Toxicol*. 2001;(20 suppl 3):23-50.
2. Wibbertmann A, Kielhorn J, Koennecker G, Mangelsdorf I, Melber C; International Programme on Chemical Safety (IPCS), a joint venture of the United Nations Environment Programme (UNEP), the International Labour Organization (ILO), and the World Health Organization (WHO). *Concise International Chemical Assessment Document 26: Benzoic Acid and Sodium Benzoate*. Geneva, Switzerland: World Health Organization; 2000.
3. Bateman B, Warner JO, Hutchinson E, et al. The effects of a double blind, placebo controlled, artificial food colourings and benzoate preservative challenge on hyperactivity in a general population sample of preschool children. *Arch Dis Child*. 2004;89:506-511.
4. Farenholz JM, Keegan MS. Adverse reactions to benzoates and parabens. In: Metcalfe D, Sampson H, Simon RA, eds. *Food Allergy: Adverse Reactions to Foods and Food Additives*. 4th ed. Malden, MA: Blackwell Science; 2008:394-402.
5. Pacor ML, Di Lorenzo G, Martinelli N, et al. Monosodium benzoate hypersensitivity in subjects with persistent rhinitis. *Allergy*. 2004;59(2):192-197.
6. White A, Nunes C, Escudier M, et al. Improvement in orofacial granulomatosis on a cinnamon- and benzoate-free diet. *Inflamm Bowel Dis*. 2006;12(6):508-514.
7. Haapasaari K, Niinimaki A. Allergic contact dermatitis from alkylammonium amidobenzoate (Osmaron B). *Contact Dermatitis*. 2001;44(2):133-134.

8. Worm M, Vieth W, Ehlers I, Sterry W, Zuberbier T. Increased leukotriene production by food additives in patients with atopic dermatitis and proven food intolerance. *Clin Exp Allergy*. 2001;31(2):265-273.

9. Jacobsen DW. Adverse reactions to benzoates and parabens. In: Metcalfe DD, Sampson HS, Simon RA, eds. *Food Allergy: Adverse Reactions to Foods and Food Additives*. 2nd ed. Cambridge, MA: Blackwell Science; 1997:375-386.

10. Winter R. *A Consumer's Dictionary of Food Additives*. 7th ed. New York, NY: Three Rivers Press; 2009:100-105.

11. Heimhuber B, Herrmann K. Benzoe-, Phenylessig-, 3-Phenylpropan- und Zimtsäure sowie Benzoylglucosen in einigen Obst- und Fruchtgemüsearten. *Deutsche Lebensmittel-Rundschau* 1990;86: Jahrg. Heft 7. [Article in German].

12. Ishiwata H, Nishijima M, Fukasawa, Ito Y, Yamada T. Evaluation of preservatives contents in foods and the daily intake deduced from the results of the official inspection in Japan in F.Y. 1994. *J Food Hyg Soc Jpn*. 1997;38:145-154.

CHAPTER **26**

Salicylate Intolerance

The only form of salicylate definitively demonstrated to trigger an adverse response is acetylsalicylic acid (ASA). This drug is known as *aspirin* in the United States, although this term is a registered trade name in Canada (Aspirin) and a few other countries. Salicylates, but not acetylsalicylic acid,[1] occur naturally in many foods. Research studies have not yet proven that food sources of salicylates cause adverse reactions even in persons sensitive to acetylsalicylic acid, but they are suspected.

Up to 25% of persons sensitive to acetylsalicylic acid also react adversely to the azo dye tartrazine (refer to Chapter 27), but it is not known whether the mechanism of action of the two chemicals is similar.[2] Sensitivity to acetylsalicylic acid has also been linked to sensitivities to benzoates and sulfites. Cross-reactivity between these substances has not yet been confirmed by research studies, but a similar mechanism of action is suspected.[3] (See "Mechanism of Action of Acetylsalicylic Acid" later in this chapter.)

The level of salicylic acid may be the determining factor in salicylate sensitivity. Dietary consumption of salicylate is estimated to be 10 to 200 mg daily,[4] whereas the usual dose in a regular aspirin is 325 mg; in extra-strength or arthritis pain relief aspirins, the dose is 600 to 650 mg of acetylsalicylic acid; and in a children's aspirin, it is 80 mg.

Absorption may also play a role in the amount of salicylate available. In a medication, ASA is in the "free form"—that is, it is not linked to another compound and is immediately available for action within the body. When the salicylate is in a food, it is complexed with many other compounds, so it will not become active until released in its free form, which will take a certain length of time and will reduce the body's immediate response to the chemical.

Symptoms Associated with Salicylate Intolerance

Sensitivity to acetylsalicylic acid (aspirin) is more common in persons with asthma. Aspirin sensitivity is estimated to be in a range of incidence of 2% to 23% of asthmatics, with sensitivity being more common in adults and rare in children.[5] However,

249

persons with asthma who are sensitive to acetylsalicylic acid can usually ingest the salicylates in foods without difficulty. No carefully controlled research has been undertaken to study how reducing dietary salicylates affects the course of asthma. Aspirin sensitivity has frequently been implicated in causing urticaria (hives) and angioedema (tissue swelling); respiratory symptoms, including rhinitis and possibly nasal polyps; and digestive tract disturbances.[4]

Some investigators have ascribed the hyperactivity experienced by some children to salicylate sensitivity,[6] but the role of salicylates in the attention-deficit hyperactivity disorder has not been proven by controlled studies. Recent studies indicate a role for benzoates and food dyes in triggering hyperactivity in children; salicylates were not implicated as triggers in these studies.[7]

Mechanism of Action of Acetylsalicylic Acid

The key event that leads to sensitivity to ASA is the same process that gives aspirin its ability to reduce pain. ASA inhibits the cyclooxygenase pathway of arachidonic acid metabolism; this is an important pathway in the production of some essential mediators that cause inflammation and that also contribute to the symptoms of allergy.[8]

In an allergic reaction, preformed inflammatory mediators are released from mast cells, which act on tissues to produce symptoms (see Chapter 1). In addition, some of these preformed mediators are enzymes that promote additional steps in the process. An essential enzyme in this respect is phospholipase A2. This enzyme breaks down phospholipids in cell membranes and releases arachidonic acid (AA) in the process. AA is a key 20-carbon chain omega-6 fatty acid that is the precursor (provides the building blocks) for more inflammatory mediators to augment the protective inflammatory response.

Two key enzyme pathways then act on AA to produce two groups of powerful inflammatory mediators: (a) the cyclooxygenase pathway that leads to the production of the prostanoids (prostaglandins; prostacyclins and thromboxane) and (b) the lipoxygenase pathway that leads to the production of leukotrienes. Each of these groups plays an extremely important role in body processes such as smooth muscle contraction and relaxation and in the widening and narrowing of blood vessels.

Some of these mediators also lead to symptoms such as pain (the prostaglandins) and the bronchospasm of asthma (the leukotrienes). A high level of leukotrienes is found in the inflamed tissues of allergic conditions in the skin such as eczema[9] and urticaria. Antileukotriene drugs are increasingly being used to treat these conditions.[10]

In the treatment of pain, reducing the level of the prostaglandins involved in the process is required. Aspirin achieves this by inhibiting the cyclooxygenase enzyme pathway which leads from AA to prostaglandins. Other analgesics—for example, ibuprofen, acetaminophen, and paracetamol—have a similar effect.

However, by inhibiting one enzyme pathway, a buildup of substrate (AA) leads to enhancement of the other. So inhibition of the cyclooxygenase pathway results in an increased production of leukotrienes via the lipoxygenase pathway. Leukotrienes cause the bronchoconstriction of asthma, thus explaining the observation that many

FIGURE 26.1

Salicylate effect on the level of secondary inflammatory mediators. Compare to release of secondary inflammatory mediators (see Chapter 1, Figure 1.2). Phospholipase A2 acts on cell membranes and releases arachidonic acid. Arachidonic acid is metabolized by two pathways: (a) the cyclooxygenase pathway and (b) the lipoxygenase pathway. The cyclooxygenase pathway produces the prostanoids, which include prostaglandins (PG_2), prostacyclin (PGI_2), and thromboxane (TX). The lipoxygenase pathway produces leukotrienes (LT_4), which include several different leukotrienes in a sequence (A, B, C, D), as shown by the arrows. Each of these mediators (prostanoids and leukotrienes) has different effects on body systems, as discussed in the text. Salicylic acid inhibits the cyclooxygenase pathway (lightning bolt). More of the substrate (arachidonic acid) is available; this causes an enhancement of the lipoxygenase pathway (block arrow), which results in an increase in leukotrienes and augments their effect on body systems as indicated by solid arrows.

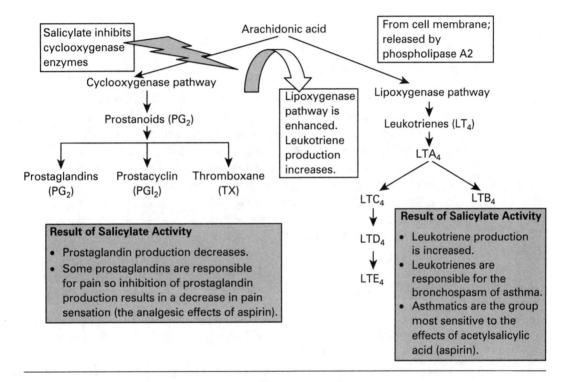

asthmatics are aspirin intolerant. (See Figure 26.1 for a pictorial representation of the process.) Research also indicates that an additional effect of the process is the release of histamine from mast cells and other granulocytes (eg, basophils, eosinophils, macrophages, platelets) in a non-immunologically mediated reaction.[4,11]

Diagnosis and Management of Salicylate Intolerance

There are no laboratory tests available for diagnosing salicylate intolerance. A clear medical history and analysis of a food and symptom record that indicates symptom development following intake of salicylate-rich foods are the best indicators that a trial of elimination and challenge of salicylates would be worthwhile.

A diagnosed sensitivity to aspirin is sometimes taken as a sign of possible salicylate sensitivity. However, because the levels of salicylic acid in aspirin and foods are so different (see earlier discussion), it is not valid to assume that an aspirin-sensitive person requires a salicylate-restricted diet.

Some practitioners in the field of food intolerance[4] believe that, although avoiding foods high in salicylates is unlikely to diminish the symptoms of most persons sensitive to acetylsalicylic acid, a salicylate-restricted diet may benefit those individuals who have a pronounced sensitivity and achieve no relief from other treatment modalities. Since salicylate intolerance, as in all food intolerances (as opposed to food allergies), is dose-related, it is probably sufficient that a person with suspected salicylate sensitivity avoid foods with the highest levels of salicylate.

Sensitivity to Ingredients with Similar Reactivity to Salicylates

The symptoms that develop from sensitivity to benzoates, azo dyes, and sulfites are often indistinguishable from those resulting from salicylate intolerance, because the mechanism of action of these substances is quite similar.[3] Frequently, salicylate sensitivity has been blamed when the sensitivity is actually to one or more of these other food components. Since a low-salicylate diet is so restrictive and may pose unnecessary nutritional risk, it is often a worthwhile exercise to restrict benzoates, azo dyes, and sulfites (predominantly foods with artificial food additives) for a time-limited trial before complete salicylate avoidance is attempted. For information on these sensitivities, refer to Chapters 21, 25, and 27.

Food Sources of Salicylates

Salicylates are a natural component of a wide range of food plants. It would be extremely difficult, if not impossible, to formulate a nutritionally adequate diet by avoiding *all* foods that contain salicylate.

Several researchers have developed tables to indicate the level of salicylate in foods.[12–14] However, the reported levels are not entirely consistent between data banks, because the level of salicylate in a food will vary according to plant variety, conditions in the growing environment, and methods of analysis in the laboratory.

Furthermore, the level of salicylate detected in the body (by analysis of a research subject's serum) varies, probably depending on individual absorption patterns and metabolism of salicylate within the body.[4,15,16] There is still a great deal to learn before we can diagnose and manage either aspirin or salicylate intolerance effectively.

Some foods have consistently lower levels of salicylates than others. Table 26.1 indicates those with relatively high and low levels. A more complete list of salicylate levels in foods compiled from several published sources is provided in Table 26.2.[12–14]

TABLE 26.1

Comparative Levels of Salicylates in Foods

Food Category	Restricted Foods (High Salicylate Content)	Allowed Foods (Low Salicylate Content)
Herbs	Mint	Poppy seed
	Thyme	Chives (fresh)
	Tarragon	Parsley
	Rosemary	
	Dill	
	Sage	
	Oregano	
	Marjoram	
	Basil	
	Celery seed	
	Sesame seed	
Spices	Aniseed	Saffron (dry powder)
	Cayenne	
	Cinnamon	
	Cumin	
	Curry powder	
	Fenugreek	
	Mace	
	Mustard	
	Paprika	
	Turmeric	
Fruits	Most (especially high levels in pineapple, apricot, raspberry, loganberry, cherry, date, dried currant, raisin)	Banana
		Pear (peeled)
		Pomegranate
		Mango
		Papaya
		Golden delicious apple
Vegetables	Most (especially high levels in cucumber, olives, endive, potato skin, sweet corn, sweet potato)	Cabbage (green)
		Cabbage (red)
		Brussels sprout
		Bean sprout
		Celery
		Leek
		Lettuce
		Pea
		Potato (skin has a high level)

Continues

TABLE 26.1
Comparative Levels of Salicylates in Foods (*Continued*)

Food Category	Restricted Foods (High Salicylate Content)	Allowed Foods (Low Salicylate Content)
		Bamboo shoot (canned)
		Chayote squash
		Shallot
Nuts	Almond	Cashew
	Brazil nut	
	Macadamia nut	
	Peanut	
	Pine nut	
	Pistachio	
	Walnut	
	Water chestnut	
	Coconut	
Beverages	Coffee	Gin
	Tea	Vodka
	Cola	Whiskey
	Peppermint tea	Cocoa (powder)
	Fruit juice	Decaffeinated coffee powder
	Most alcoholic drinks	Ovaltine powder
		Camomile herbal tea (bag)
Sweeteners and candies	Honey	Granulated sugar
	Licorice	Maple syrup
	Peppermint candy	
Flavorings, condiments, and sauces	Yeast-rich products	Soy sauce
	Marmite	Malt vinegar
	Stock cubes	
	Tomato sauce	
	Worcestershire sauce	
Meats, fish, and egg	None	Meat
		Fish
		Shellfish
		Egg
Milk and milk products	None	Milk
		Cheese
Grains	None	Wheat
		Rye
		Oats
		Barley
		Rice

Continues

TABLE 26.1
Comparative Levels of Salicylates in Foods (*Continued*)

Food Category	Restricted Foods (High Salicylate Content)	Allowed Foods (Low Salicylate Content)
Dried peas and beans (legumes)	Broad bean (fava bean)	Yellow split pea
		Brown bean
		Soy bean
		Mung bean
		Lima bean
		Green split pea
		Chickpea (garbanzo)
		Brown lentil
		Red lentil
		Black-eyed pea
Other	Processed foods	
	Instant (prepared) meals	

TABLE 26.2
Level of Salicylates in Some Commonly Eaten Foods and Beverages[a]

Food	Salicylate, mg/100 g	Serving Size	Salicylates, mg/serving
Vegetables (Fresh and Canned)			
Asparagus, fresh	4	½ cup (83 g)	3.32
Green pepper, fresh	1.2	1 large (100 g)	1.2
Mushroom, canned	1.26	¼ cup (90 g)	1.13
Endive, fresh leaves	1.9	10 (50 g)	0.95
Eggplant (with peel) fresh	0.88	½ cup (100 g)	0.88
Zucchini, fresh	1.04	½ cup (76 g)	0.79
Tomato, canned	0.53	½ cup (125 g)	0.66
Broccoli, fresh	0.65	1 stalk (100 g)	0.65
Baby squash, fresh	0.63	½ cup (100 g)	0.63
Red small radish, fresh	1.24	5 small (50 g)	0.62
Okra, canned	0.59	8–9 pods (100 g)	0.59
Spinach, fresh	0.58	3½ oz (100 g)	0.58
Chicory, fresh leaves	1.02	15–20 small (l50 g)	0.51
Potato (white), fresh	0.50	1 small (100 g)	0.5
Creamed corn, canned	0.39	½ cup (125 g)	0.49

Continues

TABLE 26.2
Level of Salicylates in Some Commonly Eaten Foods and Beverages (*Continued*)

Food	Salicylate, mg/100 g	Serving Size	Salicylates, mg/serving
Sweet potato, fresh	0.48	1 small (100 g)	0.48
Parsnip, fresh	0.45	½ cup (100 g)	0.45
Cucumber (no peel), fresh	0.78	½ medium (50 g)	0.39
Asparagus, canned	0.32	½ cup (100 g)	0.32
Mushroom, fresh	0.24	10 small (100 g)	0.24
Carrot, fresh	0.23	1 large (100 g)	0.23
Corn niblet, canned	0.26	½ cup (83 g)	0.22
Green olive, canned	1.29	2 medium (13 g)	0.17
Spinach, frozen	0.16	½ cup (100 g)	0.16
Green bean, fresh	0.11	½ cup (125 g)	0.14
Tomato, fresh	0.13	1 small (100 g)	0.13
Turnip, fresh	0.16	½ cup (76 g)	0.12
Pumpkin, fresh	0.12	2/5 cup (100 g)	0.12
Corn on the cob, fresh	0.12	½ cup (100 g)	0.12
Potato white with peel, fresh	0.12	1 medium (100 g)	0.12
Watercress, fresh	0.84	10 sprigs (10 g)	0.08
Red cabbage, fresh	0.08	1 cup shred (100 g)	0.08
Leek, fresh	0.08	3–4 medium (100 g)	0.08
Cauliflower, fresh	0.16	½ cup (50 g)	0.08
Brussels sprout, fresh	0.07	8 medium (100 g)	0.07
Black olive, canned	0.34	2 large (20 g)	0.07
Green pea, fresh	0.04	½ cup (67 g)	0.03
Onion, fresh	0.16	1 Tbsp (10 g)	0.02
Shallot, fresh	0.03	1¾ oz (50 g)	0.02
Chayote squash, fresh	0.01	½ medium (100 g)	0.01
Green cabbage, fresh	0	1 cup shred (100 g)	0
Celery, fresh	0	1 stalk (50 g)	0
Bamboo shoot, canned	0	1 cup (133 g)	0
Tomato Soup, Juice, Sauce, and Paste			
Heinz tomato sauce	2.28	2/5 cup (100 g)	2.48
Heinz tomato soup	0.54	1 cup (240 g)	1.29
Heinz tomato juice	0.12	½ cup (122 g)	0.15
Campbell tomato paste	0.57	1 Tbsp (15 g)	0.09
Dried Beans and Peas (Legumes)			
Broad (fava) bean	0.73	½ cup (112 g)	0.82
Yellow split pea	0.02	½ cup (125 g)	0.03

Continues

TABLE 26.2

Level of Salicylates in Some Commonly Eaten Foods and Beverages (*Continued*)

Food	Salicylate, mg/100 g	Serving Size	Salicylates, mg/serving
Brown bean	0.002	½ cup (112 g)	0.002
Soy bean	0	½ cup (112 g)	0
Mung bean	0	½ cup (112 g)	0
Lima bean	0	½ cup (112 g)	0
Green split pea	0	½ cup (112 g)	0
Chickpea (garbanzo)	0	½ cup (112 g)	0
Brown lentil	0	½ cup (112 g)	0
Red lentil	0	½ cup (112 g)	0
Black-eyed pea	0	½ cup (112 g)	0
Fruit: Fresh, Frozen, Canned, Dried, and Juiced			
Sultana raisin, dried	7.80	½ cup (76 g)	5.93
Letona prune, canned	6.87	5 medium (86 g)	5.91
Raisin, dried	6.62	½ cup (76 g)	5.03
Currant, dried	5.80	½ cup (72 g)	4.18
Date, dried	4.50	10 (83 g)	3.74
Blueberry, canned	2.76	½ cup (128 g)	3.53
Cherry, canned	2.78	½ cup (125 g)	3.48
Orange, fresh	2.39	1 medium (140 g)	3.35
Raspberry, fresh	5.14	½ cup (61 g)	3.14
Red currant, frozen	5.06	½ cup (56 g)	2.83
Apricot, fresh	2.58	3 medium (106 g)	2.74
Boysenberry, canned	2.04	½ cup (128 g)	2.61
Blackberry, canned	1.86	½ cup (128 g)	2.38
Raspberry, frozen	3.88	½ cup (61 g)	2.37
Black currant, frozen	3.06	½ cup (56 g)	1.71
Pineapple, canned	1.36	½ cup (125 g)	1.70
Strawberry, fresh	1.36	½ cup (125 g)	1.70
Pineapple, fresh	2.10	½ cup (78 g)	1.64
Ardmona apricot, canned	1.42	4 halves (90 g)	1.28
Tangelo, fresh	0.72	1 medium (170 g)	1.22
Guava, canned	2.02	½ cup (60 g)	1.21
Cantaloupe, fresh	1.50	½ cup (80 g)	1.20
Kalamata fig, dried	0.64	10 figs (187 g)	1.20
Grape juice	0.88	½ cup (126 g)	1.11
Red plum, canned	1.16	3 medium (95 g)	1.10

Continues

TABLE 26.2

Level of Salicylates in Some Commonly Eaten Foods and Beverages (*Continued*)

Food	Salicylate, mg/100 g	Serving Size	Salicylates, mg/serving
Cranberry sauce	1.44	¼ cup (69 g)	0.99
Sweet cherry, fresh	0.85	15 (102 g)	0.87
Grape, fresh	1.88	½ cup (46 g)	0.86
Peach, canned	0.68	½ cup (124 g)	0.84
Cranberry, canned	0.64	½ cup (50 g)	0.82
Granny Smith apple, fresh	0.59	1 medium (138 g)	0.81
Grapefruit, fresh	0.68	½ cup (118 g)	0.80
Mandarin orange, fresh	0.56	1 (135 g)	0.76
Nectarine, fresh	0.49	1 medium (136 g)	0.67
Ardmona apple, canned	0.55	½ cup (102 g)	0.56
Jonathan apple, fresh	0.38	1 medium (138 g)	0.52
Avocado, fresh	0.60	½ medium (87 g)	0.52
Grapefruit juice	0.42	½ cup (123 g)	0.52
Bartlett pear (with skin), fresh	0.31	1 medium (166 g)	0.52
Peach, fresh	0.58	1 medium (87 g)	0.51
Kiwi fruit, fresh	0.32	2 medium (152 g)	0.49
Packham pear (with skin), fresh	0.27	1 medium (166 g)	0.45
Red malaita grape, fresh	0.94	½ cup (46 g)	0.43
Watermelon, fresh	0.48	½ cup (80 g)	0.38
Sour cherry, canned	0.30	½ cup (125 g)	0.38
Lychee, canned	0.36	10 medium (100 g)	0.36
Red plum, fresh	0.21	2 medium (132 g)	0.28
Red delicious apple, fresh	0.19	1 medium (38 g)	0.26
Kadota fig, canned	0.25	3 figs (85 g)	0.21
Light seedless grape, canned	0.16	½ cup (128 g)	0.21
Pineapple juice	0.16	½ cup (125 g)	0.20
Fig, fresh	0.18	2 figs (100 g)	0.18
Persimmon, fresh	0.18	3 medium (75 g)	0.14
Green plum, fresh	0.095	2 medium (132 g)	0.13
Mango, fresh	0.11	½ medium (103 g)	0.11
Golden delicious apple, fresh	0.08	1 medium (138 g)	0.11
Pomegranate, fresh	0.07	1 medium (154 g)	0.11
Lemon, fresh	0.18	1 medium (58 g)	0.10
Rhubarb, fresh	0.13	½ cup (68 g)	0.09
Papaya, fresh	0.08	3½ oz (100 g)	0.08
Passion fruit, fresh	0.14	1 medium (18 g)	0.03

Continues

TABLE 26.2

Level of Salicylates in Some Commonly Eaten Foods and Beverages (*Continued*)

Food	Salicylate, mg/100 g	Serving Size	Salicylates, mg/serving
Packham pear (no skin)	0	1 medium fresh (166 g)	0
Letona bartlett pear	0	½ cup canned (125 g)	0
Banana, fresh	0	1 medium (114 g)	0
Nuts and Seeds			
Water chestnut, canned	2.92	8 medium (50 g)	1.46
Almond, fresh	3.0	12–15 (15 g)	0.45
Peanut, unshelled, fresh	1.12	1 oz (28 g)	0.31
Pistachio nut, fresh	0.55	30 nuts (15 g)	0.08
Macadamia nut, fresh	0.52	6 nuts (15 g)	0.08
Pine nut, fresh	0.51	2 Tbsp (15 g)	0.08
Brazil nut, fresh	0.46	4 medium (15 g)	0.07
Walnut, fresh	0.30	8–15 halves (15 g)	0.05
Peanut butter	0.23	1 Tbsp (15 g)	0.04
Sunflower seed, dry	0.12	3 Tbsp (28 g)	0.03
Desiccated coconut, dry	0.26	2 Tbsp (11 g)	0.03
Hazelnut, fresh	0.14	10–12 (15 g)	0.02
Sesame seed, dry	0.23	1 Tbsp (8 g)	0.02
Pecan nut, fresh	0.12	12 halves (15 g)	0.02
Cashew nut, fresh	0.07	6–8 (15 g)	0.01
Poppy seed, dry	0	1 tsp (3 g)	0
Seasonings			
Curry powder	218	1 tsp (2 g)	4.36
Hot paprika, dry powder	203	1 tsp (2 g)	4.06
Worcestershire sauce	64.3	1 tsp (5 g)	3.22
Dill, dry powder	94.4	1 tsp (2 g)	1.89
Thyme, dry leaves	183	1 tsp (1 g)	1.83
Tumeric, dry powder	76.4	1 tsp (2 g)	1.53
Rosemary, dry powder	68	1 tsp (2 g)	1.36
Garam masala, dry powder	66.8	1 tsp (2 g)	1.34
Oregano, dry powder	66	1 tsp (2 g)	1.32
Mixed herbs, dry leaves	55.6	1 tsp (2 g)	1.11
Cumin, dry powder	45.0	1 tsp (2 g)	0.90
Tarragon, dry powder	34.8	1 tsp (2 g)	0.70
Mace, dry powder	32.2	1 tsp (2 g)	0.64
Five spice, dry powder	30.8	1 tsp (2 g)	0.62
Fenugreek, dry powder	12.2	1 tsp (4 g)	0.49

Continues

TABLE 26.2
Level of Salicylates in Some Commonly Eaten Foods and Beverages (*Continued*)

Food	Salicylate, mg/100 g	Serving Size	Salicylates, mg/serving
Aniseed, dry powder	22.8	1 tsp (2 g)	0.46
Mustard, dry powder	26	1 tsp (1.5 g)	0.39
Cayenne, dry powder	17.6	1 tsp (2 g)	0.35
Cinnamon, dry powder	15.2	1 tsp (2 g)	0.30
Sage, dry leaves	21.7	1 tsp (1 g)	0.22
Celery, dry powder	10.1	1 tsp (2 g)	0.20
White vinegar, liquid	1.33	1 Tbsp (14 g)	0.19
Cardamom, dry powder	7.7	1 tsp (2 g)	0.15
Black pepper, dry powder	6.2	1 tsp (2 g)	0.12
Clove, whole dry	5.74	1 tsp (2 g)	0.12
Sweet paprika, dry powder	5.7	1 tsp (2 g)	0.11
Allspice, dry powder	5.2	1 tsp (2 g)	0.10
Mint, fresh	9.4	1 tsp (1 g)	0.09
Ginger root, fresh	4.5	1 tsp (2 g)	0.09
Caraway, dry powder	2.82	1 tsp (2 g)	0.06
Nutmeg, dry powder	2.4	1 tsp (2 g)	0.05
Red chili pepper, fresh	1.2	1 tsp (3 g)	0.04
Vegemite, spread	0.81	1 tsp (5 g)	0.04
Chili, dry powder	1.3	1 tsp (3 g)	0.04
Marmite, spread	0.71	1 tsp (5 g)	0.04
Dill, fresh	6.9	1 tsp (0.5 g)	0.04
Basil, dry powder	3.4	1 tsp (1 g)	0.03
Chili, dry flakes	1.38	1 tsp (2 g)	0.03
Bay leaf, dry leaves	2.52	1 tsp (1 g)	0.03
Horseradish, canned	0.18	1 Tbsp (18 g)	0.03
Green chili pepper, fresh	0.64	1 tsp (3 g)	0.02
Yellow-green chili pepper	0.62	1 tsp fresh (3 g)	0.02
Tabasco sauce	0.45	1 tsp (5 g)	0.02
White pepper, dry powder	1.1	1 tsp (2 g)	0.02
Fennel, dry powder	0.8	1 tsp (2 g)	0.02
Vanilla essence, liquid	1.44	1 tsp (1 g)	0.01
Coriander, fresh leaves	0.2	1 tsp (2 g)	0.004
Chives, fresh	0.031	1 Tbsp (10 g)	0.003
Parsley, fresh leaves	0.08	1 tsp (3 g)	0.002
Garlic, fresh	0.1	1 tsp (2 g)	0.002
Malt vinegar, liquid	0	1 Tbsp (14 g)	0

Continues

TABLE 26.2
Level of Salicylates in Some Commonly Eaten Foods and Beverages (*Continued*)

Food	Salicylate, mg/100 g	Serving Size	Salicylates, mg/serving
Soy sauce, liquid	0	1 Tbsp (18 g)	0
Saffron, dry powder	0	1 tsp (1 g)	0
Tandoori spice, dry powder	0	1 tsp (2 g)	0
Sweeteners			
Honey, liquid, assorted	2.2–11.24	1 Tbsp (20 g)	0.50–2.25
Molasses, liquid	0.22	1 Tbsp (20 g)	0.04
Golden syrup, liquid	0.10	1 Tbsp (20 g)	0.02
Camp maple syrup, liquid	0	1 Tbsp (20 g)	0
White granulated sugar	0	1 Tbsp (12 g)	0
Candy			
Licorice	7.96–9.78	20 g	1.59–1.96
Peppermint candy	0.77–7.58	3 pieces (12 g)	0.09–0.91
Lifesavers peppermint	0.86	5 pieces (10 g)	0.09
Pascall cream caramel	0.12	3 pieces (28 g)	0.03
Beverages			
Coca-Cola	0.25	½ cup (125 g)	0.31
Twinings lemon-scented tea	7.34	1 bag (1 g)	0.07
Tetley tea	5.57	1 bag (1 g)	0.06
Twinings Irish breakfast tea	3.89	1 bag (1 g)	0.04
Twinings Earl Grey tea	3	1 bag (1 g)	0.03
Twinings English breakfast tea	3	1 bag (1 g)	0.03
Burmese green tea	2.97	1 tsp leaves (1 g)	0.03
Indian green tea	2.97	1 tsp leaves (1 g)	0.03
Twinings orange pekoe tea	2.75	1 bag (1 g)	0.03
Twinings lapsang souchong tea	2.40	1 bag (1 g)	0.02
Old Chinese tea	1.9	1 tsp leaves (1 g)	0.02
Peony jasmine tea	1.9	1 tsp leaves (1 g)	0.02
Maxwell House instant coffee, powder	1	2 tsp (2 g)	0.02
Nescafé instant coffee, granules	0.59	2 tsp (2 g)	0.01
Peppermint herbal tea	1.10	1 bag (1 g)	0.01
Rose hip herbal tea	0.40	1 bag (1 g)	0.004
Fruit herbal tea	0.36	1 bag (1 g)	0.004
Camomile herbal tea	0.06	1 bag (1 g)	0
Cocoa, dry powder	0	1 Tbsp (21 g)	0
Carob, dry powder	0	1 Tbsp (21 g)	0
Nescafé decaf coffee	0	2 tsp powder (2 g)	0
Ovaltine, powder	0	3 heaping tsp (19 g)	0

Continues

TABLE 26.2
Level of Salicylates in Some Commonly Eaten Foods and Beverages (*Continued*)

Food	Salicylate, mg/100 g	Serving Size	Salicylates, mg/serving
Alcoholic Beverages			
Beer and ale	0.32–1.26	12 fl oz (360 g)	1.15–4.54
Benedictine liqueur	9.04	1 fl oz (28 g)	2.53
Champagne (1 example)	1.02	4 fl oz (120 g)	1.22
Port	1.4–4.2	1 fl oz (28 g)	0.39–1.18
Wine	035–0.90	4 fl oz (120 g)	0.42–1.08
Cider (sweet and dry)	0.16–0.19	12 fl oz (360 g)	0.58–0.68
Drambuie liqueur	1.68	1 fl oz (28 g)	0.47
Captain Morgan rum	1.28	1 fl oz (28 g)	0.36
Tia Maria liqueur	0.83	1 fl oz (28 g)	0.23
Cointreau liqueur	0.66	1 fl oz (28 g)	0.19
Sherry (sweet and dry)	0.46–0.56	1 fl oz (28 g)	0.13–0.16
Dry vermouth	0.46	1 fl oz (28 g)	0.13
Hennessy brandy	0.4	1 fl oz (28 g)	0.11
Smirnoff vodka	0	1 fl oz (28 g)	0
Johnnie Walker whiskey	0	1 fl oz (28 g)	0
Gilbey's gin	0	1 fl oz (28 g)	0

[a] In each food category, salicylate levels are listed from highest to lowest per serving size.

Source: Data are compiled from references 12, 13, and 14.

A salicylate-restricted diet should not be followed for longer than 4 weeks initially. After this time, sequential incremental dose challenge of salicylate-rich foods (see Table 26.1) should be undertaken to confirm salicylate intolerance.

References

1. Janssen PL, Katan MB, van Staveren WA, Hollman PC, Venema DP. Acetylsalicylate and salicylates in foods. *Cancer Lett.* 1997;19(1-2):163-164.
2. Ros AM, Juhlin L, Michaelsson G. A follow-up study of patients with recurrent urticaria and hypersensitivity to aspirin, benzoates and azo dyes. *Br J Dermatol.* 1976;96:19-24.
3. Juhlin L, Michaelsson G, Zetterstrom O. Urticaria and asthma induced by food and drug additives in patients with aspirin sensitivity. *J Allergy Clin Immunol.* 1972;50:92-98.
4. Baenkler HW. Salicylate intolerance. *Dtsch Arztebl Int.* 2008;105(8):137-142.
5. Obase Y, Matsuse H, Shimoda T, Haahtela T, Kohno S. Pathogenesis and management of aspirin-intolerant asthma. *Treat Respir Med.* 2005;4(5):325-336.
6. Feingold B. Hyperkinesis and learning disabilities linked to artificial food flavors and colors. *Am J Nurs.* 1975;75(5):797-803.

7. Bateman B, Warner JO, Hutchinson E, et al. The effects of a double blind, placebo controlled, artificial food colourings and benzoate preservative challenge on hyperactivity in a general population sample of preschool children. *Arch Dis Child.* 2004;89:506-511.

8. Willis AL, Smith DL. Metabolism of arachidonic acid. In: Cunningham FM, ed. *The Handbook of Immunopharmacology and Lipid Mediators.* London, UK: Academic Press; 1994:1-32.

9. Ruzicka T. Leukotrienes in atopic eczema. *Acta Derm Venereol Suppl (Stockh).* 1989; 144:48-49.

10. Nettis E, D'Erasmo M, Di Leo E, et al. The employment of leukotriene antagonists in cutaneous diseases belonging to allergological field. *Mediators Inflamm.* 2010; pii: 628171. Epub Sept 22, 2010.

11. Farooque S, Lee T. Mechanisms of aspirin-sensitive respiratory disease: a two component model. *Int Arch Allergy Immunol.* 2007;142:59-63.

12. Swain AR, Dutton S, Truswell AS. Salicylates in foods. *J Am Diet Assoc.* 1985; 85(5):950-960.

13. Margen S. *The Wellness Encyclopedia of Food and Nutrition.* New York, NY: Random House Press; 1992.

14. Pennington JAT, Douglass JS. *Bowe's and Church's Food Values of Portions Commonly Used.* 18th ed. Baltimore, MD: Lippincott Williams & Wilkins; 2005.

15. Blacklock CJ, Lawrence JR, Wiles D, et al. Salicylic acid in the serum of subjects not taking aspirin. Comparison of salicylic acid concentrations in the serum of vegetarians, non-vegetarians and patients taking low-dose aspirin. *J Clin Pathol.* 2001;54:553-555.

16. Baenkler M, Leykauf M, John S. Functional analysis of eicosanoids from white blood cells in sepsis and SIRS. *J Physiol Pharmacol.* 2006;57:25-34.

CHAPTER **27**

Intolerance of Tartrazine and Other Food Colors

Color is one of the most important aspects of food presentation. Unless foods are the right color, they are unacceptable to many people. As a result, various colors are added to manufactured foods to enhance their market appeal and consumption.

Most of the colors used in foods are considered "safe" (ie, they receive the Generally Recognized as Safe [GRAS] designation) and have not been cited as a cause of adverse reactions. However, tartrazine and some other azo (nitrogen-containing) dyes, such as sunset yellow (FD&C yellow #6), ponceau (FD&C red #4), and amaranth (FD&C red #5), have been implicated in adverse reactions. As a result, regulations in the United States require that artificial colors added to foods or medications should be listed separately on the product label.[1] In other countries, including Canada, this listing may be voluntary on the part of the manufacturer.

Tartrazine is a commonly used color all over the world, mainly for yellow, but it can also be used with brilliant blue FCF (FD&C Blue 1, E133) or green S (E142) to produce various green shades.

Conditions Caused by Tartrazine in Sensitive People

Tartrazine appears to cause the most frequently reported intolerance reactions of all the azo dyes, with urticaria and asthma being the most frequently reported symptoms,[2] particularly when there is also intolerance to aspirin.[3]

Tartrazine (FD&C #5) can cause symptoms resembling an allergic reaction. Tartrazine-sensitive individuals with asthma tend to experience triggering or exacerbation of asthma. A 1990 Cochrane review on the association between tartrazine and asthma concluded that although exclusion of tartrazine from the diet may not benefit most people with asthma, those who are actually sensitive to tartrazine would benefit from avoiding the food color in their diet and medications.[4] Other symptoms reported to be associated with tartrazine intolerance include urticaria (hives),[5] itching, nasal congestion and runny nose, blurred vision, purple patches on the skin, and migraine headaches.

Not all people with asthma, urticaria, and other symptoms previously listed react adversely to tartrazine and therefore will not benefit from avoiding dietary tartrazine. A 2010 study in Brazil reported that in their study population of 26 atopic adults with symptoms of allergic rhinitis, asthma, urticaria, or pseudo-allergic reactions to nonsteroidal anti-inflammatory drugs, none reacted adversely to tartrazine in double-blind, placebo-controlled, cross-over challenge.[6] However, the study population in this report is too small to draw any conclusions as to the effects of tartrazine in the population as a whole.

Tartrazine and five other food dyes, together with the preservative benzoate, have recently been implicated as triggers of hyperactivity in children.[7] For more information on this topic, see Chapter 45.

Symptoms caused by tartrazine sensitivity can occur by either ingestion or cutaneous exposure to a substance containing tartrazine.

Mechanism of Action of Tartrazine in Intolerance Reactions

There is no evidence that an immunologically mediated allergic reaction is involved in tartrazine sensitivity. However, tartrazine has been demonstrated to raise plasma histamine levels even in normal healthy adults when doses in excess of 50 mg are consumed.[8] It is thought that tartrazine triggers this rise as it initiates the release of histamine from mast cells by a non-immunologically mediated process.

Histamine-sensitive individuals with deficient levels of diamine oxidase (see Chapter 31 for details) react at much lower levels of tartrazine than subjects without histamine intolerance.[9] Some people who are sensitive to acetylsalicylic acid (aspirin) also experience an adverse reaction to tartrazine. It is unclear whether dietary salicylates, which are naturally present in a large number of foods (primarily fruits and vegetables), also are involved in this cross-reactivity (see Chapter 26 for more information on salicylates). Other azo dyes have also been implicated in adverse reactions.

Since tartrazine-induced symptoms are similar to those induced by acetylsalicylic acid, tartrazine might have an inhibitory effect on the cyclooxygenase pathway for converting arachidonic acid to prostanoids (see Chapter 26). However, this mechanism of action has not been proven.

Management of Tartrazine Intolerance

There are no diagnostic tests for tartrazine intolerance. The only way to determine a person's sensitivity to the food dye is to remove it from the diet for a trial period (ideally 4 weeks) and then reintroduce tartrazine-rich foods and monitor for the return of symptoms. Tartrazine and any other suspect food dyes can then be reintroduced to determine a person's sensitivity to them.

Double-blind placebo-controlled food challenge, although considered by many to be the "gold standard" for diagnosing food sensitivities (allergy and intolerance), does not work well for intolerance reactions to foods and food additives; tartrazine intolerance is no exception. A single dose is rarely adequate to induce a reaction, because the response depends on both a person's limit of tolerance and the level of the food component in the body at the time of testing.[10] Incremental buildup of the food component to a person's "reactive level" is the only effective way to determine a person's sensitivity to tartrazine. Details of sequential incremental dose challenge (SIDC) of food additives are discussed in more detail in Chapter 7.

Sources of Food Coloring Agents

Natural Sources

Many food colors are derived from natural sources:

- Saffron and turmeric as a source of yellow
- Beetroot as a red color
- Caramel from burned sugar as a brown color
- Titanium oxide as a white color
- Silver, gold, and aluminum as their natural colors
- Chlorophyll from green vegetables as a green color

These are not included as causes of food intolerance. However, certain sensitive people may experience an allergic reaction to the plant from which the color was derived. A much greater number of colors are derived synthetically from chemicals in the laboratory. These are the artificial food dyes.

Artificial Food Dyes

In the United States, the Food and Drug Administration (FDA) allows nine artificial colors derived from coal tar under the Food Dye and Coloring Act (FD&C; see Table 27.1.[1] Many other countries have similar regulations. In Canada, several colors are listed as "permitted" for use in foods (see Box 27.1[11] for the artificial food dyes in common use). In Britain and Europe, it is somewhat easier for the consumer to identify artificial ingredients on food labels, because an efficient system of numbering (E numbers) has been developed. Each food additive has a designated number, and a person who knows which food ingredient to avoid simply needs to identify their specific number on the label, which is much easier than looking through a long list of unpronounceable chemical terms. Table 27.2 provides a list of the most common artificial colors and their E numbers in the European labeling system. Table 27.3 is an example of the use of artificial colors in commercial food products.

TABLE 27.1
Artificial Food Dyes Permitted in the United States

Food and Drug Administration Name	Common Name	Color
FD&C Yellow #5	Tartrazine	Lemon yellow
FD&C Yellow #6	Sunset yellow	Orange
FD&C Red #3	Erythrosine	Cherry red
FD&C Red #40	Allura red	Orange-red
FD&C Citrus red #2[a]	Citrus red #2	Red
Orange B[b]	Orange B	Orange
FD&C Blue #1	Brilliant blue	Bright blue
FD&C Blue #2	Indigotine	Royal blue
FD&C Green #3	Fast green	Sea green

[a] Citrus red #2 is restricted to coloring orange skins in fruit not used for manufacture of food products (such as orange juice).
[b] Orange B is restricted to the casings and surfaces of frankfurters and sausages. It is similar in chemical structure to amaranth, which is not allowed in the United States but is permitted for use in other countries including Canada.
Source: Data are from reference 1.

BOX 27.1   Artificial Food Dyes Permitted in Canada

Alkanet	Erythrosine[a]
Allura red[a]	Fast green FCF[a]
Aluminum metal	Indigotine[a]
Amaranth	Iron oxide
Anthocyanin	Orchil
Brilliant blue FCF[a]	Ponceau SX
Canthaxanthine	Saunderswood
Carbon black	Sunset yellow FCF[a]
Citrus red #2[a]	Tartrazine[a]
Cochineal	

[a] Corresponds to a color in U.S. FD&C list in Table 26.1.
Source: Data are from reference 11.

TABLE 27.2
Artificial Food Dyes Permitted in the European Union (EU)

E Number	Name
E102	Tartrazine
E104	Quinoline yellow
E107	Yellow 2G
E110	Sunset yellow
E120	Cochineal
E122	Carmoisine
E123	Amaranth
E124	Ponceau 4R
E127	Erythrosine BS
E128	Red 2G
E129	Allura red
E131	Patent blue V
E132	Indigo carmine
E133	Brilliant blue FCF
E142	Green S
E151	Black PN
E153	Carbon black
E154	Brown FK
E155	Brown HT
E180	Pigment rubine

TABLE 27.3
Artificial Colors Used in Commercial Food Products
Note: Not all manufacturers of the foods use the artificial colors indicated. Some countries ban the use of certain colors. The regulations change frequently, so users of this information should check details before any policy is implemented.

Color Name	Examples of Foods Containing the Color	Prohibited In
Tartrazine	Fruit punch and cordials; colored carbonated drinks	Austria, Norway
	Instant puddings	
	Packaged convenience foods	
	Cake mixes	
	Soups (dried and canned)	
	Bottled sauces	
	Pickles	
	Commercial salad dressings	
	Ice creams and sherbets	
	Candies	

Continues

TABLE 27.3
Artificial Colors Used in Commercial Food Products (*Continued*)
Note: Not all manufacturers of the foods use the artificial colors indicated. Some countries ban the use of certain colors. The regulations change frequently, so users of this information should check details before any policy is implemented.

Color Name	Examples of Foods Containing the Color	Prohibited In
	Chewing gum	
	Jams and jellies	
	Smoked fish	
	Gelatin dessert mixes (Jell-O)	
	Mustard	
	Yogurt	
Sunset yellow	Typically used for fermented foods that must be heat-treated, such as hot chocolate mix, dried soup mixes, candies, yogurts, commercial breadcrumbs, cheese sauce mixes, jams and marmalades, canned shrimps and prawns, pickled cucumbers (dill pickles)	Finland, Norway
Erythrosine	Glacé cherries	Norway, United States
	Canned red cherries, strawberries, and rhubarb	
	Scotch eggs	
	Packaged dessert mixes	
	Stuffed olives	
	Chocolates	
	Crab meat	
	Salmon spread and pâté	
	Garlic sausage	
	Luncheon meat	
	Danish salami	
Ponceau	Cake mixes	Norway, United States
	Dried soup mixes	
	Dessert toppings	
	Canned strawberries	
	Canned cherry, raspberry, and red currant pie fillings	
	Gelatin dessert mixes (Jell-O)	
	Salami	
Allura red[a]	Dried soup mixes	Austria, Norway, Sweden, Japan, Finland
	Cake mixes	
	Gravy mixes	
	Canned pie fillings	
	Jams and jellies	
	Canned applesauce	

Continues

TABLE 27.3

Artificial Colors Used in Commercial Food Products (*Continued*)

Note: Not all manufacturers of the foods use the artificial colors indicated. Some countries ban the use of certain colors. The regulations change frequently, so users of this information should check details before any policy is implemented.

Color Name	Examples of Foods Containing the Color	Prohibited In
Allura red[a] (Continued)	Canned shrimp and prawns	
	Canned pears	
	Liquid vitamin C preparations	
Amaranth[a]	Dried soup mixes	Norway, United States (in France and Italy, use is limited to caviar)
	Cake mixes	
	Gravy mixes	
	Canned pie fillings	
	Jams and jellies	
	Canned applesauce	
	Canned shrimp and prawns	
	Canned pears	
	Liquid vitamin C preparations	
Indigotine	Cookies	Norway
	Candies	
	Savory convenience food mixes	
Brilliant blue	Canned processed peas	Austria, Belgium, Denmark, France, Germany, Greece, Italy, Norway, Spain, Sweden, Switzerland
Carmoisine	Foods that are heat-treated after fermentation, such as dried soup mixes, packaged breadcrumbs, packaged gelatin desserts, candies, cake and cheesecake mixes, bottled condiments, savory convenience food mixes, almond paste, flavored yogurts, ice cream, jams, preserves	Japan, Norway, Sweden, United States

[a] As indicated in table, amaranth and allura red are used in similar foods.

References

1. Code of Federal Regulations—Title 21: Food and Drugs. http://cfr.vlex.com/source/code-federal-regulations-food-drus-1070#ixzz1Cjo2GySD. Accessed April 25, 2012.
2. Dipalma JR. Tartrazine sensitivity. *Am Fam Phys*. 1990;42(5):1347-1350.
3. Ros A, Juhlin L, Michaëlsson G. A follow-up study of patients with recurrent urticaria and hypersensitivity to aspirin, benzoates and azo dyes. *Br J Dermatol*. 1976;96:19-24.
4. Ardern KD, Ram FS. Tartrazine exclusion for allergic asthma. *Cochrane Database Syst Rev*. 2001;(4):CD000460.
5. Michaëlsson G, Juhlin L. Urticaria induced by preservatives and dye additives in food and drugs. *Br J Dermatol*. 2006;88(6):525-532.

6. Pestana S, Moreira M, Olej B. Safety of ingestion of yellow tartrazine by double-blind placebo controlled challenge in 26 atopic adults. *Allergol Immunopathol (Madr)*. 2010;38(3):142-146.

7. Bateman B, Warner JO, Hutchinson E, et al. The effects of a double blind, placebo controlled, artificial food colourings and benzoate preservative challenge on hyperactivity in a general population sample of preschool children. *Arch Dis Child*. 2004;89:506-511.

8. Murdoch RD, Pollock I, Naeem S. Tartrazine induced histamine release in vivo in normal subjects. *J Roy Coll Phys Lond*. 1987;21(4):257-261.

9. Schaubschläger WW, Zabel P, Schlaak M. Tartrazine-induced histamine release from gastric mucosa. *Lancet*. 1987;2(8562):800-801.

10. Bunselmeyer B, Laubach HJ, Schiller M, Stanke M, Luger TA, Brehler R. Incremental build-up food challenge—a new diagnostic approach to evaluate pseudoallergic reactions in chronic urticaria: a pilot study. *Clin Exper Allergy*. 2009:39:116-126.

11. Canadian Food Inspection Agency. Food Colours: Permitted Synthetic Colours in Canada and Corresponding United States and European Names. http://www.inspection.gc.ca/english/fssa/labeti/decisions/coloure.shtml. Accessed June 25, 2012.

CHAPTER 28

Intolerance of Butylated Hydroxyanisole (BHA) and Butylated Hydroxytoluene (BHT)

The antioxidants BHA (butylated hydroxyanisole) and BHT (butylated hydroxytoluene) are used to prevent fat from becoming rancid and giving foods an objectionable taste and odor. BHA and BHT do not occur in nature. BHA is a mixture of 2- and 3-tert-butyl-4-methoxy-phenol, made from p-methoxyphenol and isobutylene. BHT is made from p-cresol and isobutylene; it was originally developed as an antioxidant for use with petroleum and rubber products. Both products are effective antioxidants and, for most people, have proven to be safe as a food additive (U.S. Food and Drug Administration [FDA] Generally Recognized as Safe [GRAS] designation).[1]

BHA and BHT are often used in combination with other antioxidants such as a gallate (where this is allowed), citric acid, or phosphoric acid.[2] Because a large percentage of the antioxidant is lost during the processing of food (eg, potato chips and similar snack foods lose 90% of the antioxidant; cookies lose about 35%), the quantity consumed is actually much less than that added to the product during its manufacture. However, when BHA and BHT are used in the same product, 20 times the usual amount of BHA is stored in the body's fat.

Sensitivity to BHA and BHT

Extremely high doses of BHA and BHT in experimental animals have consistently resulted in liver enlargement. Both kidney and liver functions have been affected. In addition, adverse effects on the brain have resulted in abnormal behavior patterns in experimental animals.[3] In humans, BHA and BHT have caused rashes and hives (urticaria) in sensitive individuals.[4] Some reports indicate that BHA and BHT may exacerbate asthma in sensitive individuals with asthma, but confirmation of this response in subsequent studies failed to substantiate the findings.[3] The group most frequently affected are people who are sensitive to aspirin. Therefore, the intolerance to BHA and BHT theoretically might be due to inhibition of the cyclooxygenase pathway of arachidonic acid metabolism, similar to the inhibition suspected for salicylate sensitivity (see Chapter 26). Some reports have implicated BHA and BHT in childhood hyperactivity disorders, but this association has not been substantiated in well-controlled trials.

In 1978, the United Nations Joint FAO/WHO Expert Committee on Food Additives suggested that daily ingestion of BHA and BHT should not exceed 0.5 mg per kg body weight (ie, 34 mg for a 68-kg adult).[5] However, intake should be much lower for individuals who are sensitive to these chemicals. Their goal should be to eliminate BHA and BHT by reading food labels carefully and avoiding all possible sources of these preservatives. In many countries, BHT is not permitted in foods intended specifically for babies and young children.

Double-blind placebo-controlled randomized trials have not substantiated the role of BHA and BHT in triggering intolerance reactions in humans, except in a few cases. However, whenever additives are suspected to be involved in an individual's adverse reactions to foods, it is worthwhile to undertake appropriate investigation. A time-limited trial on a BHA- and BHT-restricted diet (eg for 4 weeks), followed by challenge with the suspect additive, should determine a person's response to it. Many manufactured foods may contain BHT and BHA; these should be avoided.

Food Products That May Contain BHA or BHT

In the United States, BHA and BHT will usually appear on food labels when they are added to manufactured foods, although labeling in this case is voluntary on the part of the producer. Foods likely to contain BHA and BHT are:

■ Vegetable oils
■ Margarines
■ Foods cooked in or containing vegetable oils, such as potato chips, nuts, doughnuts, pastries and pie crusts, breakfast cereals, baked goods, salted roasted peanuts
■ Dehydrated potatoes and sweet potatoes (ie, potato and sweet potato flakes)
■ Dry breakfast cereals
■ Dried fruits
■ Dry yeast
■ Packaged convenience foods

Additional foods that may contain BHA and BHT are:

■ Beverages
■ Ice cream
■ Candies

- Chewing gum
- Gelatin desserts
- Soup bases
- Lard and shortening
- Animal fats
- Unsmoked dry sausage
- Enriched rice
- Cake and dessert mixes
- Glacé fruits

BHA and BHT in Food Packaging

BHA and/or BHT may be added to the packaging of cereals, crackers, and other foods to help maintain freshness of the food. BHA and BHT will appear on the label if the food contains the preservatives or if they are present in the packaging materials.

References

1. US Food and Drug Administration Generally Recognized as Safe (GRAS). Sections 201(s) and 409 of the Federal Food, Drug, and Cosmetic Act (the Act), http://www.fda.gov/Food/FoodIngredientsPackaging/GenerallyRecognizedasSafeGRAS/default.htm. Accessed April 24, 2012.
2. Branen AL. Toxicology and biochemistry of butylated hydroxyanisole and butylated hydroxytoluene. *J Am Oil Chem Soc.* 1975;52(2):59-63.
3. Weber RW. Adverse reactions to the antioxidants butylated hydroxyanisole (BHA) and butylated hydroxytoluene (BHT). In: Metcalfe DD, Sampson HA, Simon RA, eds. *Food Allergy: Adverse Reactions to Foods and Additives.* 4th ed. Cambridge, MA: Blackwell Science; 2008:386-393.
4. Goodman DI, McDonnell JT, Nelson HS, Vaughan TR, Weber RW. Chronic urticaria exacerbated by the antioxidant food additives, butylated hydroxyanisole (BHA) and butylated hydroxytoluene (BHT). *J Allergy Clin Immunol.* 1990;86:570-575.
5. Llaurado JP. The saga of BHT and BHA in life extension myths. *J Am Coll Nutr.* 1985;4:481-484.

CHAPTER 29

Nitrate and Nitrite Sensitivity

Nitrates and nitrites are used in foods as preservatives, particularly as protection against the deadly bacterium *Clostridium botulinum*, the cause of botulism. They are also used to impart flavor and color to manufactured foods, especially processed meats.[1] An acceptable daily intake (ADI) for nitrate of 3.7 mg/kg body weight, equivalent to 222 mg nitrate per day for a 60-kg adult, was established by the Scientific Committee on Food (SCF). In 2002, this was reconfirmed by the Joint FAO/WHO Expert Committee on Food Additives (JECFA).[2]

Nitrites and nitrates represent one of the oldest and most effective ways of preserving meats. Without nitrites and nitrates, there would be many deaths from the growth of toxic microorganisms. However, the mechanisms that allow the chemicals to kill bacteria may also cause adverse effects in the human body when nitrate or nitrite is consumed in excessive quantities.

Nitrate is a normal component of plant tissues.[3] Nitrite, in contrast, is not normally found in plants unless microbial spoilage has converted the nitrate to nitrite. Nitrate can be detected in natural foods such as vegetables, fruits, cereals, fish, milk, and milk products. It can also be found in water that has been contaminated by nitrogen-containing fertilizers and animal waste. Nitrate in the soil is taken up by plants as a nitrogen source in the formation of proteins. Nitrate accumulation in plants is determined by genotype, growing conditions, light levels, soil temperature, and nitrogen fertilizers. Consequently, the level of nitrates and nitrites in plant and animal foods differs widely between samples taken during different growing seasons and from diverse locations worldwide.[4]

Symptoms of Sensitivity

Nitrites preserve the red color of meat by changing the nature of the hemoglobin of the red blood corpuscles. The function of hemoglobin is to carry oxygen throughout the body. When nitrites enter the bloodstream, the person's hemoglobin is likewise changed if the nitrite level is excessive. This may lead to a condition known as *methemoglobinemia*, with symptoms such as anemia, breathing difficulty, pallor, dizziness, and headaches.[5] Because of their small size, infants and young children are more susceptible to nitrite poisoning than adults, and nitrites are not permitted in foods intended for babies under the age of 6 months.

Nitrites are also capable of reacting with substances called *amines* in the digestive tract to form nitrosamines, which may be carcinogenic if exposure is excessive and prolonged. There is evidence that consumption of vitamins A, C, and E (antioxidants) in the form of fresh yellow and green vegetables, fish, and plant oils is protective against stomach and intestinal cancer in this situation.

Prolonged exposure to nitrate may cause anemia and inflammation of the kidneys, and ingestion of a large quantity may result in gastrointestinal inflammation with severe abdominal pain, vomiting, vertigo, muscular weakness, and irregular pulse (nitrate toxicity). A lethal dose of nitrite for adults is reported to be 1 g.[6]

Nitrates may be converted to nitrites during food spoilage[2] or by intestinal bacteria after consumption. They then have the same effect as nitrites, as previously discussed.

In low doses, symptoms such as flushing of the face and extremities, digestive tract discomfort, and headache have been reported.[3] Other symptoms reported to be triggered by nitrates and nitrites include recurrent hives[7] and migraine and non-migraine headaches.[8]

There is one report of anaphylaxis associated with nitrate consumption[9] in a 22-year-old man. The patient in this case was also sensitive to artificial food colorings and metabisulphite, so his recurrent anaphylactic-type reactions to takeout food could have involved a variety of mechanisms. Further research needs to be conducted on the possibility of such episodes.

Nitrates and Nitrites in Foods

The presence of nitrates or nitrites in manufactured foods will be indicated on the label as one of the following:

- Sodium nitrate
- Potassium nitrate
- Sodium nitrite
- Potassium nitrite

High levels are found in processed meats such as pepperoni, frankfurters, sausages, salami, bologna, luncheon meats, bacon, ham, smoked fish, and some imported cheeses. Plants can contain naturally occurring nitrates derived mainly from nitrate-containing fertilizers. Nitrite toxicity has been reported in people who have

BOX 29.1	Plant Species Most Likely to Accumulate Nitrates

Beet and beet greens	Lettuce
Cabbage	Parsley
Carrot	Potato
Celery	Radish
Collards	Spinach
Eggplant	Strawberry
Fennel	String bean (green bean; French bean)
Leek	Turnip greens

Source: Data are from Allergy Advisor; Zing Solutions. Allergy and Intolerance software. http://AllergyAdvisor.com. Accessed April 25, 2012.

consumed overfertilized spinach.[10] Box 29.1 lists the plant species that accumulate nitrates at fairly high levels.[11]

Table 29.1 provides details about the use and function of nitrate and nitrite additives used in the preservation of foods. Tables 29.2 and 29.3 list *estimated* nitrite and nitrate levels in commonly consumed foods. Because the levels of nitrates and nitrites vary according to how much is added to a processed meat or how much is in the soil in which a plant is grown, it is not possible to provide an accurate measure of the chemicals in each food. The disparity in reported levels in similar foods is evident from the tables where conflicting values are from data collected from different references.[12–15]

TABLE 29.1
Summary of the Use and Effects of Nitrates and Nitrites in Manufactured Foods

Compound (E Number)	Description, Effect, and Function	Used in
Potassium nitrite (E249)	• Potassium salt of nitrous acid. Occurs naturally. Manufactured by reacting nitrous oxide and nitric oxide with potassium hydroxide. • Converts the iron-containing pigments in the flesh to stable bright pink compounds. • Preservative in meat, particularly in preventing the development of spores of *Clostridium botulinum,* the bacterium responsible for botulism.	Cooked meats Canned meats Corned meat Liver sausage Meat pâté Pickled meats Sausages Smoked fish

Continues

TABLE 29.1

Summary of the Use and Effects of Nitrates and Nitrites in Manufactured Foods (*Continued*)

Compound (E Number)	Description, Effect, and Function	Used in
Sodium nitrite (E250)	• Does not occur naturally. Derived from sodium nitrate by bacterial or chemical action. • Preservative, especially by inhibition of *Clostridium botulinum.* • Used in meat curing to impart a red color.	Cured meats Cured meat products Salted meats Pork sausage Bacon Turkey and ham loaf Smoked frankfurters Wieners Tongue Pressed meats Canned meats Frozen pizza Smoked fish
Sodium nitrate (E251)	• Naturally occurring mineral, especially in the Chilean desert (known as *Chile saltpeter*). Formed by reaction between nitric acid and sodium carbonate. • Preservative; added to salt in curing meats. • Fixes color in meats.	Bacon Pressed meats Ham Tongue Beef Canned meats Cheese, other than cheddar, cheshire, grana padano, and provolone Frozen pizza
Potassium nitrate (E252)	• Commonly known as *saltpeter*. • Naturally occurring mineral formed by reaction of potassium chloride and concentrated nitric acid. May be manufactured artificially from waste animal and vegetable material. • Inhibits growth of *Clostridium botulinum.* • Added to salt in curing of meat products. Color fixative.	Cured meats Sausages Smoked frankfurters Wieners Bacon Ham Tongue Pressed meats Canned meats Dutch cheeses Fish products Spirits

TABLE 29.2
Estimated Level of Nitrites in Selected Meats and Vegetables[a]

Food	Mean Level (mg/100 g) or Range (mg/100 g) of Nitrites
Meats	
Bacon	1.3
Bacon, smoked	3.1
Luncheon meat	0.3
Ham, smoked	3
Salami	0.3
Salami, kosher	38
Vegetables	
Carrot, raw	0.002–0.023
Cabbage, raw	0–0.041
Chinese cabbage, raw	0–0.065
Bok choy, raw	0.009–0.242
Cucumber, raw	2.4
Cucumber, raw	0–0.011
Green bean, raw	25.3
Eggplant, raw	30.2
Eggplant, raw	0.007–0.049
Lettuce, raw	85
Lettuce, raw	0.008–0.215
Lima beans, raw	5.4
Melon, raw	43.3
Mustard greens, raw	0.012–0.064
Onion, raw	13.4
Peas, raw	2.8
Pepper, sweet, raw	12.5
Pickles	5.9
Potato, raw	11.9
Pumpkin, raw	41.3
Sauerkraut	19.1
Spinach, raw	186
Spinach, raw	0–0.073
Sweet potato, raw	5.3
Tomato, raw	6.2

[a] This table provides available published estimates of nitrites in foods. Levels of nitrates and nitrites vary according to how much is added to a processed meat or how much is in the soil in which a plant is grown. Therefore, it is not possible to provide an accurate measure of the chemicals in each food. The disparity in reported levels in similar foods is evident from the tables where conflicting values are data from different references.

Source: Data are from references 12 through 15.

TABLE 29.3
Estimated Level of Nitrates in Selected Vegetables[a]

Food	Mean Level (mg/100 g) or Range (mg/100 g) of Nitrates
Asparagus, raw	2.1
Beet, raw	276
Beans, dry	1.3
Broccoli, raw	78.3
Cabbage, raw	63.5
Cabbage, raw	25.9–125
Chinese cabbage, raw	42.9–161
Carrot, raw	11.9
Carrot, raw	92–195
Cauliflower, raw	84.7
Corn, raw	4.5
Eggplant, raw	25–42.4
Mustard greens, raw	70–95
Lettuce	12.3–267.8
Spinach, raw	23.9–387.2

[a] This table provides available published estimates of nitrates in foods. Levels of nitrates and nitrites vary according to how much is added to a processed meat or how much is in the soil in which a plant is grown. Therefore, it is not possible to provide an accurate measure of the chemicals in each food. The disparity in reported levels in similar foods is evident from the tables where conflicting values are data from different references. In addition, nitrates may be converted to nitrites in the mouth and intestine. Thus, the level of the chemical in food does not always reflect the level in the body after digestion.

Source: Data are from references 12 through 15.

Management of Nitrate and Nitrate Sensitivity

Persons will vary in their tolerance of nitrates and nitrites. It is therefore difficult to give directives concerning how much of a food can be eaten without eliciting symptoms. In general, if a person is suspected to be intolerant to nitrites and nitrates, he or she should avoid the foods that have the highest levels of these chemicals for a period of 4 weeks. An appropriate diet can be developed from that data. If the symptoms resolve, challenge with nitrate- and nitrite-rich foods can be undertaken. If symptoms recur, an intolerance is confirmed.

References

1. Winter R. *A Consumer's Dictionary of Food Additives*. 7th ed. New York, NY: Random House; 2009:382-385.
2. European Food Safety Authority. Nitrate in vegetables—scientific opinion of the Panel on Contaminants in the Food Chain: Question No. EFSA-Q-2006-071. *EFSA J.* 2008;689:1-79.

3. Dennis MJ, Wilson LA. Nitrates and nitrites. In: Caballero B. Trugo L, Finglas PM, eds. *Encyclopedia of Food Sciences and Nutrition.* 2nd ed. Cambridge, MA Elsevier Science; 2003:4136-4141.

4. Petersen A, Stoltz S. Nitrate and nitrite in vegetables on the Danish market: content and intake. *Food Addit Contam.* 1999;16(7):291-299.

5. Keating JP, Lell ME, Straus AW, Zarkowsky H, Smith GE. Infantile methemoglobinemia caused by carrot juice. *N Engl J Med.* 1973;288:825-826.

6. Fasset DW. Nitrates and nitrites. In: *Committee on Food Protection. Toxicants Occurring Naturally in Foods.* 2nd ed. Washington, DC: National Academy of Sciences; 1973:7-25.

7. Gibson A, Clancy R. Management of chronic idiopathic urticaria by the identification and exclusion of dietary factors. *Clin Allergy.* 1980;10:699-704.

8. Millichap JG, Yee MM. The diet factor in pediatric and adolescent migraine. *Pediatr Neurol.* 2003;28(1):9-15.

9. Hawkins CA, Katelaris CH. Nitrate anaphylaxis. *Ann Allergy Asthma Immunol.* 2000;85(1):74-76.

10. Simios A. Methemoglobinemia von nitrate gehalt in spinat. *Munch Med Wochenschr.* 1964;1180-1182.

11. Allergy Advisor; Zing Solutions. Allergy and Intolerance software. http://AllergyAdvisor .com. Accessed April 25, 2012.

12. Leszczyńska T, Filipiak-Florkiewicz A, Cieślik E, Sikora E. Effects of some processing methods on nitrate and nitrite changes in cruciferous vegetables. *J Food Compost Anal.* 2009;22(4):315-321.

13. Correia M, Barroso A, Fátima Barroso M, Soares D, Oliveira MBPP, Delerue-Matos C. Contribution of different vegetable types to exogenous nitrate and nitrite exposure. *Food Chem.* 2010;120(4):960-966.

14. Wang ZHTX, Wei YS, Li SX. Nitrate accumulation and its regulation by nutrient management in vegetables. In: *Balanceable Fertilization and High Quality Vegetables.* Beijing, China: China Agricultural University Press; 2000.

15. Hord NG, Tang Y, Bryan NS. Food sources of nitrates and nitrites: the physiologic context for potential health benefits. *Am J Clin Nutr.* 2009;90(1):1-10.

CHAPTER **30**

Monosodium Glutamate (MSG) Sensitivity

Monosodium glutamate (MSG), a traditional flavor enhancer in Chinese and other types of Asian cooking, is used increasingly to flavor Western foods. In addition, some foods such as tomatoes, mushrooms, some canned meat, soy sauce, and some cheeses (eg, Parmesan) contain natural glutamates that resemble MSG.[1]

People sensitive to MSG report a variety of symptoms previously known as the *Chinese restaurant syndrome* or sometimes *Kwok's syndrome*. Symptoms may include facial flushing, pain in the face and the back of the neck, headache, tingling and burning sensations, blurred vision, nausea and vomiting, increased heartbeat, chills, and shaking.[2] Depression, irritability, and other mood changes have also been reported, and some people with asthma report MSG triggering or worsening their asthma.[3]

Experts are widely divided on the subject of MSG sensitivity. A 1993 study concluded that "'Chinese restaurant syndrome' is an anecdote applied to a variety of postprandial illnesses: rigorous and realistic scientific evidence linking the syndrome to MSG could not be found."[4] On the other hand, some clinicians have confirmed the sensitivity using double-blind placebo-controlled challenge protocols on randomized sensitive and non-sensitive subjects.[5] According to some estimates, the prevalence of *MSG symptom complex* (the designation recommended by the U.S. Food and Drug Administration [FDA]) may be as high as 1.8% of the adult population.[6]

Several incidents of severe asthma have been attributed to the ingestion of MSG; however, a 1999 study of subjects with and without a perceived sensitivity to MSG failed to induce signs or symptoms of asthma. The authors state that "in view of the poorly conducted studies that proposed that MSG induced asthma and the subsequent studies that failed to confirm those findings, it is important to maintain a healthy skepticism about the existence of MSG sensitivity in individuals with asthma."[7]

Symptoms Reported to Be Caused by MSG

The following symptoms have been reported to be caused by MSG in various studies:

- Flushing
- Tightness around face, jaw, and chest; numbness of face
- Tingling, burning of face and chest
- Rapid heartbeat
- Nausea, diarrhea, stomach cramps
- Headache, especially at back of head and neck
- Weakness, dizziness, balance problems, staggering
- Confusion, slurred speech
- Blurring of vision, difficulty focusing, seeing shining lights
- Chills and shaking, excessive perspiration
- Difficulty in breathing
- Symptoms of asthma (in persons with asthma)
- Water retention, thirst
- Insomnia, sleepiness
- Stiffness, heaviness of arms and legs
- Mood changes, such as irritability, depression, and paranoia

Symptoms of the MSG symptom complex are reported to usually occur within 30 minutes of eating a meal high in MSG. Symptoms of asthma, however, have been reported to occur 1 to 2 hours after MSG ingestion, and even as long as 12 hours later.[3]

Mechanism of Action of MSG

The mechanism responsible for provocation of symptoms by MSG is largely unknown. One proposed theory to explain sensitivity to MSG links its action to abnormally high levels of acetylcholine, a neurotransmitter that acts on the brain and central nervous system. MSG is the sodium salt of the amino acid glutamic acid; glutamate is the active ingredient in acetylcholine. Glutamate acts as a precursor in the synthesis of acetylcholine and other physiological chemicals. So theoretically, the symptoms ascribed to MSG sensitivity may be caused by excessive levels of acetylcholine that rise rapidly after ingesting glutamate in a readily available form.[8]

The usual source of exogenous glutamate is food proteins, where it is combined with other amino acids. Before glutamate is free to be absorbed, the peptide bonds in these proteins must be broken by enzymes. Because this process is gradual, it controls the level of free glutamate in the body. According to the theory of "neurotransmitter toxicity," when MSG is eaten, glutamate enters the bloodstream rapidly because no peptide linkages need to be broken.

Level of MSG That May Trigger Symptoms in Sensitive Individuals

Clinical studies have shown that an MSG dose of 0.1 g per kg of body weight can induce plasma glutamate levels to peak to 15 times the basal concentration in approximately 1 hour.[4] However, a correlation between plasma glutamate levels and symptoms has not been demonstrated.

A report on MSG by the FDA indicated that healthy individuals may respond to an oral intake of 3 g MSG within an hour in the absence of food.[9] The dietary intake of naturally occurring free glutamate has been estimated to average approximately 1 g/d in Europe and the United States, with an additional 0.3 to 1 g per day from food-additive sources of glutamate.[10]

Some practitioners have noticed a deficiency of vitamin B-6 (pyridoxine) in several people who are sensitive to MSG.[11] This factor could retard hepatic catabolism of glutamate, thus prolonging high plasma glutamate levels and exacerbating symptoms.

Management of MSG Sensitivity

A "safe level" of MSG in foods cannot be set because several factors contribute to plasma levels of glutamate, only one of which is the MSG added to food. Glutamate is a natural constituent of the body, where it plays an essential role in metabolism. Enzymes called *transaminases* in the liver allow glutamate to interact in a variety of reactions, and free glutamate is also found in muscle and in the brain, kidneys, and other organs. The average person weighing 70 kg has the equivalent of about 12 g of MSG in the body.[6] Whether any particular plasma level can be considered "safe" is not known.

Milk contains natural free glutamate. The daily intake of a 3-kg infant obtained from 480 g of mother's milk is 3.75 g (1.25 g/kg body weight).[4] The Joint Food and Agriculture Organization of the United Nations (FAO) and World Health Organization (WHO) Expert Committee on Food Additives has evaluated MSG and has judged that no restriction is necessary for the use of MSG in food.[12] This means that MSG can be added to any prepared food to the level that the manufacturer considers optimum for enhancing the flavor of its product.

Because MSG is a food additive that appears on the Generally Recognized as Safe (GRAS) list, food manufacturers are not required by law to include MSG on a list of ingredients on product labels. Persons sensitive to MSG should be advised to restrict their intake of MSG as much as possible.

Factors That Might Contribute to the Uptake of MSG in Foods

Because alcohol seems to increase the rate of absorption of many foods as well as MSG, drinking alcoholic beverages while eating MSG-containing foods probably increases both the severity and rate of onset of symptoms. In addition, eating foods containing MSG on an empty stomach seems to increase the adverse effects of MSG.

Sources of MSG

MSG as a food additive is derived from proteins that contain glutamic acid by acid or enzymatic hydrolysis. When plant protein is hydrolyzed, it yields MSG. When the hydrolysate is incorporated into a food, it is usually indicated by terms such as *hydrolyzed plant protein* (HPP) or *hydrolyzed vegetable protein* (HVP), or it uses the plant source name (eg, hydrolyzed soy protein [HSP]). These terms on food labels indicate the presence of MSG when MSG as a term may be absent.

The following flavorings contain MSG and may appear on food labels:

- Accent
- Ajinomoto
- Zest
- Vetsin
- Gourmet powder
- Subu
- Chinese seasoning
- Glutavene
- Glutacyl
- Hydrolyzed vegetable protein (HVP)
- Hydrolyzed plant protein (HPP)
- Natural flavoring (may be HVP)
- Flavorings
- Kombu extract
- Mei-jing
- Wei-jing
- RL-50

Many prepared foods contain MSG or one of the flavorings mentioned earlier. Foods containing these additives include:

- Canned meats
- Prepared dinners and side dishes
- Canned soups
- Dry soup mixes
- Gravy and seasoning mixes
- Cookies and crackers
- Cured meats
- Smoked meats and sausages
- Diet foods
- Freeze-dried foods
- Frozen foods
- Potato chips
- Prepared snacks
- Prepared salads, salad dressings, and mayonnaise

- ■ Croutons
- ■ Bottled and canned sauces
- ■ Spices and seasonings

Glutamate is also present in monopotassium glutamate, monoammonium glutamate, calcium glutamate, and other salts of glutamic acid. Some persons sensitive to
MSG may also react to these salts.

MSG Sensitivity and Diet

When MSG sensitivity has been determined, the only way individuals can avoid their
symptoms is to reduce their intake of all sources of MSG, both naturally occurring
and as an additive to manufactured foods, to a level below their "limit of tolerance."
An MSG-restricted diet should be followed carefully for a minimum of 4 weeks. If
symptoms have not occurred within that time, gradual reintroduction of some of the
foods may be possible. Careful monitoring of MSG intake and the onset of symptoms should enable individuals to determine their tolerance threshold.[1] Maintaining
the total daily intake of MSG within their safe limit should allow individuals to
remain symptom free for the long term.

References

1. Williams AN, Woessner KM. Monosodium glutamate "allergy": menace or myth? *Clin Exper Allergy.* 2009;39:640-646.
2. Raiten DJ, Talbot JM, Fisher KD. Executive summary from the report: analysis of adverse reactions to monosodium glutamate (MSG). *J Nutr.* 1995;125(suppl): 2892S-2906S.
3. Allen DH, Baker GJ. Chinese restaurant asthma. *New Engl J Med.* 1981;305(19): 1154-1155.
4. Tarasoff L, Kelly MF. Monosodium L-glutamate: a double-blind study and review. *Food Chem Toxicol.* 1993;31(12):1019-1035.
5. Yang W, Drouin MA, Herbert M, Yang M, Karsh J. The monosodium glutamate symp-tom complex: assessment in a double-blind placebo-controlled randomized study. *J Allergy Clin Immunol.* 1997;99(6 part 1):757-762.
6. Kerr G, Wu-Lee M, El-Lozy M. Prevalence of the "Chinese restaurant syndrome." *J Am Diet Assoc.* 1979;75:29-33.
7. Woessner KM, Simon RA, Stevenson DD. Monosodium glutamate sensitivity in asthma. *J Allergy Clin Immunol.* 1999;104:305-310.
8. Ghadimi J, Kumar S, Abaci F. Studies on monosodium glutamate ingestion: biochemical explanations of Chinese restaurant syndrome. *Biochem Med.* 1971;5:447-456.
9. US Food and Drug Administration. FDA and monosodium glutamate (MSG). *FDA Back-grounder.* August 31, 1995.
10. Beyreuther K, Biesalski HK, Fernstrom JD, et al. Consensus meeting: monosodium glutamate—an update. *Eur J Clin Nutr.* 2007;61:304-313.

11. Rand MJ. The international status of MSG. ILSI MSG Symposium. *Food Australia.* 1991;43(7):S4-S5.

12. Joint FAO/WHO Expert Committee on Food Additives. JECFA L-glutamic acid and its ammonium, calcium, monosodium and potassium salts. In: *Toxicological Evaluation of Certain Food Additives.* WHO Food Additive Series. Cambridge, UK: Cambridge University Press; 1987:97-161.

PART IV

Conditions Associated with Specific Food Components

CHAPTER 31

Histamine Sensitivity

Histamine sensitivity results from a reduced capacity for the body to break down histamine in a timely and efficient manner. As a result, histamine levels rise and symptoms typical of histamine excess develop

Excessive histamine, from a variety of different sources, will result in symptoms usually indistinguishable from allergy. This is not surprising, because the early symptoms of an allergic reaction are mediated by the histamine released during the progress of the allergic response.

Approximately 1% of the population suffers from histamine intolerance, and 80% of those affected are middle-aged.[1] Because the symptoms are diverse, often closely mimic allergy, and are often misinterpreted, the existence of histamine sensitivity (often referred to as *histamine intolerance*) is frequently unsuspected; therefore, the condition is generally underdiagnosed.

What Is Histamine?

Histamine is a bioactive chemical (specifically, a biogenic amine) that is indispensable in the efficient functioning of many body systems. It is a critical messenger molecule that, in times of bodily stress, promotes alertness, blood flow, and healing. It is a *neurotransmitter* (a chemical that conveys messages between cells of the nervous system) and is involved in several essential bodily processes, such as the regulation of gastric acid, the permeability of blood vessels, muscle contraction, and brain function. Histamine plays an essential role in defending the body against invasion by potential disease-causing agents such as bacteria, viruses, and other foreign bodies.

Histamine is made and stored within the intracellular granules in leukocytes, called *granulocytes,* such as mast cells in tissues and basophils that circulate in blood. When the immune system is activated in response to foreign material entering the body, histamine is the first "defense chemical," or more correctly, *inflammatory mediator* released in the process of inflammation. Inflammation is the clinical evidence that the immune system is responding to a potential threat to the body. Histamine is always present when inflammation occurs, and excess histamine will result in symptoms that resemble inflammation.

In addition to its role in controlling vital body processes and defending against foreign invaders, histamine is a key mediator in the symptoms of an allergic reaction. Since allergy is essentially an inflammatory reaction, histamine, together with other protective inflammatory mediators, is released in response to the allergen (see Chapter 1).

Effects of Histamine

Histamine has several effects in the body. It:

- Causes widening of blood vessels (vasodilation or vasodilatation)
- Induces reddening of the skin (erythema)
- Increases permeability of cell membranes, allowing the cell's internal fluid to leak out into adjacent tissues
- Causes itching (pruritus)
- Causes release of gastric (stomach) secretions, especially an increase in gastric acid
- Acts as a neurotransmitter

As the level of histamine rises in the body, these effects become apparent as symptoms.

How Much Histamine Is Excessive?

Basal histamine levels of 0.3 to 1 ng/mL are considered normal.[2] Histamine in excess of these quantities will produce symptoms in sensitive people, depending on their level of tolerance. Even healthy people with normal histamine-degrading enzymes will develop severe headaches or flushing after ingesting massive amounts of histamine in foods.[3] Increasing levels of histamine give rise to symptoms of increasing severity, up to and including cardiac arrest at levels of 100 ng/mL or more.[1]

Everyone has a level of histamine that they tolerate without symptoms. Exceeding that level (called a person's *limit of tolerance* or *tolerance threshold*) can result in symptoms. It has been speculated that the differences in the level of histamine that people can tolerate may be of genetic origin. In addition, various conditions can reduce the tolerance threshold of any individual. These situations include:

- Infectious diseases of various types, especially some viral diseases
- Autoimmune diseases
- Various abnormal physiological conditions

▪ Hormone changes, especially in women at various stages in the menstrual cycle and at menopause

▪ Medications

What Causes an Individual to Be Histamine Sensitive?

Several abnormal physiological conditions may lead to histamine intolerance, in particular a defect in the process of histamine breakdown (*catabolism*). Under normal physiological conditions, excess histamine is degraded by two enzyme systems:[4] (a) histamine N-methyl transferase (HNMT) mainly at cell surfaces; and (b) diamine oxidase (DAO) in serum and in the intestine.[5] Often the two enzymes occur in the same tissues and act at sites throughout the body.[6] Of the two systems, the deficiency in the DAO enzyme system has received most attention as the probable cause of "histamine intolerance."

Under normal conditions, when histamine levels from any source rise above a certain level, these enzymes rapidly degrade the excess. However, when the rate of breakdown of histamine is insufficient to deal with the excess, the total level of histamine in the body rises. At a certain critical level, signs and symptoms occur that are the result of histamine coupling with histamine receptors on specific cells, producing a clinical picture that is often indistinguishable from allergy.

Symptoms of Histamine Excess

Whatever the source of histamine, when the total body level exceeds the enzymes' capacity to break it down, symptoms of histamine excess occur. Histamine intolerance manifests itself in a variety of signs and symptoms, such as the following:[1]

▪ Itching (pruritus) especially of the skin, eyes, ears, and nose
▪ Hives (urticaria; sometimes diagnosed as *idiopathic urticaria* when a cause is not obvious)
▪ Tissue swelling (angioedema), especially of facial and oral tissues and sometimes of the throat, the latter causing the feeling of throat tightening (sometimes diagnosed as *idiopathic angioedema* when a cause is not obvious)
▪ Drop in blood pressure (hypotension)
▪ Increased pulse rate, "heart racing" (tachycardia)
▪ Symptoms resembling an anxiety or panic attack
▪ Chest pain
▪ Nasal congestion (rhinitis) and runny nose (rhinorrhea)
▪ Irritated, watery, reddened eyes (conjunctivitis)
▪ Headache
▪ Fatigue, confusion, irritability

- Loss of consciousness usually lasting for 1 or 2 seconds (this symptom happens rarely)
- Digestive tract upset, especially heartburn, indigestion, and reflux (gastro-esophageal reflux)

Not all of these symptoms occur in any single individual, and the severity of symptoms varies, but the pattern of symptoms seems to be consistent for each person. In addition to the symptoms listed here, excess histamine can make some existing conditions worse; for example, allergy, anaphylaxis, inflammation, eczema, mastocytosis, symptoms related to hormonal fluctuations, and adverse reactions to medications.

Histamine and Allergy

In an allergic reaction, inflammatory mediators, designed to defend the body from the perceived threat of the foreign allergen, are released from the granules within the mast cells in which they are stored—a process called *degranulation*. This process begins when the IgE antibodies produced in response to the allergen, coupled to specific IgE receptors on the surface of mast cells, encounter the allergens against which they were produced. The allergen attaches to two adjacent IgE molecules, thus forming a bridge between them. This bridging process initiates a series of reactions that disrupt the cell membrane and release the granules and their contents, the inflammatory mediators. Histamine is the most important of these inflammatory mediators in the initial response to the allergen. More details of the process are provided in Chapter 1.

Histamine and Anaphylaxis

If a person has an allergy and also has a deficiency in DAO, the symptoms of the allergic reaction will be significantly worse, up to and including anaphylaxis. Some evidence suggests that people who are prone to recurrent anaphylactic reactions may be experiencing histamine intolerance in addition to their allergies. In such situations, the histamine released in the allergic response quickly rises to a dangerously high level, uncontrolled by the body's enzyme systems (DAO and HNMT) that normally keep histamine at a tolerable level; this leads to a situation that may be life-threatening.[7]

Histamine and Inflammation

Histamine is an important mediator whenever the immune system is activated. In inflammation, whether produced in defending the body from injury or infection or as a result of an allergic reaction, lymphocytes, cytokines, and antibodies signal the release of inflammatory mediators, including histamine. Therefore, whenever there is infection, trauma, or some other health-threatening condition, histamine levels rise.

This can be seen most obviously in a local response; for example, after a scratch, scrape, or injury to the skin. The site becomes red, swollen, hot, and painful—all results of the release of inflammatory mediators, especially histamine. Such a response can happen anywhere in the body; when the injury is internal, the signs are not so obvious, but the effects are felt in various tissues and organs. When the infection or injury is a threat to the body's health or survival, histamine is an essential mediator; it is only when histamine levels rise above the body's immediate requirements that it becomes a problem. In conditions that result in chronic inflammation, sometimes caused by autoimmune processes, excess histamine can make the symptoms considerably worse.

Histamine and Eczema

Histamine does not cause eczema, but it may exacerbate the condition. Eczema is an inflammatory condition in the skin, sometimes called *atopic* (allergic) *dermatitis*. When high-histamine foods are consumed, people with less-than-efficient histamine tolerance may experience an increase in the severity of their eczema.[8]

Histamine and Mastocytosis

Mastocytosis is a group of diseases characterized by the accumulation of mast cells in various tissues, especially the skin, bone marrow, gastrointestinal tract, liver, spleen, and lymph nodes.[9] In this disease, the body makes an excessive number of mast cells that infiltrate tissues and organs. These white blood cells are one of the most important in making and storing histamine. So when there are large numbers of these cells in any tissues, histamine, together with other inflammatory mediators, is released in enormous quantities in response to any event that causes them to be degranulated. When this happens, the sufferer experiences all the symptoms of histamine excess (see earlier).

The vast majority of people with mastocytosis do not show reactions to many routine allergy tests but often demonstrate an exaggerated response to histamine, which is used as the positive control in allergy skin tests.[10]

Histamine and Hormones

Women who are intolerant to histamine often suffer from the symptoms listed previously, especially headaches and menstrual pain, during certain phases of their menstrual cycle. Histamine levels tend to fluctuate with the level of hormones, especially estrogen and progesterone, at ovulation and just prior to the onset of menstruation. Fluctuation in hormone levels, especially progesterone,[11] may affect histamine levels and therefore affect the reactions that are triggered by histamine.

In contrast, many women with both allergies and histamine intolerance find significant relief of their symptoms during pregnancy; this is because the placenta makes a great deal of DAO, the enzyme that breaks down histamine.[12] The result is that the level of histamine no longer exceeds the woman's tolerance threshold, and she may remain blissfully free from her symptoms throughout her pregnancy. Unfortunately, the symptoms tend to recur once the DAO from the placenta is no longer available after the birth of her child.

Histamine and Medications

Some medications can release histamine; others can reduce the effectiveness of the DAO that breaks down histamine. As a result, the level of histamine rises and may cause symptoms, even in a person who has shown no signs of histamine intolerance in the past. Common painkillers such as aspirin, nonsteroidal anti-inflammatory drugs (NSAIDs), some diuretics, antibiotics, and antidepressants are among the medications that can affect the functioning of DAO. A list of medications that either release histamine or decrease the effectiveness of DAO can be found in reference 1.

How Can Histamine Intolerance Be Distinguished from Food Allergy?

As previously discussed, food allergy is a hypersensitivity reaction of the immune system that occurs when antibodies of the IgE type are produced against a specific food allergen. When the allergenic food is consumed by someone whose immune system has produced IgE to the food on a previous occasion (ie, someone who is sensitized to the allergen), inflammatory mediators are immediately released. This results in the usually rapid (minutes to a few hours) onset of symptoms. Thus, an allergic reaction to a food leads to the appearance of symptoms in response to the mere presence of the allergen, however small the dose might be.

In contrast, symptoms of histamine intolerance, although they may be the same in type, take time to appear and are not usually evident immediately after histamine-rich foods and beverages are consumed. This is because the level of histamine needs to reach a certain critical level before the tissues respond. Thus, a small amount of histamine will not cause a response—it is the total amount of histamine in the body, in excess of the body's requirements, that causes the reaction. Figure 31.1 illustrates the overflow of histamine as it builds up as a result of:

■ Basal histamine (essential for body functions)
■ Exposure to histamine-releasing events (allergy)
■ Consumption of histamine-associated foods (eg, cheese, tomato, strawberries, and wine)—a meal of pizza with cheese, tomato, and pepperoni; a strawberry dessert; and a glass or two of wine would achieve this result!

It is the overflowing of histamine that results in symptoms. For this reason, tests designed to provoke and measure an immediate response, such as a double-blind, placebo-controlled food challenge (DBPCFC)—considered to be the "gold standard

FIGURE 31.1

Buildup of histamine in the body. Histamine excess is dose related. Each function and food adds its own level of histamine up to the individual's limit of tolerance. Once the limit is reached, histamine "overflows" and symptoms result. The severity of the symptoms depends on the amount of excess histamine in the system. The diagram represents a person with allergies to pollen and cat dander who has eaten a meal containing histamine-rich foods (ie, cheese, tomato, strawberries) with wine.

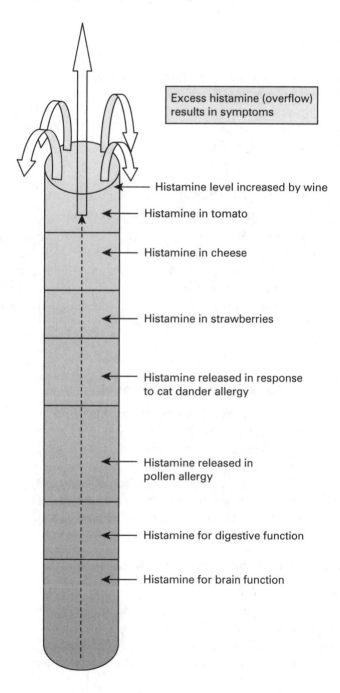

Excess histamine (overflow) results in symptoms

Histamine level increased by wine

Histamine in tomato

Histamine in cheese

Histamine in strawberries

Histamine released in response to cat dander allergy

Histamine released in pollen allergy

Histamine for digestive function

Histamine for brain function

for allergy testing"—will not detect histamine intolerance. Often symptoms will appear several hours after consumption of histamine-rich foods, as the total level of histamine in the body gradually rises and overwhelms the enzymes' capacities to break it down. Thus the association between cause and effect is often difficult to demonstrate in histamine intolerance.

Sources of Histamine

Histamine is a biogenic amine (sometimes referred to as a *vasoactive amine*) that, in mammals, is produced primarily by the action of the enzyme histidine decarboxylase on the amino acid histidine. Histidine is one of the 20 or so amino acids that combine together to make a protein. So whenever histidine decarboxylase is present, histidine in the associated protein will be converted to histamine.

Body Cells and Systems (Intrinsic Histamine)

Histidine decarboxylase is present in large quantities in granulocytes, especially in tissue mast cells and blood basophils (see "What Is Histamine," earlier in this chapter). In these cells, it converts histidine to histamine. The newly formed histamine is then stored in structures within the cell (the intracellular granules) in readiness for release in response to signals from a variety of body systems. In humans, the highest histamine concentrations are found in the skin, lungs, and stomach, with smaller amounts in the brain and heart. However, this is not the only source of histamine in the body.

Microorganisms in the Large Bowel

A large number of microorganisms are capable of producing histamine. Many of the bacteria that colonize the large bowel produce histidine decarboxylase and can convert the histidine in any protein that enters the bowel into histamine. Therefore, the more histidine decarboxylase–producing microorganisms that are present in the colon, and the greater the amount of histidine-containing protein that enters the bowel, the higher the level of histamine in the digestive tract. From here, histamine can be conveyed through the bowel wall to various sites in the body.

Histamine in Food (Extrinsic Histamine)

Histamine in Natural Foods

Another source of preformed histamine is commonly eaten foods. Microorganisms capable of converting histidine to histamine exist ubiquitously in nature, so histamine can arise from various sources. For example, histidine decarboxylase–producing bacteria colonize the gut of fish. As soon as a fish dies, the gut bacteria start to break down the tissue proteins, releasing histidine, which is then rapidly converted to histamine. Since bacteria multiply rapidly, it is possible that the level of histamine in the ungutted fish can double every 20 minutes. The longer a fish remains ungutted after it dies, the higher the level of histamine in its tissues. Furthermore, since shellfish are not gutted after harvesting, the bacteria in their gut will produce histamine as long as the fish remain uncooked. Many a reaction to fish or shellfish has been blamed on allergy, when in reality it was a reaction to an exceedingly high level of histamine in an incorrectly processed fish.

Histamine in Manufactured Foods

A number of food-manufacturing processes depend on the production of amines and similar chemicals for the flavor and nature of the food. Any process that requires microbial fermentation will result in the production of relatively high levels of amines, especially histamine. Cheese of all types; alcoholic beverages; vinegar; fermented vegetables such as sauerkraut; fermented soy products such as soy sauce; and processed meats such as pepperoni, bologna, salami, and frankfurters that are processed by fermentation all contain substantial levels of histamine.

Other Food Sources of Histamine

Certain foods seem to contain high levels of histamine in conditions where microbial fermentation is an unlikely event. Histamine has been consistently detected in citrus fruits; berries such as strawberries and raspberries; tomatoes; several types of tree fruits, such as apricot, cherry, and plums; a few vegetables, particularly eggplant; and pumpkin. Some preliminary research studies have indicated that histamine may be produced during ripening in tomatoes, and it may be that some other fruits that go through a similar process produce histamine in the course of ripening. In general, the riper the fruit, the higher its histamine content. It remains for future research to explain this phenomenon.

Histamine Derived from Foods by Unknown Mechanisms

Traditionally, certain foods have been said to have "histamine-releasing" properties because ingestion of the food tends to result in symptoms of histamine. For example, egg white is frequently referred to as "histamine-releasing," separate and distinct from its activity as an allergen. Strawberries, raspberries, and shellfish were previously similarly designated, but more recent research has uncovered evidence of physiological and biochemical processes as the origin of histamine from these foods (see previous discussion). However, a nonallergic mechanism of histamine release by egg white remains to be determined.

Food Additives

Another mode of histamine release associated with food materials is suggested by research into the mechanisms of intolerance associated with additives and similar naturally occurring chemicals in foods. Azo (nitrogen-containing) food dyes such as tartrazine (Chapter 27), preservatives such as benzoates (Chapter 25), and sulfites (Chapter 21) have been shown to release histamine by a process that is not yet entirely understood. Clinical experiments have demonstrated that persons sensitive to these chemicals experience an increase in plasma histamine that remains elevated long after histamine levels in the nonreactive person have returned to normal. Salicylates (see Chapter 26) may induce a similar pattern of reactivity, but this remains to be proven by appropriate investigation. A precise understanding of the way in which histamine is released in such reactions will depend on future research.

How Can Diet Help in Reducing Excess Histamine?

The degree of improvement or resolution of the symptoms of histamine excess that can be achieved by diet alone will depend on whether the food sources of histamine can be reduced below a person's limit of tolerance.[13] The histamine-restricted diet detailed here is designed to exclude all known food sources of histamine. However, some people will not achieve relief by diet alone because even by excluding all of the histamine-rich foods, their total level of histamine still exceeds their enzymes' capacity to break it down. In these cases, taking antihistamines sometimes helps.

A person with histamine intolerance will typically experience a constant fluctuation in the signs and symptoms of histamine excess in response to changing conditions. For example, when a person is experiencing allergy to airborne allergens such as seasonal pollens, the histamine released in the allergic response alone might put them into the symptom range. In such a case, avoiding histamine-associated foods will no longer relieve their symptoms, because their total level of histamine will remain above their limit of tolerance. This explains the observation that during "pollen allergy season," many people find themselves reacting to foods (usually histamine-rich foods) that they could normally eat with impunity.

As a result of the multiple factors contributing to excess histamine, combined with each individual's capacity to deal with histamine excess, symptoms of histamine intolerance are constantly changing in incidence and severity. Unlike an allergy in which the presence of the antigen results in an immunological response and development of typical symptoms, histamine intolerance is frequently baffling because a specific food does not always result in clinical symptoms.[14] Therefore, it is not possible to eliminate just those foods that cause a reaction. It is necessary to restrict a person's intake of histamine-associated foods to a total that remains below their personal limit of tolerance. This usually requires following the histamine-restricted diet for the long term if a histamine-intolerant person wishes to remain symptom free.

The guidelines for the histamine-restricted diet are provided in Box 31.1. It is imperative that anyone following a diet that restricts important nutrients obtain complete balanced nutrition by substituting foods of equal nutritional value (see Chapter 8 for details).

BOX 31.1 Managing Histamine Intolerance: The Histamine-Restricted Diet

Lists of histamine content of foods differ widely between testing laboratories. It is difficult to determine the accurate histamine content of food, especially of fruits and vegetables, because of variations in the foods, such as degree of ripeness, time and method of harvesting, storage conditions, degree of contamination, and differences in analytical techniques used by the testing lab. Peeled, packaged fruits, salads, and vegetables often have a higher histamine content than fresh. Fresh, whole fruits and vegetables are protected from microbial invasion (and therefore histamine production) by their peels or skins. Products with cut surfaces (eg, shredded or sliced packaged salads) are more susceptible to bacterial invasion and are therefore more likely to contain histamine. For example, packaged mung bean, lentil, and radish sprouts contain double the histamine content compared to homegrown sprouts. Fresh is best!

The restricted foods in this management program also include foods that release histamine by unknown mechanisms, such as egg white; some plant foods; and additives, such as azo dyes, sulfites, and benzoates whose adverse effects include an increase in histamine (for details, see earlier discussion). Therefore, these lists are not limited to foods reported as containing a high level of histamine when measured in the laboratory. Not all people will react to the additives, so judicious challenge after the initial trial will determine whether these need to be avoided in the long term.

The lists provided here have been compiled from a variety of resources and reflect the foods and additives that are most consistently associated with higher levels of histamine.

Histamine-Restricted Diet Guidelines
The following foods and additives are *avoided* during the 4-week trial elimination period.

Fish, Eggs, Meat
- Fish and shellfish whether fresh, frozen, smoked, or canned, if processing is unknown. Note: If the fish is freshly caught, gutted, and cooked within ½ hour, it may be eaten.
- Eggs. Note: A small quantity of cooked egg in a baked product such as pancakes, muffins, cakes is usually tolerated.
- Processed, smoked, and fermented meats of all types such as luncheon meat, sausage, wiener, bologna, salami, pepperoni, smoked ham, cured bacon.
- Leftovers. Note: freeze any uneaten protein-based food. Bacteria will quickly act on protein at room and refrigerator temperatures, resulting in histamine production.

Milk and Milk Products
- All fermented milk products and those containing bacterial culture, including:
  - Cheese: any kind of fermented cheese such as cheddar, Colby, blue cheese, Brie, Camembert, feta, Romano, and so on
  - Cheese products such as processed cheese, cheese slices, cheese spreads
  - Cottage cheese
  - Ricotta cheese
  - Yogurt
  - Buttermilk
  - Kefir

Continues

BOX 31.1 **Managing Histamine Intolerance: The Histamine-Restricted Diet (*Continued*)**

Fruits
- Apricots
- Cherries
- Citrus fruits: Orange, grapefruit, lemon, lime
- Cranberries
- Currants (fresh or dried)
- Dates
- Grapes
- Loganberries
- Pineapple
- Prunes
- Raisins
- Raspberries
- Strawberries

Vegetables
- Avocado
- Eggplant
- Olives
- Pickles, relishes, and other foods containing vinegar
- Pumpkin
- Spinach
- Tomatoes, tomato sauces, ketchup

Legumes
- Red beans
- Soy and soy products

Food Additives
- Tartrazine and other artificial food colors
- Preservatives, especially benzoates and sulfites
- Medications and vitamin pills that contain artificial food colors, benzoates, or sufites (a pharmacist will be able to recommend additive-free supplements and medications)

Seasonings
- Chili powder
- Cinnamon
- Cloves
- Curry powder
- Nutmeg
- Thyme
- Vinegar

Continues

BOX 31.1   **Managing Histamine Intolerance: The Histamine-Restricted Diet (*Continued*)**

Miscellaneous
- Fermented soy products (such as soy sauce, miso)
- Fermented foods (such as sauerkraut)
- Tea (regular or green)
- Chocolate, cocoa, and cola drinks
- Alcoholic beverages of all types
- Nonalcoholic versions of alcoholic beverages (eg, nonalcoholic beer, ale, wine, etc)

Are There Nondietary Methods of Reducing Histamine?

At this time, a limited amount of research is being undertaken to determine whether increasing the level of diamine oxidase will increase a person's ability to break down histamine. Some people intolerant of histamine have found that taking DAO in a pill form,[a] together with a histamine-restricted diet, greatly relieves their symptoms. Further research is required to investigate the efficacy of this therapy in evidence-based controlled trials.

Theoretically, another approach to reducing histamine from extrinsic sources would be to reduce the numbers of histidine decarboxylase–producing microorganisms in the colonic microflora. This should reduce the amount of histamine arising from conversion of dietary histidine in food residue in the large bowel to histamine that might be absorbed into circulation. At the present time, specific methods to achieve this have not been investigated.

Future management of histamine involving manipulation of the colonic microflora might use specific strains of probiotic microorganisms. Several strains of bacteria are known to be capable of producing diamine oxidase, so it might be possible to deliver these strains to the digestive tract in the form of a probiotic and thereby increase the level of DAO available for histamine breakdown in the digestive tract of a histamine-intolerant person. However, this possibility is not currently under investigation, and the strains of bacteria being used in commercially available probiotic foods and supplements are not those that produce DAO. More research in this area is required before a safe probiotic as a source of DAO can be developed.

Currently, the only method available to reduce the symptoms of histamine intolerance is to carefully follow a histamine-restricted diet[15] (see Box 31.1), possibly in combination with a DAO supplement. A DAO supplement alone would be unlikely to reduce histamine to a tolerable level, because, in addition to the amount of

---

[a] DAO from pig kidney is currently available as a dietary supplement, marketed as DAOSin in Europe and Histame and Daosin in the United States and Canada.

available DAO, other factors such as the activity of histamine N-methyl transferase (HNMT) contribute to the control of histamine levels in the body.

References

1. Maintz L, Novak N. Histamine and histamine intolerance. *Am J Clin Nutr.* 2007;85:1185-1196.
2. Dyer J, Warren K, Merlin S, Metcalfe DD, Kaliner M. Measurement of plasma histamine: description of an improved method and normal values. *J Allergy Clin Imunol.* 1982;70:72-87.
3. Wohrl S, Hemmer W, Focke M, Rappersberger K, Jarische R. Histamine intolerance-like symptoms in healthy volunteers after oral provocation with liquid histamine. *Allergy Asthma Proc.* 2004;25:305-311.
4. Rangachari PK. Histamine: mercurial messenger in the gut. *Am J Physiol.* 1992;262:G1-G13.
5. Jarisch R, Wantke F. Wine and headache. *Int Arch Allergy Immunol.* 1996;110:7-12.
6. Huertz G-N, Schwelberger HG. Simultaneous purification of the histamine degrading enzymes diamine oxidase and histamine N-methyltransferase from the same tissue. *Inflamm Res.* 2003;52(suppl 1):S65-S66.
7. Hershko AY, Dranitzki Z, Ulmanski R, Levi-Schaffer F, Naparstek Y. Constitutive hyperhistaminaemia: a possible mechanism for recurrent anaphylaxis. *Scand J Clin Lab Invest.* 2001;61:449-452.
8. Worm M, Fiedler EM, Dolle S, et al. Exogenous histamine aggravates eczema in a subgroup of patients with atopic dermatitis. *Acta Derm Venereol.* 2009;89(1):52-56.
9. Castells MC: Mastocytosis: classification, diagnosis, and clinical presentation. *Allergy Asthma Proc.* 2004;25:33-36.
10. Payne V, Kam PCA. Mast cell tryptase: a review of its physiology and clinical significance. *Anaesthesia.* 2004;59:659-703.
11. Vasiadi M, Kempuraj D, Boucher W, Kalogeromitros D, Theoharides TC. Progesterone inhibits mast cell secretions. *Int J Immunopathol Pharmacol.* 2006;19:787-794.
12. Maintz L, Schwartzer V, Bieber T, van der Ven K, Novak N. Effects of histamine and diamine oxidase activities on pregnancy: a critical review. *Hum Reprod Update.* 2008;14(5):485-495.
13. Joneja JMV, Carmona Silva C. Outcome of a histamine-restricted diet based on chart audit. *J Nutr Environ Med.* 2001;11(4):249-262.
14. Wantke F, Gotz M, Jarisch R. Histamine-free diet: treatment of choice for histamine-induced food intolerance and supporting treatment for chronic headaches. *Clin Exper Allergy.* 1993;23:982-985.
15. Schwelberger HG. Histamine intolerance: a metabolic disease? *Inflamm Res.* 2010; 59(2):219-221.

CHAPTER 32

Tyramine Sensitivity

Dietary tyramine does not usually cause any ill effects, except in people who are (a) taking monoamine oxidase inhibitors (MAOI) drugs or (b) tyramine intolerant, probably due to a deficiency of monoamine oxidase. Tyramine (4-hydroxyphenethylamine) is produced from the amino acid tyrosine by the action of the enzyme tyrosine decarboxylase. Tyrosine is present in many food proteins and is readily converted to tyramine by the action of tyrosine decarboxylase-producing microorganisms during fermentation or bacterial spoilage. In the body, tyramine acts as a weak catecholamine and also triggers release of the more powerful catecholamines, dopamine, epinephrine (adrenaline) and norepinephrine (noradrenaline). Catecholamines are modulating chemicals in the central nervous system; they act as neurotransmitters in the sympathetic nervous system and as hormones in the blood.

Tyramine and Monoamine Oxidase

Tyramine levels in the body are controlled by the enzyme system monoamine oxidase (MAO). There are two subtypes of MAO: MAO-A and MOA-B. These control the levels of various biogenic amines (ie, amines involved in neural functions) in the body. Tyramine (and dopamine) can be metabolized by both subtypes.

MAOI drugs impair the ability of MAO enzymes to regulate tyramine in the body, which can lead to a dramatic increase in tyramine levels. High levels of catecholamines, particularly norepinephrine, resulting from excess tyramine can cause high blood pressure, severe headache, and cardiac arrhythmia (hypertensive crisis). Tyramine can also act directly to affect the regulation of blood pressure.

To reduce the amount of tyramine in the body, people taking MAOI drugs need to follow a tyramine-restricted diet. However, the list of foods that are recommended for a tyramine-restricted diet in this population[1] is more liberal than that recommended for individuals with tyramine sensitivity (discussed in this chapter).

MAOI Medications

The first types of drugs developed to treat depression were monoamine oxidase inhibitors (MAOIs). Although still effective, they have been largely replaced by safer antidepressants with fewer adverse effects. The newer (non-MAOI) antidepressant drugs do not require any dietary restrictions. However, MAOIs may still be used in patients for whom other antidepressants seem to be ineffective.

MAOIs approved by the Food and Drug Administration to treat depression, with their generic names followed by available brand names in parentheses, include:[2]

- Isocarboxazid (Marplan)
- Phenelzine (Nardil)
- Selegiline (Emsam, Eldepryl, Zelapar)
- Tranylcypromine (Parnate)

Research indicates that when an MAOI is administered by a transdermal route in a patch applied to the skin, rather than taken by mouth, a tyramine-restricted diet may not be required.[3]

Foods Restricted for People Taking MAOI Drugs

The requirement for a tyramine-restricted diet for persons using MAOI drugs usually will be decided by the prescribing physician on an individual basis.

There has been a great deal of debate over the years regarding which foods should be allowed for those taking MAOI drugs.[4] It has been suggested that many tyramine-restricted diets for control of symptoms arising from MAO inhibition are excessively restrictive and founded on inadequate science.[5] Current recommendations are to restrict tyramine-containing foods that have the highest risk for inducing a hypertensive crisis in people taking MAOI drugs.[6] A safe level of tyramine in food for people taking MAOI drugs is considered to be less than 6 mg.[1] Foods to be completely avoided include:[1]

- Aged and hard cheeses
- Aged and cured meats
- Banana peel
- Broad bean pods
- Improperly stored or spoiled meats, poultry, and fish
- Concentrated yeast extracts (eg, Marmite, Vegemite, Bovril)
- Sauerkraut
- Tofu
- Soy sauce and other soybean condiments
- Beer from a tap

Foods to be consumed only in moderate amounts include:

■ Red or white wine
■ Bottled or canned beer (including nonalcoholic varieties)

Tyramine Intolerance (Without MAOI Drug Therapy)

Not much is known about the causes of tyramine sensitivity in people not taking MAOIs. Presumably the problem lies in a relative deficiency of the monoamine oxidase enzyme system that normally breaks down tyramine in the body. An excess of undegraded tyramine is responsible for the symptoms. As a result of excess tyramine, norepinephrine levels rise, leading to the development of symptoms.

Symptoms

Symptoms reported to be due to a tyramine sensitivity include:[7,8]

■ Increase in blood pressure
■ Rapid heartbeat
■ Migraine headache
■ Nonmigraine headache
■ Light-headedness
■ Hot feeling
■ Sweating
■ Clamminess
■ Chills
■ Redness of skin
■ Urticaria (hives)
■ Itchiness

In one study, tyramine sensitivity was demonstrated in cases of atopic dermatitis (eczema) in children with food allergies.[9] A trial on a reduced tyramine diet would be worthwhile for people who are experiencing chronic urticaria or migraine headaches, with or without the additional symptoms listed earlier, which are suspected to be the result of tyramine sensitivity. For further discussion of the role of tyramine in urticaria, see Chapter 36; for more informaion about tyramine and migraine, see Chapter 38. The response to tyramine is dose-dependent, and the amount of tyramine in foods that causes an adverse reaction will depend on individual tolerance. The number of foods to be restricted initially is more extensive than that recommended for people taking MAOI drugs, since foods containing lower levels of tyramine may trigger symptoms in highly sensitive individuals.

Tyramine in Foods

Tyramine is produced from the amino acid tyrosine by the action of the enzyme tyrosine decarboxylase. Tyrosine is present in many proteins and is readily converted to tyramine by the action of tyrosine decarboxylase–producing microorganisms. Like histamine, tyramine is found in foods where microbial fermentation is used in their manufacture and in food spoilage where vigorous microbial activity is taking place.

People with tyramine sensitivity need to avoid foods with a particularly high level of tyramine. In addition to the foods listed previously in the section "Foods Restricted for People Taking MAOI Drugs," high-tyramine foods to avoid include the following:

- Aged cheeses
- Fermented meats and sausages
- Chicken liver
- Yeast extract
- Wine (especially red)
- Beer
- Other fermented beverages
- Fermented vegetables (eg, sauerkraut)
- Fermented soy products
- Vinegar and pickles
- Raspberries
- Red plums
- Figs
- Avocado
- Eggplant
- Bananas
- Tomato

Improperly stored or spoiled food can create an environment where tyramine concentrations increase. The freshness of food has been identified as a factor in the amount of tyramine present; the longer a food containing tyrosine is stored, the higher the tyramine content. The tyrosine in the food is converted to tyramine by microorganisms that synthesize tyrosine decarboxylase. This phenomenon has been noted in meat, especially chicken liver and air-dried sausages; beer; and cheese.[10]

Determining Tyramine Sensitivity

There are no tests available for determining a person's sensitivity to tyramine. When tyramine intolerance (or sensitivity) is suspected to be causing an individual's symptoms, a time-limited trial (usually 4 weeks is adequate) on a tyramine-restricted diet is the best way to determine the role that the amine is playing in the etiology of their symptoms. Following the trial period, judicious reintroduction of tyramine-rich foods and monitoring the recurrence of symptoms should determine a person's sensitivity to tyramine. This diet is unnecessarily restrictive for individuals who are taking MAOI drugs and are not otherwise tyramine intolerant.

References

1. Gardner DM, Shulman KI, Walker SE, Tailor SAN. The making of a user-friendly MAOI diet. *J Clin Psychiatry*. 1996;57(3):99-104.
2. Mayo Clinic Health Information. Monoamine oxidase inhibitors (MAOIs) http://www.mayoclinic.com/health/maois/MH00072. Accessed April 25, 2012.
3. Amsterdam JD. A double-blind, placebo-controlled trial of the safety and efficacy of selegiline transdermal system without dietary restrictions in patients with major depressive disorder. *J Clin Psychiatry*. 2003;64(2):208-214.
4. Marcason W. What is the bottom line for dietary guidelines when taking monoamine oxidase inhibitors? *J Am Diet Assoc*. 2005;105(1):163.
5. Shulman KI, Walker SE. Refining the MAOI diet. *J Clin Psychiatry*. 1999;60(3):191-193.
6. Sweet RA, Brown EJ, Heimberg RG, et al. Monoamine oxidase inhibitor dietary restrictions: what are we asking patients to give up? *J Clin Psychiatry*. 1995;56(5):196-201.
7. Smith I, Kellow AH, Hanington E. A clinical and biochemical correlation between tyramine and migraine headache. *Headache*. 1970;10:43-51.
8. Forsythe WI, Redmond A. Two controlled trials of tyramine in children with migraine. *Dev Med Child Neurol*. 1974;16:794-799.
9. Van Bever HP, Docx M, Stevens WJ. Food and food additives in severe atopic dermatitis. *Allergy*. 1989;44:588-594.
10. Walker SE, Shulman KI, Tailor SA, Gardner D. Tyramine content of previously restricted foods in monoamine oxidase inhibitor diets. *J Clin Psychopharmacol*. 1996;16(5):383-388.

CHAPTER **33**

Oral Allergy Syndrome

The term *oral allergy syndrome* (OAS), which is sometimes referred to as *pollen-food allergy syndrome*, describes a complex of clinical symptoms in the mucosa of the mouth and throat that result from direct contact with food allergens in a sensitized individual[1] who also exhibits respiratory allergy to inhaled allergens, usually tree, weed, or grass pollens (*pollinosis*).[2]

There are no authoritative data on the real prevalence of OAS, since the cross-reactivity patterns show geographical and climatic differences, depending on the exposure to inhaled and ingested allergens.[3] For example, in central and northern Europe, allergies to fruits such as apples and stone fruits (eg, peaches) of the *Rosaceae* family are closely associated with birch tree pollinosis, while they are also associated with grass or ragweed pollen in North America, wormwood in Europe, and cedar in Japan.[4]

Symptoms of OAS

Symptoms include itching, tingling, and irritation of oral tissues; swelling of the lips, palate, tongue and sometimes papules or blistering of these tissues; occasional sensation of tightness in the throat; and rarely systemic symptoms.[5] Most people with this allergy exhibit symptoms within 5 minutes of eating the offending food, and almost all individuals show symptoms within 30 minutes after contact with the food.[1]

Although some reports in the literature suggest that OAS may result in anaphylaxis, most researchers and clinicians in the field recognize that anaphylaxis to a food should not be considered as OAS but should be treated as classic food allergy that presents with symptoms in the mouth in addition to other organs.[6,7]

Oral symptoms following ingestion of fruits, vegetables, and nuts have been described in individuals with coexisting allergy to trees of the birch/alder group,[5,8–17] weeds such as mugwort,[18,19] ragweed,[20,21] grasses,[22,23] and other pollens.[24] Table 33.1 provides a summary of frequently reported pollen and food associations.[7,12,13,15–17,24–27]

TABLE 33.1
Frequently Reported Cross-Reacting Foods, Pollens, and Other Allergens

Pollen Allergen	Fruits	Legumes and Grains	Nuts and Seeds	Vegetables, Herbs, and Spices
Birch pollen	Apple	Beans	Almond	Anise
Mugwort pollen	Apricot	Lentils	Chestnut	Asparagus
Grass pollens	Cherry	Peanut	Hazelnut	Cabbage
Timothy grass	Kiwi fruit	Peas	Walnut	Carrot
	Melon	Soy	Caraway seed	Celery
	Nectarine	Rye	Poppy seed	Coriander
	Orange		Sesame seed	Cumin
	Peach		Sunflower seed	Dill
	Pear			Fennel
	Plum			Green pepper
	Prune			Parsley
	Watermelon			Parsnips
				Potato
				Tomato
Ragweed	Banana			Cucumber
	Cantaloupe			Zucchini
	Honeydew			
	Melon			
	Peach			
	Watermelon			

Source: Data are from references 7, 12, 13, 15, 16, 17, 24, 25, 26, and 27.

Cause of OAS

OAS symptoms are caused by a rapid response of the mast cell–bound IgE to allergens released from raw fruits and vegetables as the allergens enter the mouth and come into contact with saliva. There are unusually high concentrations of mast cells, which release the inflammatory mediators responsible for the symptoms of the allergy, in the oral and pharyngeal tissues. It is thought that the high reactivity of these mast cells results from continual exposure to the pollen allergens as they are inhaled.[8]

As defined, the syndrome has two important aspects:

■ Symptoms appear in the mucosa of the oral cavity and arise immediately after contact with the allergenic food.
■ There is a coexisting allergy to inhaled plant materials, usually pollens (pollinosis) that are serologically related to the food responsible for the oral symptoms. Pollinosis typically precedes the onset of oral allergy syndrome, sometimes for as long as several years.

This type of response is called *class 2 food allergy*, in contrast with class 1 food allergy, where the sensitization process occurs via the oral route, usually leading to more severe reactions.[25] Refer to Chapter 2 for more information.

Characteristics of Allergenic Food Protein in Relation to OAS

Analysis of many food proteins at the molecular level has tremendously facilitated the understanding of clinical signs and symptoms of food allergy. This is particularly true of OAS.[1,8,28] The OAS is due to similarities between amino acid sequences (cross-reactivity) of food allergens (eg, apple, carrot, or hazelnut) and pollen proteins (eg, birch pollen). Over 70% identity in amino acid sequence is generally needed for cross-reactivity. Other syndromes due to cross-reactivity between respiratory allergens and foods include the latex food syndrome (Chapter 34), the house mite/seafood syndrome, and the bird/egg syndrome.[29] In investigations of OAS, birch pollen and its associated food allergens have been the most extensively studied.

Birch Pollen Allergens and OAS

At present, at least seven birch pollen antigens have been well identified (designated *Bet v 1* through *Bet v 7*) that may have an allergenic effect.[30] Bet v 1 was the first of these allergens to be identified and is thought to be the most significant in birch pollen allergy.[31] There is a considerable degree of similarity between the structure of Bet v 1 and the main apple allergen (*Mal d 1*), which is thought to account for the potential for raw apple to trigger OAS in individuals with birch allergies.

Bet v 2 and Bet v 4 are two other allergens that seem to be involved in the birch pollen–associated OAS (but at probably lower reaction levels).[30] Bet v 2 has lower allergenicity than Bet v 1 (ie, has a reduced tendency to induce allergy, and the allergy it triggers is less severe). However, in persons who are sensitized to Bet v 1 (ie, have produced IgE antibodies to the allergen) and to Bet v 2, there is a stronger tendency for food allergy to develop and manifest as OAS.[30] This may be true of other birch allergens, such as Bet v 4, that have a tendency to trigger IgE in individuals allergic to birch during birch pollen immunotherapy.[32]

There are indications that the severity of an allergic reaction to a food depends on the allergen responsible for the sensitization. By studying the IgE reactivity profiles against hazelnut extract of individuals with severe anaphylactic reactions, Pastorello and colleagues[33] demonstrated that anaphylactic subjects reacted only to an allergenic hazelnut lipid transfer protein (see the next section of this chapter, "Allergenicity of Plant-derived Proteins"). On the other hand, individuals sensitized to the major hazelnut allergen (*Cor a 1*), which is 70% similar to birch pollen (Bet v 1), presented only OAS.[34,35] In the same context, the major allergen responsible for cross-reactivity between birch and cherry has been identified as *Pru av 1*.[36]

Allergenicity of Plant-derived Proteins

One of the most important groups of plant-derived proteins that are responsible for allergies are the pathogenesis-related (PR) proteins. PRs are proteins that are induced by environmental stresses on the plant such as infection by pathogens, wounding, and other adverse events such as dehydration, pollution, or noxious chemicals.[29]

Pathogenesis-related proteins have been classified into 14 families. Examples of plant food allergens homologous[a] to PRs include:

---

[a] *Homology* refers to structural identity: a *homologue* is closely similar in structure to another.

- Chitinases (PR-3 family) from avocado, banana, and chestnut
- Antifungal proteins such as the thaumatin-like proteins (PR-5) from cherry and apple
- Proteins homologous to the major birch pollen allergen Bet v 1 (PR-10) from vegetables and fruits
- Lipid transfer proteins (PR-14) from fruits and cereals.

Allergens other than PR homologs can be allotted to other well-known protein families, including:

- Inhibitors of alpha-amylases and trypsin from cereal grain seeds
- Profilins from fruits and vegetables
- Seed storage proteins from nuts and mustard seeds
- Proteases from fruits

Properties of Plant-Derived Proteins and Associated Food Allergy

Different properties of these groups of plant-derived proteins may account for differences observed in the clinical presentation of individuals with food allergies. Classification of allergens into groups with structural similarities may help to predict cross-reactivities, thus providing useful information to individuals with food allergies.

To distinguish between those causes of oral symptoms not definable as OAS and those fitting the definition of OAS, it is essential that the allergen responsible be identified and its presence established in each of the allergenic materials.[7,26,37] Ideally, each antigen that could be responsible for apparent cross-reactivity between inhaled and ingested matter should be isolated and identified to confirm the specificity of the cross-reacting component.[27] Perhaps over time, such analyses will help to elucidate the elusive element that confers the property of allergenicity on an antigen.

Management of Oral Allergy Syndrome

A list of the foods that most frequently trigger symptoms of OAS in individuals allergic to pollen is provided in Table 33.1. It is important for a person with any allergy to consume the widest possible range of foods from all food groups in order to avoid nutritional deficiencies. It is therefore essential that the foods that do cause symptoms are correctly identified. Only those causing an immediate reaction should be avoided; all foods that do not cause symptoms should be included in the diet.

People who develop OAS should avoid only the foods that cause symptoms. Individuals allergic to pollen who do not exhibit symptoms of OAS should not restrict their diet in order to avoid the possibility of developing OAS. It is unnecessary for a person with OAS to avoid other pollen-associated foods if they have not become sensitized to them.[38]

In most cases, the allergen responsible for OAS is a class 2 allergen (see Chapter 2) and is therefore likely to be heat-labile.[25] This means that individuals with OAS can usually consume the plant foods with impunity after the foods have been cooked. Cooking the food frequently allows a person to eat the food without a reaction even when symptoms develop in contact with the raw food.

Identification of the Foods That Cause Symptoms

Very often it is clear which foods trigger OAS, because the reaction is immediate on contact with the raw food. Individuals often report exactly which foods cause a problem and record the reaction in their food and symptom records (see Chapter 6 for details). However, when the foods responsible are not obvious, or if the list of suspect foods is extensive, an OAS elimination diet is useful. This would then be followed by challenge to identify the foods responsible.

Open Food Challenge

An open food challenge with incremental doses of the test food will usually identify the foods that need to be avoided. Sequential incremental dose challenge (SIDC) is a very effective method of challenge in which a small quantity of the test food is consumed and symptoms monitored for an initial 4-hour period. If no symptoms develop, the test dose of the food is doubled, and again symptoms are monitored for another 4 hours. If symptoms again do not occur, a further doubled dose of the food is consumed. This method of challenge is usually very effective in demonstrating food allergy when symptoms occur both in the oral tissues and at diverse sites in the body, and when the quantity of food is an important factor in triggering a response. Details of the open SIDC are provided in Chapter 7.

Topical Application of the Food

When the symptoms occur predominantly in the oral tissues and on immediate contact with the food, applying a little of the test food to the lip may be all that is needed to elicit a response. The site of application is observed for the development of overt signs of a reaction, such as itching, reddening, blistering, or swelling. Twenty minutes is usually a sufficient length of time for the reaction to develop. If topical application does not elicit an adverse response, SIDC as described previously should confirm whether the food is indeed responsible for symptoms.

The Final Diet

When the culprit foods have been identified by challenge, they should be carefully eliminated from the diet. Complete balanced nutrition must be supplied from alternate foods, especially when the foods restricted are important sources of essential nutrients.

References

1. Webber CM, England RW. Oral allergy syndrome: a clinical, diagnostic, and therapeutic challenge. *Ann Allergy Asthma Immunol.* 2010;104(2):101-108.
2. Kelso JM. Oral allergy syndrome? *J Allergy Clin Immunol.* 1995;96(2):275.
3. Ausukua M, Dublin I, Echebarria MA, Aquirre JM. Oral allergy syndrome (OAS). General and stomatological aspects. *Med Oral Patol Oral Cir Bucal.* 2009;14(11):e568-e572.
4. Lázaro M, Cuesta J, Igea JM. Alergia a rosáceas: el melocotón. *Alergol Immunol Clin.* 1999;14:234-240.
5. Sicherer SH, Sampson HA. Food allergy. *J Allergy Clin Immunol.* 2006;117(2 suppl Mini-Primer):S470-S475.
6. Nash S, Burks AW. Oral allergy syndrome. *Curr Allergy Asthma Rep.* 2007;7:1-2.
7. Joneja JMV. Oral allergy syndrome, cross-reacting allergens and co-occurring allergies. *J Nutr Environ Med.* 1999;9(4):289-303.
8. Amlot PL, Kemeny DM, Zachary C, Parkes P, Lessof MH. Oral allergy syndrome (OAS): symptoms of IgE-mediated hypersensitivity to foods. *Clin Allergy.* 1987;17:33-42.
9. Eriksson NE, Formgran H, Svenonius E. Food hypersensitivity in patients with pollen allergy. *Allergy.* 1982;37:437-443.
10. Eriksson NE, Wihl JA, Arrendhal H. Birch pollen-related food hypersensitivity: influence of total and specific IgE levels: a multicenter study. *Allergy.* 1983;38:353-357.
11. Halmepuro L, Vuontela K, Kalimo K, Bjorksten F. Cross-reactivity of IgE antibodies with allergens in birch pollen, fruits and vegetables. *Int Arch Allergy Apl Immunol.* 1984;74:235-240.
12. Halmepuro I, Lowenstein H. Immunological investigations of possible structural similarities between pollen antigens and antigens in apple, carrot, and celery tuber. *Allergy.* 1985;40:264-272.
13. Calkhoven PG, Aalbers M, Koshte VL, Pos O, Oei HD, Aalberse RC. Cross-reactivity among birch pollen, vegetables and fruits as detected by IgE antibodies is due to at least three distinct cross-reactive structures. *Allergy.* 1987;42:382-390.
14. Lahti A, Bjorksten F, Hannuskela M. Allergy to birch pollen and apple and cross-reactivity of the allergens studies with RAST. *Allergy.* 1980;35:297-300.
15. Lowenstein H, Eriksson N. Hypersensitivity to foods among birch pollen allergic patients. *Allergy.* 1983;38:577-578.
16. Pauli G, Bessot JC, Dietemann-Molard A, Braun PA, Thierry R. Celery sensitivity: clinical and immunological correlations with pollen allergy. *Clin Allergy.* 1985;15(3):273-279.
17. Dreborg S, Foucard T. Allergy to apple, carrot and potato in children with birch pollen allergy. *Allergy.* 1983;38:167-172.
18. Vallier P, Dechamp C, Vial O, Deviller P. A study of allergens in celery with cross-sensitivity to mugwort and birch pollens. *Clin Allergy.* 1988;18:491-500.
19. Wuthrich B, Staeger J, Johansson SGO. Celery allergy associated with birch and mugwort pollinosis. *Allergy.* 1990;45:566-571.
20. Anderson LB, Dreyfuss EM, Logan J. Melon and banana sensitivity coincident with ragweed pollinosis. *J Allergy.* 1970;45:310.
21. Enberg RN, Leickly FE, McCullough S, Bailey J, Ownby DR. Watermelon and ragweed share allergens. *J Allergy Clin Immunol.* 1987;79:867-875.
22. Ekramoddoullah AK, Kisil FT, Sehon AH. Allergenic cross-reactivity of cytochromes c of Kentucky bluegrass and perennial ryegrass pollens. *Molec Immunol.* 1982;19:1527-1534.

23. Heiss S, Fischer S, Muller W-D, et al. Identification of a 60 kd cross-reactive allergen in pollen and plant-derived food. *J Allergy Clin Immunol*. 1996;98(5 part 1):938-947.

24. Bircher AJ, van Melle G, Haller E, Curty B, Frei PC. IgE to food allergens are highly prevalent in patients allergic to pollens, with and without symptoms of food allergy. *Clin Exp Allergy*. 1994;24(4):367-374.

25. Kondo Y, Urisu A. Oral allergy syndrome. *Allergol Int*. 2009;58:485-491.

26. UTMB University of Texas Medical Branch. SDAP—Structural Database of Allergenic Proteins. http://fermi.utmb.edu/SDAP. Accessed April 25, 2012.

27. Hiller R, Laffer S, Harwanegg C, et al. Microarrayed allergen molecules: diagnostic gatekeepers for allergy treatment. *FASEB J*. 2002;16(3):414-416.

28. Breiteneder H, Ebner C. Molecular and biochemical classification of plant-derived food allergens. *J Allergy Clin Immunol*. 2000;106(1 pt 1):27-36.

29. Ortolani C, Pastorello EA, Farioli L, et al. IgE-mediated allergy from vegetable allergens. *Ann Allergy*. 1993;71(5):470-476.

30. Modrzynski M, Zawisza E. Possible induction of oral allergy syndrome during specific immunotherapy in patients sensitive to tree pollen. *Med Sci Monit*. 2005;11(7): CR351-355.

31. Holm J, Baerentzen G, Gajhede M, et al. Molecular basis of allergic crossreactivity between group 1 major allergens from birch and apple. *J Chromatogr B Biomed Sci Appl*. 2001;25:307-313.

32. Movérare R, Elfman L, Vesterinen E, Metso T, Haahtela T. Development of new IgE specificities to allergenic components in birch pollen extract during specific immunotherapy studied with immunoblotting and Pharmacia CAP System. *Allergy*. 2002;57:423-430.

33. Pastorello EA, Vieths S, Pravettoni V, et al. Identification of hazelnut major allergens in sensitive patients with positive double-blind, placebo-controlled food challenge results. *J Allergy Clin Immunol*. 2002;109(3):563-570.

34. Ortolani C, Ballmer-Weber BK, Hansen KS, et al. Hazelnut allergy: a double-blind, placebo-controlled food challenge multicenter study. *J Allergy Clin Immunol*. 2000; 105(3):577-581.

35. Papageorgiou PS. Clinical aspects of food allergy. *Biochem Soc Trans*. 2001;30:901-906.

36. Holm J, Baerentzen G, Gajhede M, et al. Molecular basis of allergic cross-reactivity between group 1 major allergens from birch and apple. *J Chromatogr B Biomed Sci Appl*. 2001;756(1-2):307-313.

37. Vieths S, Scheurer S, Ballmer-Weber B. Current understanding of cross-reactivity of food allergens and pollen. *Ann NY Acad Sci*. 2002;964:47-68.

38. Aser R, Massironi F, Velati C. Detection of prognostic factors for oral allergy syndrome in patients with birch pollen hypersensitivity. *J Allergy Clin Immunol*. 1996;97(2): 611-616.

CHAPTER **34**

Latex Allergy and Latex-Fruit Syndrome

Allergy to natural rubber latex (NRL) is an IgE-mediated hypersensitivity reaction that is frequently seen in health care workers and workers in the rubber industry. An additional high-risk group includes individuals who have undergone multiple surgical procedures where internal organs have been exposed to the rubber in surgical gloves and appliances; a particularly vulnerable group includes children with spina bifida, due to the number of surgical procedures they often undergo.[1]

Some foods, unrelated botanically to latex-producing trees, synthesize proteins that are structurally almost identical to those in latex rubber. When latex-allergic individuals consume these foods, the homologous antigens couple with the IgE antibodies formed against the latex allergens on the surface of mast cells. This causes degranulation of the mast cell and release of the inflammatory mediators stored within. Symptoms of allergy, including anaphylaxis, result. The condition has been designated *latex-fruit syndrome*, although foods other than fruits may also be involved.

Symptoms of Latex Rubber Allergy

Symptoms of NRL allergy arise from direct contact with a latex product such as gloves, tubing, or other rubber products or by inhalation of airborne NRL allergens in powder—for example, from latex gloves. Symptoms include:

- Contact dermatitis
- Eczema, especially of the hands
- Angioedema (swelling of tissues)
- Rhinoconjunctivitis (hay fever–like symptoms with itchy, watery eyes)
- Asthma (in asthmatics)
- Anaphylaxis in extremely severe cases

In adults with NRL allergy, the prevalence of hand eczema has been reported to be as high as 82%.[2]

Incidence of Natural Rubber Latex Allergy

The incidence of NRL has been estimated to be:[2]

- 1% in the general population
- 2.8% to 17% of hospital workers
- 5% to 11% in workers using latex rubber gloves (eg, hairdressers, greenhouse workers, housekeepers, latex glove manufacturers)
- 23% to 65% of children with spina bifida and other conditions requiring multiple surgical procedures

Allergens in Natural Rubber Latex

The raw material of natural rubber products is obtained from the rubber tree *Hevea brasiliensis*. Proteins from rubber products are responsible for NRL allergy. Of the more than 200 different proteins or polypeptides in NRL, about 25% have been shown to be allergenic—that is, sensitized individuals form IgE antibodies to them.

To determine the allergenicity of NRL and define the nature of the cross-reactivity of allergens in plant foods associated with the latex-fruit syndrome, several of the antigenic proteins in NRL have been identified and analyzed. The World Health Organization (WHO) International Union of Immunological Societies Allergen Nomenclature Committee provides information on those that have been characterized:[3]

- Hev b 2, Hev b 5, Hev b 6, and Hev b 13 together were identified in over 80% of health care workers with latex allergy.
- Hev b 6 with Hev b 1 or Hev b 3 were identified in sera from spina bifida patients with latex allergy.
- Hev b 2, Hev b 6, Hev b 7, and Hev b 8 and class I chitinases of several plant-derived foods are associated with latex-fruit syndrome.

Table 34.1 summarizes characteristics and functions of the most important of these proteins.[1-4]

Natural Rubber Latex Allergens in Unrelated Plants

Allergen cross-reactivity is due to IgE antibodies that recognize structurally similar epitopes[a] on proteins from different, often unrelated, plants.[5] Consequently, people

---

[a]An epitope is the piece of a molecule that elicits a response of the immune system, which results in the production of antibody specifically structured to couple with it.

TABLE 34.1
Characteristics of Antigenic Proteins in Natural Rubber Latex

Allergen	Common Name	Function
Hev b 1	Rubber elongation factor	Biosynthesis of polyisoprene
Hev b 2	β-1,3-glucanase	Defense protein
Hev b 3	Small rubber particle protein	Biosynthesis of polyisoprene
Hev b 4	Microhelix component	Structural component
Hev b 5	Acidic protein	Structural protein
Hev b 6.01	Prohevein	Plant defense
Hev b 6.02	Hevein	Plant defense
Hev b 6.03	C-terminal domain of hevein	Plant defense
Hev b 7	Patatin-like protein	Esterase of polyisoprene
Hev b 8	Profilin	Cell growth regulation
Hev b 9	Enolase	Enzyme
Hev b 10	Manganese superoxide dismutase	Enzyme
Hev b 11	Class I chitinase	Enzyme
Hev b 12	Lipid transfer protein	Plant defense
Hev b 13	Esterase	Enzyme

Source: Data are from references 1 through 4.

may experience hypersensitivity reactions to allergens without previous sensitization to the food itself.[5] The antibodies are formed against the latex, not against the food.[6,7] When certain individuals allergic to latex consume a food containing the structurally homologous antigen, symptoms develop. This type of reaction has been named *latex-fruit syndrome*.[8] Not all people allergic to latex have latex-fruit syndrome, but many do, and the specific foods to which these people react differ between individuals.

Latex-Fruit Syndrome Incidence

It is estimated that 50% to 70% of people with latex allergies have IgE antibodies that cross-react with antigens of plant-derived foods. In many cases, this leads to symptoms of allergy when the foods are consumed. Fruits are especially notorious for their frequent cross-reactivity with latex, and the first foods to be identified as causing this type of allergic reaction were all fruits. This explains the name *latex-fruit syndrome*. Now that other foods have been identified as cross-reacting with latex allergens, a more accurate name probably would be *latex-food syndrome*.

The type and number of reported food allergies associated with NRL allergy vary among studies.[9] The most severe reaction is anaphylaxis, which may be life-threatening. The incidence of NRL-related food anaphylaxis varies from 50% to less than 5% in different studies.[8,10] The number of foods to which a person with NRL reacts may increase over time.

Diagnosis of Latex Fruit Syndrome

Diagnostic tests for latex allergy are fairly straightforward: Both skin tests and blood tests for latex-specific IgE are usually diagnostic for latex rubber allergy. However, testing for foods that might cause a reaction when eaten by the individual allergic to latex is far from easy.

Because the primary allergen is a latex protein, the IgE will be formed against that protein. Frequently there is no food-specific IgE in the person's serum. Therefore, an important aspect of food allergy testing in people with NRL allergy is that neither blood tests for allergen-specific IgE nor skin tests correlate well with the results of provocation (challenge) tests when the suspect food is consumed. Furthermore, there is often a discrepancy between the results of skin tests and tests for allergen-specific IgE in blood. In research studies, food-specific IgE antibodies were detected in serum samples from only a small number of the individuals who reported symptoms after eating the food. Thus, serological tests are of low significance for predicting food allergy in people with latex allergy.[1]

This result occurs because there is an important difference between an allergy in which primary sensitization is to food (class 1 allergy) and that in which primary sensitization is to material other than food (class 2 allergy; see Chapter 2 for details). With NRL allergy, the primary sensitization is to latex, and IgE antibodies to latex antigens are present in the blood of latex-allergic individuals,[6] but antibodies against homologous foods are not.

When there is a positive skin test to a food or proven presence of food-specific IgE, it means that the person has been independently sensitized to the food allergen *in addition* to latex. The presence or absence of the anti-food IgE does not predict reactivity (or nonreactivity) to the latex-associated food when it is consumed. This is a characteristic of the person's immune response (idiosyncrasy), not of the food or latex allergen.

Management of the Latex-Fruit Syndrome

The management of food hypersensitivity associated with NRL allergy is based solely on exclusion diets. However, clinicians and researchers are undecided on specific dietary recommendations for people with documented NRL allergy.

Individuals with a history of developing symptoms after consuming foods with allergens that cross-react with latex must avoid their reactive foods. However, recommendations for people with NRL allergy with and without food-specific IgE (detected by skin tests or blood tests for allergen-specific IgE such as RAST), and without symptoms after consumption of associated foods, have not been agreed upon. The following is a summary of the most frequently cited recommendations for NLR allergic individuals:[6]

■ Foods involved in the latex-fruit syndrome should be avoided if they elicit a positive skin test and the foods are not regularly consumed.

■ NRL-associated foods tolerated and regularly consumed should not be avoided, even if the NRL skin test is positive, although individuals should be advised of the potential risks.

■ Foods showing negative skin tests should not be avoided.

■ When in doubt, an oral challenge test of the food should be performed.

Box 34.1 provides a list of the foods associated with NRL allergy and the basis for their association in clinical practice (note that the list of potential foods with cross-reactivity to latex will likely expand as the molecular structure of more allergens in latex are discovered in other plants).[1–8,11-14] As the data in the box show, the strongest evidence for potential reactions to the NRL-associated food allergens (type III) comes from a combination of clinical evidence (ie, development of symptoms when the food is consumed) and proven presence of the allergen in both latex and the food. Evidence for the possibility of reactions to NRL-associated food allergens

---

BOX 34.1 Categorization of Plant Foods with Potential to Produce Cross-Reactivity with Latex Based on Level of Investigation[a]

Type I Foods
- Apricot
- Carrot
- Cherry
- Coconut
- Eggplant
- Loquat
- Spinach
- Strawberry
- Walnut
- Watermelon

Type II Foods
- Apple
- Fig
- Melon
- Peach
- Pineapple
- Pistachio

Type III Foods (with known cross-reactive allergens)
- Avocado (class I chitinase)
- Banana (class I chitinase)
- Cassava (class I chitinase)
- Cherimoya (class I chitinase)
- Chestnut (class I chitinase)
- Kiwi fruit (class I chitinase)
- Mango (class I chitinase)
- Papaya (class I chitinase)
- Passion fruit (class I chitinase)
- Tomato (class I chitinase)
- Turnip (Hev b 6.01)
- Zucchini (Hev b 6.01)
- Bell pepper (profilin)
- Celery (profilin)
- Potato (patatin-like protein Hev b 7)
- Custard apple (Hev b 6.02)

[a] Key: *Type I* is based on clinical evidence alone; *type II* indicates moderate but limited evidence (ie, clinical findings plus characterization of cross-reactive components by extract inhibition assays); *type III* has the strongest level of evidence for cross-reactivity (ie, clinical findings plus identification of cross-reactive allergens).

Source: Data are from references 1 through 13.

(type II) comes from a combination of clinical evidence and indirect evidence of the presence of the latex-associated allergen in the food. The weakest evidence for the possibility of a person with NRL allergy reacting to the listed food comes from NRL-allergic individuals reacting to the food, mostly in published case study reports (type I).

Many reports of clinical reactivity to allergens do not differentiate between the reactions triggered by cross-reacting allergens to latex and those in which the allergy is due to independent sensitization to other foods in an allergic individual. Therefore, reports of allergic reactions to cereal grains, fish, shellfish, and other nonplant foods based solely on clinical studies must be viewed with caution. Because a person is allergic to latex does not mean the individual does not have independent allergies to other foods at the same time.

In practice, the most important fact to keep in mind is that every NRL-allergic person reacts differently to foods with latex cross-reacting allergens. It is an individual characteristic as to which food will trigger a reaction. So the bottom line is this: The foods to which a person has reacted at any time must be avoided carefully. In various reports, several foods seemed to elicit allergic reactions in NRL-allergic individuals more frequently than others. The most frequently reported foods include:

- Avocado
- Banana
- Chestnut
- Fig
- Kiwi fruit
- Melon
- Mango
- Papaya
- Passion fruit
- Peach
- Pineapple
- Tomato
- Walnut

Consequently, many clinicians advise patients who are allergic to latex to avoid these foods in the interest of safety. However, it cannot be assumed that everyone in this group will react to these foods or that other foods will not trigger a reaction.

References

1. Wagner S, Breitenender H. The latex-fruit syndrome. *Biochem Soc Trans.* 2001;30(pt 6):935-940.
2. Alenius H, Turjanmaa K, Palosuo T. Natural rubber latex allergy. *Occup Environ Med.* 2002;59:419-424.

3. The World Health Organization (WHO) International Union of Immunological Societies Allergen Nomenclature Committee list of NRL allergens. www.allergen.org. Accessed April 25, 2012.

4. Kurup VP, Sussman GL, Yeang HY, et al. Specific IgE response to purified and recombinant allergens in latex allergy. *Clin Mol Allergy*. 2005;3:11-20.

5. Kurup VP, Fink JN. The spectrum of immunologic sensitization in latex allergy. *Allergy*. 2001;56(2):2-12.

6. Blanco C. Latex-fruit syndrome. *Curr Allergy Asthma Rep*. 2003;3(1):47-53.

7. Perkin JE. The latex and food allergy connection. *J Am Diet Assoc*. 2000;100(11): 1381-1384.

8. Blanco C, Carrillo T, Castillo R, Quiralte J, Cuevas M. Latex allergy: clinical features and cross-reactivity with fruits. *Ann Allergy*. 1994;73:309-314.

9. Kim KT, Hussain H. Prevalence of food allergy in 137 latex-allergic patients. *Allergy Asthma Proc*. 1999;20:95-97.

10. Poley GE, Slater JE. Latex allergy. *J Allergy Clin Immunol*. 2000;105:1054-1062.

11. Gamboa PM, Sanchez-Monge R, Diaz-Perales A, Salcedo G, Ansotegui J, Sanz ML. Latex-vegetable syndrome due to custard apple and aubergine: new variations of the hevein symphony. *J Investig Allergol Clin Immunol*. 2005;15(4):308-311.

12. Ibero M, Castillo MJ, Pineda F. Allergy to cassava: a new allergenic food with cross-reactivity to latex. *J Investig Allergol Clin Immunol*. 2007;17(6):409-412.

13. Pereira C, Tavares B, Loureiro G, Lundberg M, Chieira C. Turnip and zucchini: new foods in the latex-fruit syndrome. *Allergy*. 2007; 62(4):452-453.

14. Latex allergy and plant chitinases. In: Clare Mills EN, Shewry PR, eds. *Plant Food Allergens*. Hoboken, NJ: Wiley-Blackwell; 2003:87-105.

PART V

Selected Conditions Often Associated with Adverse Reactions to Foods

CHAPTER 35

Eczema and Diet

E czema, or atopic dermatitis (AD), is one of the most troublesome allergic conditions in infants and is the most common skin disease of childhood. It may start as early as the first few weeks of life, and occasionally may even be present at birth. In many cases, eczema appears within the first 3 months. The baby is obviously distressed by the condition—he or she seems irritable and uncomfortable, rubs or scratches the affected areas, making the situation appear worse, and often has restless and disturbed sleep. Parents and caregivers are frequently even more distressed than the baby. Eczema is unsightly, and when a baby is obviously uncomfortable, everyone is anxious to relieve the problem in any way possible. The fact that food allergy is often an important factor in the condition creates a situation in which food restrictions for both the baby and the breastfeeding mother are often undertaken, sometimes creating nutritional deficiencies in both.

Symptoms of Eczema

Eczema tends to appear in a fairly typical pattern that changes at different ages. The symptom presentation in different age groups are summarized in the following sections.

Infantile Eczema

Infantile eczema usually starts between 2 and 6 months of age, although it often appears earlier if the baby is highly allergic to foods. The baby develops a red rash, which may weep. It appears on the cheeks and may spread to the forehead and the backs of arms and legs. In severe cases, it may involve the whole body. Heavy scaling may occur. This early eczema is often associated with food allergy and tends to disappear between the ages of 3 and 5 years as food allergies are outgrown.

Childhood Eczema

Childhood eczema may follow the infantile phase almost immediately, or it may start for the first time between the ages of 2 and 4 years. In childhood eczema, the rash is found in the creases of the elbows, behind the knees, and across the ankles, and it may involve the face, ears, and neck. This form of eczema is frequently associated with allergy to airborne and contact allergens such as dust mites, animal dander, mold spores, and plant pollens. It often disappears by the age of 10 but may continue into adult life.

Adult Eczema

Adult eczema usually appears as large areas of very itchy, reddened, weeping skin with the elbow creases, wrists, neck, ankles, and behind the knees being especially affected. It may also be troublesome on the palms of the hands and between the fingers. The condition tends to improve in middle life and is unusual in the elderly.

Causes of Eczema

There is a great deal of debate about the causes of eczema and whether eczema is associated with food allergy, either as a cause or an effect. There is increasing evidence that a major risk factor for eczema involves filaggrin gene defects, indicating a genetic origin for the condition.[1] Filaggrins are proteins that bind to keratin fibers in epithelial cells. In the skin it is thought that defects in filaggrin proteins result in abnormalities in the structure of the skin, and individuals with the defect are predisposed to dry skin and eczema.[2]

Eczema and Food Allergy

Food allergy and eczema often occur in the same individual, especially in childhood. Clinical reports from the past few decades indicate that foods such as cow's milk, hen's eggs, soy, wheat, and a few other foods can directly provoke eczema flare-up in children, especially if the child is sensitized to the food.[3] Those at greatest risk for food-induced eczema are young children in whom eczematous lesions are severe or resistant to treatment.[4]

More than 50% of all children with atopic dermatitis have been reported to experience exacerbation of their eczema alone or in addition to immediate symptoms in other organ systems when exposed to their allergenic food.[3] Adolescents and adults with atopic dermatitis may also react to foods, but not as frequently as children. Reactions to environmental allergens such as dust mites and molds are more common in the older age groups.

Experts differ considerably in their opinions as to the value of food-exclusion diets for the treatment of childhood eczema.[5] A 2008 literature review of the topic found that up to 40% of children hospitalized for treatment had a flare-up of the atopic eczema in reaction to certain food allergens,[6] but the report indicated that these children were likely to be sensitized to the food allergen and that the eczema exacerbation was part of the overall food allergy response rather than an isolated symptom. A cautionary note is provided by a 2010 publication that states, "Only a small portion of cutaneous reactions to food in the form of late, eczematous eruptions will directly exacerbate AD in young infants who have moderate to severe AD,"[7] and warns against the uncontrolled elimination of foods from a child's diet in attempts to prevent and control the symptoms of eczema.

However, a 2010 study involving a literature search of PubMed and Medline to review the epidemiology and pathophysiology of AD, with special focus on the role of food allergy in the development of AD,[8] indicated that food allergens readily provoked AD in 35% of patients, as proven through double-blind placebo-controlled food challenge studies. Milk, egg, wheat, soy, and peanut accounted for 75% of the cases of food-induced AD.

In infancy, eczema may be one of the earliest signs that a baby might have food allergy. Of course, not all babies with eczema have food allergy; a figure of one-third is usually quoted as the number of young children whose atopic dermatitis can be attributed to food allergy. For example, in one typical study, 33.8% (25 of 74) of the pediatric patients with AD were diagnosed with food allergy.[9] The foods most frequently identified as allergens in this group were eggs, milk, and peanuts.

Infantile eczema can also occur as a response to an allergic reaction to environmental allergens such as dust mites, mold spores, animal dander, and plant pollens, among others. These allergens are usually a problem as the baby gets older, and the allergens gain access to the immune cells through the nonintact skin of the eczematous patches of inadequately controlled AD.[5]

Eczema as a Route for Allergic Sensitization to Foods

An additional connection between AD and food allergy is becoming more widely recognized in food allergy prevention and management. Understanding of the potential for allergic sensitization to foods via the transdermal route is becoming of increasing importance in food allergy prevention and management. The skin barrier defect in AD may allow for easier and earlier sensitization to food and airborne allergens; therefore, exposure to food proteins in AD skin may act as a risk factor for development of food allergies.[7]

Foods Associated with Food Allergy in Babies and Children with Eczema

Eczema as a symptom of food allergy seems to be much more common in early childhood than later in life. The first symptoms that alert health care providers and parents that a baby is allergic (or atopic) are in the digestive tract (often exhibited as prolonged coliclike symptoms) and in the skin (eczema and hives). In babies under the age of 6 months, eliminating the foods that are triggering symptoms often leads to a significant improvement in the eczema, and in some cases, total remission. These foods may be in the diet of the breastfeeding mother or in the baby's diet if he or she is formula-fed or has started to consume solid foods.

The food allergens that most frequently trigger the onset of eczema in babies and children are reported to be:

■ Egg
■ Milk and milk products
■ Peanut
■ Soy
■ Wheat

Occasionally, green peas and tomatoes are added to the list of frequently identified food allergies in children with eczema, usually after they have been introduced as solid foods.[10] In another study, the authors found that all the children who were allergic to sesame seed had atopic dermatitis.[11]

When the baby is being breastfed, this means the mother avoids these foods (and includes nutritionally equivalent substitutes in her diet to ensure complete balanced nutrition for herself and her baby). For the formula-fed baby, an extensively hydrolyzed casein-based formula may be necessary to avoid the milk proteins in conventional milk-based infant formulas.

Of course, every baby is an individual and may have been sensitized to foods other than those previously mentioned. If elimination of these foods does not result in complete resolution of the baby's eczema, others may be eliminated, based on careful analysis of records of the baby's diet and symptoms, and the diet of the mother if the baby is being breastfed.

Reintroducing each food into the mother's diet and monitoring the baby's response will usually provide the information required to formulate a diet that is free from the baby's eczema triggers and provides complete balanced nutrition from alternate sources, both for the baby and for the breastfeeding mother.

When environmental allergens such dust mites, mold spores, pollens, and animal dander trigger or exacerbate AD in a sensitized individual, diet manipulation may not have a significant effect on the condition, so this should be considered when evaluating the role of food allergy in a person's AD.

It is not uncommon for eczema in a 2-year-old child to increase in severity and at the same time symptoms such as rhinitis and wheezing suddenly appear, especially when the child is in an environment where airborne allergens, typically dust mites and animal dander, are unusually high. This scenario is typical of the atopic child who starts out with eczema as a symptom of food allergy and becomes sensitized to allergens in the environment as he or she becomes older. Up to the age of about 5 years, but more commonly at age 2 or 3 years, it is not unusual for food and inhalant allergy to coexist, so any symptoms are worse because there are now more allergens to trigger the release of inflammatory mediators and increase symptom severity and incidence.

Management of Food Allergy in a Child with Eczema

Many authorities recommend that "diagnostic evaluation of food allergy should be performed in all children" with AD.[12] Blood tests for food allergen–specific IgE are the only safe allergy tests for children with eczema. Allergy skin testing is not advisable because their skin is already highly reactive and will frequently produce false-positive reactions and create a possible route for sensitization to allergens in the test reagents.

A short trial on a diet that excludes any foods that test positive in allergen-specific IgE tests, as well as the foods that are most frequently associated with eczema (ie, eggs, milk and milk products, peanut, soy, wheat, tomato, sesame seed, and green pea), should show improvement in the child's symptoms if foods are playing a significant role in the eczema. Reintroducing these foods separately and monitoring the child's response (by looking for reddening of the skin, itching, and an obvious increase in eczema) will confirm that the specific food that triggered this response should be avoided.

When implementing an elimination diet for a child, it is extremely important that each food that is excluded from a child's or breastfeeding mother's diet be replaced by one of equal nutritional value. Neither should be put at nutritional risk as a result of removing important food groups at this critical stage of a child's development. (Chapters 10 through 19 provide more details of the foods to be avoided and their nutritional substitutes when foods other than those listed here need to be avoided as a result of allergy tests or as indicated by an analysis of the child's and mother's diet and symptom records.)

This diet should be followed for 4 weeks. If significant improvement in the child's eczema is achieved on this regimen, reintroduction of each eliminated food individually, either into the child's diet or into the mother's diet if she is breastfeeding the baby, with careful monitoring of the child's response should determine exactly which foods are contributing to the eczema. These foods should then be avoided for as long as the child has symptoms—usually at least until age 5 years—when retesting of the foods should be undertaken to determine if the child has developed tolerance to them. Details of challenge protocols for identification of offending food allergens are provided in Chapter 7.

References

1. Worth A, Sheikh A. Food allergy and atopic eczema. *Curr Opin Allergy Clin Immunol.* 2010;10(3):226-230.
2. Weidinger S, Rodríguez E, Stahl C, et al. Filaggrin mutations strongly predispose to early-onset and extrinsic atopic dermatitis. *J Invest Dermatol.* 2007;127(3):724-726.
3. Werfel T, Breuer K. Role of food allergy in atopic dermatitis. *Curr Opin Allergy Clin Immunol.* 2004;4(5):379-385.
4. Kim JS. Pediatric atopic dermatitis: the importance of food allergens. *Semin Cutan Med Surg.* 2008;27(2):156-160.

5. Werfel T, Ballmer-Weber B, Eigenmann PA, et al. Eczematous reactions to food in atopic eczema: position paper of the EAACI and GA2LEN. *Allergy*. 2007;62(7):723-728.

6. Schäfer T. The impact of allergy on atopic eczema from data from epidemiological studies. *Curr Opin Allergy Clin Immunol*. 2008;8(5):418-422.

7. Suh KY. Food allergy and atopic dermatitis: separating fact from fiction. *Semin Cutan Med Surg*. 2010;29(2):72-78.

8. Greenhawt M. The role of food allergy in atopic dermatitis. *Allergy Asthma Proc*. 2010;31(5):392-397.

9. Eigenmann PA, Calza A-M. Diagnosis of IgE-mediated food allergy among Swiss children with atopic dermatitis. *Pediatr Allergy Immunol*. 2000;11(2):95-100.

10. Eigenmann PA, Sicherer SH, Borkowski TA, Cohen BA, Sampson HA. Prevalence of IgE mediated food allergy among children with atopic dermatitis. *Pediatrics*. 1998;101:E8.

11. Caubet JC, Hofer MF, Eigenmann PA, Wassenberg J. Snack seeds allergy in children. *Allergy*. 2010;65(1):136-137.

12. Fiocchi A, Bouygue GR, Martelli A, Terracciano L, Sarratud T. Dietary treatment of childhood atopic eczema/dermatitis syndrome (AEDS). *Allergy*. 2004;59(suppl 78):78-85.

CHAPTER **36**

Urticaria, Angioedema, and Diet

U rticaria, commonly called *hives*, is a rash appearing as raised, red, itchy bumps usually surrounded by a red flattened area of various shapes and sizes. Angioedema is a related condition, which involves tissues deeper within the skin rather than on the skin surface. Both can be caused by allergic or nonallergic triggers.

Urticaria

An estimated 15% to 20% of people experience hives at some time in their lives.[1] Sixty-three percent of people with hives suspect food as the triggering factor.[2] Hives are frequently caused by allergic reactions; however, there are many nonallergic causes. For convenience, urticaria can be categorized as:

- Acute urticaria (hives lasting less than 6 weeks): commonly the result of an allergy, or in some cases can be part of a viral infection (referred to as *viral exanthema*).[3]
- Chronic urticaria (hives lasting longer than 6 weeks): rarely due to an allergy.[4] It is estimated that in 30% to 40% of cases of chronic urticaria, the cause is probably due to some autoimmune process.[5]
- Idiopathic urticaria: term given to urticaria in which the cause is entirely unknown. Identification of the agent responsible for urticaria in most studies is less than 20%.[6]
- Cholinergic urticaria: urticaria due to friction, pressure, temperature extremes,[7] exercise, and sweating.[8]

Typical Picture of Urticaria

Urticaria can appear anywhere on the skin's surface. Whether the trigger is allergic or nonallergic, there is a complex release of inflammatory mediators, including

333

histamine, from mast cells in the skin. Histamine causes several effects (see Chapter 31). In urticaria, the effects of histamine can be seen as:

- Increased permeability of the blood vessels, allowing fluid to leak from the blood vessels into tissues, causing the localized swelling (wheal). Wheals may be pinpoint in size or several inches in diameter.
- Widening of blood vessels, which brings an increased blood flow to the area, causing reddening.
- Itching—the pruritus associated with histamine—confirming its presence in the affected area.

Individual hives that are painful, last more than 24 hours, or leave a bruise as they heal are more likely to be a more serious condition called *urticarial vasculitis*.[9] This is sometimes associated with a condition such as *thrombocytopenic purpura* or as a symptom of mastocytosis in which release of inflammatory mediators from mast cells causes localized reactions in the skin.

Dermatographism is a skin condition that involves hives that result when skin is stroked or scratched. This condition is often characterized by linear hives and is benign.[10] Dermatographism is estimated to affect approximately 4% to 5% of the population.[10]

Angioedema

Angioedema is similar to urticaria but with larger edematous areas that involve swelling of the skin and mucous membranes. Swelling of the eyelids, lips, and tongue is the most common. Other parts of the body that may be affected are the face, ears, under the chin, the genitalia, hands, feet, trunk, and arms.[11] Angioedema is usually not itchy.

Headache, arthralgia, the sensation of a lump in the throat, hoarseness, shortness of breath, wheezing, nausea, vomiting, abdominal pain, and diarrhea may occur at the same time as angioedema.[12] Often the cause of angioedema is unknown, leading to a diagnosis of *idiopathic angioedema*.

Triggers of angioedema are often the same as those associated with urticaria. Angioedema may also occur after infections, especially viral infections, or with other illnesses (including autoimmune disorders such as lupus and malignancies such as leukemia and lymphoma).

Atopic disease conditions, such as asthma, rhinitis, and eczema, have been reported to be greater in urticaria and angioedema subjects than normal in some studies and no greater than normal in others.[13]

Causes of Urticaria and Angioedema

Allergy to any food or intolerance of a food additive or its naturally occurring counterpart and sensitivity to biogenic amines such as histamine and tyramine may contribute to urticaria and angioedema.

Allergy

The main immunological process involved in allergic urticaria and angioedema is an IgE-mediated hypersensitivity reaction to an allergenic food or an inhaled allergen in a sensitized individual. The symptoms typically appear approximately 30 minutes after ingestion or inhalation of an allergen. As a result, identification of the allergen is sometimes obvious.

Foods and other substances that are most frequently implicated in provoking IgE-mediated urticaria include shellfish, nuts, and drugs.[10] Although inhaled allergens are rarely reported to be the cause of urticaria,[11] a theory of "total allergy burden" has been proposed[11] in which one allergen does not result in urticaria, but the additive effect of several contact, inhaled, and ingested allergens produce urticaria as they each release a battery of inflammatory mediators from mast cells. Since several allergens are responsible, identification of each contributing allergen is often very difficult in practice.

Histamine Sensitivity

Histamine is the primary inflammatory chemical responsible for urticaria and angioedema.[14] Some subjects with urticaria/angioedema have a defect in the enzymes, especially diamine oxidase (DAO), that metabolize histamine.[15] Many factors, such as physical stimuli, drug intake, diet, and some unknown factors may contribute to an increased level of histamine.[2] Dietary sources of histamine may be a significant source of histamine in individuals with reduced DAO enzyme activity in the small bowel mucosa that would normally break down histamine and maintain total body histamine at a "normal level"[16] (see Chapter 31 for details).

Any allergic reaction will result in histamine release, so food or inhalant allergy will increase the level of histamine in the body and result in symptoms of urticaria and/or angioedema in sensitive people. In addition, food and food additives may increase the release of histamine in body tissues through immunological and/or non-immunological mechanisms.[17]

DAO and histamine N-methyltransferase (HNMT) are the two enzymes responsible for the catabolism of histamine. Hepatic HNMT enzymes ensure a consistent posthepatic level of blood histamine. DAO breaks down excess histamine, which is excreted from the body as imidazole compounds in urine. A deficiency in the catabolism of histamine would allow excess histamine to enter the circulation (see Chapter 31 for details). The excess histamine then causes the urticaria and angioedema.

Levels of histamine fluctuate constantly in the body as histamine is produced as an essential mediator required for brain function, digestive processes, and protection. It is only when the level of histamine exceeds the enzymes' capacities to maintain it at a "normal level" that symptoms result. Histamine from extrinsic sources such as foods, food additives, beverages, and supplements can contribute to the overload. People with symptoms of histamine sensitivity, such as urticaria and angioedema, usually benefit greatly from restricting their intake of histamine-associated foods and beverages. If all dietary sources of histamine can be eliminated, the symptoms of chronic urticaria/angioedema are often alleviated.

Tyramine Sensitivity

Tyramine is another important biogenic amine that has been implicated in the etiology of chronic urticaria and angioedema in a number of research reports.[18] However, where a specific role for tyramine has been investigated, the results indicate that its effects may be minor.[19]

Food and Food Additives That May Trigger Urticaria and Angioedema

Food Allergens

The highly allergenic foods most frequently reported to induce urticaria include shellfish, fish, egg, nuts, milk, and wheat. However, any food is capable of triggering an allergic reaction in a sensitized individual. Identification of food allergens responsible for urticaria or angioedema should be determined in the same way as for any food allergy: by tests for allergen-specific IgE, followed by elimination and challenge to identify the culprit food (see Chapters 5, 6, and 7).

Food Additives

Food additive elimination diets have been reported to control urticaria in approximately 20% to 50% of subjects.[13] The substances most commonly implicated in these studies have been azo dyes such as tartrazine and sunset yellow and preservatives such as benzoates and sulfites. Naturally occurring salicylates and benzoates have also been implicated as contributors to inducing urticaria. All of these additives seem to elicit an adverse reaction by releasing histamine, thus contributing to histamine overload in sensitive individuals.

Pseudoallergens

Foods that trigger urticaria or angioedema but do not elicit an IgE-mediated response may be acting in numerous ways that are not mediated by an allergic reaction.[20] Some researchers have designated these foods as *pseudoallergens* and have reported good success in controlling the symptoms by use of a pseudoallergen-restricted diet. In one study, a third of the subjects reported the diet alleviated their urticaria.[21] Interestingly, the pseudoallergens listed in the report —foods and food additives— are those that contain histamine or release histamine; basically, the pseudoallergen-restricted diet is a histamine-restricted diet.

Histamine-Containing Foods

Histamine is formed in food from the decarboxylation of histidine by bacteria that possess the enzyme histidine decarboxylase (see Chapter 31). Proteinaceous foods that are aged and fermented commonly have increased histamine levels. Other foods release histamine or contain histamine as a result of the ripening process.

The amount of histamine in a particular food may vary a great deal, depending on the conditions under which it was processed and stored. Box 36.1 lists the foods and other dietary ingredients that contain or release histamine.

BOX 36.1   Histamine-Associated Foods in Urticaria and Angioedema

Meat, Poultry, Fish
- All shellfish (mollusks and crustaceans)
- Fish, whether fresh, frozen, smoked, or canned, if the processing is unknown. However, if the fish is freshly caught, gutted, and cooked within ½ hour, or is frozen as soon as it is caught, it may be eaten.
- Egg: Only a small quantity of cooked egg in a baked product such as pancakes, muffins, cakes is allowed.
- Processed, smoked, and fermented meats such as luncheon meat, sausage, wiener, bologna, salami, pepperoni, smoked ham, cured bacon
- Leftover meat and fish

Milk and Milk Products
- All fermented milk products, including:
  - Any kind of fermented cheese such as cheddar, Colby, blue cheese, Brie, Camembert, feta, Romano, Parmesan
  - Cheese products such as processed cheese, cheese slices, cheese spreads
  - Cottage cheese
  - Ricotta cheese
  - Yogurt
  - Buttermilk
  - Kefir

Fruits
- Apricot
- Cherry
- Citrus fruits: Orange, grapefruit, lemon, lime
- Cranberry
- Currant (fresh or dried)
- Date
- Grape
- Loganberry
- Pineapple
- Plum
- Prune

Continues

BOX 36.1   Histamine-Associated Foods in Urticaria and Angioedema (*Continued*)

- Raisin
- Raspberry
- Strawberry

Vegetables
- Avocado
- Eggplant
- Olives
- Pickles, relishes, and other foods containing vinegar
- Pumpkin
- Spinach
- Tomato, tomato sauce, ketchup

Legumes
- Red beans
- Soy bean and soy products

Food Additives
- Tartrazine and other azo dyes used as artificial food colors
- Preservatives, especially benzoates and sulfites
- Note: Many medications and vitamin supplements also contain these additives

Seasonings
- Chili powder
- Cinnamon
- Clove
- Curry powder
- Nutmeg
- Thyme
- Vinegar

Miscellaneous
- Alcoholic beverages of all types
- Chocolate, cocoa, and cola drinks
- Fermented soy products (such as soy sauce, miso)
- Fermented foods (such as sauerkraut)
- Nonalcoholic versions of beer, ale, wine, and so on
- Tea (regular or green)

> **BOX 36.2   Foods with High Levels of Tyramine**
>
> - Aged cheese
> - Avocado
> - Banana
> - Chicken liver
> - Eggplant
> - Fermented beverages, such as beer and ale, wine (especially red)
> - Fermented meats and sausages
> - Fermented soy products
> - Fermented vegetables (eg, sauerkraut)
> - Fig
> - Raspberry
> - Red plum
> - Tomato
> - Vinegar and pickles
> - Yeast extract

Tyramine-Containing Foods

Although a role for tyramine in the etiology of urticaria and angioedema has not been substantiated by well-controlled research studies, some reports seem to implicate the amine as a contributing factor in their subject population.[22] Details about tyramine sensitivity can be found in Chapter 32. See Box 36.2 for foods that have high levels of tyramine.

Detecting the Offending Foods in Urticaria and Angioedema

Identifying the offending triggers can be a tedious task, especially since there are virtually no definitive tests available for diagnosis. The steps required for identifying food triggers will be the same as those employed for diagnosing any allergic or intolerance reaction to food components (see Chapters 5, 6, and 7). In addition, histamine and tyramine intolerance should be considered.

In many cases, the few foods elimination diet is a worthwhile starting point. If symptoms resolve on this diet, the offending foods should be identified by challenge with each of the suspect foods and careful monitoring of symptom development. Refer to Chapter 7 for details.

In a number of cases where evidence for food allergy or any other obvious cause is lacking, a trial on a histamine-restricted diet is worthwhile, because histamine is the major mediator of the symptoms of urticaria and angioedema, whatever the major etiological agent may be. Four weeks on the histamine-restricted diet is usually sufficient to determine whether this approach will relieve the symptoms.

The Histamine-Restricted Diet

The diet designed to manage idiopathic urticaria and angioedema restricts the intake of foods and food additives that are known to increase histamine in the body, either because of their intrinsic histamine content or by a mechanism of endogenous histamine release. This management approach has proved very effective in several cases that have not improved with any other treatment.[23]

Combined Histamine- and Tyramine-Restricted Diet

When symptoms remain on the histamine-restricted diet, it is sometimes beneficial to follow up with a short trial (1 to 2 weeks is usually adequate) on a diet that restricts both histamine- and tyramine-associated foods. Because most of the food restrictions relating to tyramine sensitivity are the same as those responsible for high levels of histamine, only a few additional foods need to be avoided on the combined diet:

■ Chicken liver
■ Fig
■ Banana
■ Yeast extract

Because reactions to food components mediated by mechanisms other than IgE-mediated allergy are mainly dose-related and require time for symptoms to develop, the "gold standard" of oral provocation by double-blind placebo-controlled food challenge is of little or no value in identifying the offending foods.[24] Sequential incremental dose challenge (SIDC) over a period of up to 4 days is the most effective method of determining the culprit food and food additives responsible for a person's reactions in cases of chronic conditions such as urticaria and angioedema when IgE-mediated allergy has been ruled out. Details about the SIDC can be found in Chapter 7.

References

1. Atkins FM. Food-induced urticaria In: Metcalfe DD, Sampson HA, Simon RA, eds. *Food Allergy: Adverse Reactions to Foods and Food Additives.* 2nd ed. Oxford, UK: Blackwell Scientific; 1997:211-219.
2. Zuberbier T. The role of allergens and psuedoallergens in urticaria. *J Investig Dermatol Symp Proc.* 2001;6:132-134.
3. Guin JD. The evaluation of patients with urticaria. *Dermatol Clin.* 1985;3:29-49.
4. Greaves MW. Chronic urticaria. *New Engl J Med.* 1995;332:1767-1772.
5. Burrall BA, Halpern GM, Huntley AC. Chronic urticaria. *West J Med.* 1990;152(3): 268-276.
6. Matthews KP. Urticaria and angioedema. *J Allergy Clin Immunol.* 1983;72:1-14.
7. Mahmoudi M. Cold-induced urticaria. *J Am Osteopath Assoc.* 2001;101(5 suppl):S1-S4.
8. Horikawa T, Fukunaga A, Nishigori C. New concepts of hive formation in cholinergic urticaria. *Curr Allergy Asthma Rep.* 2009;9(4):273-279.

9. Mehregan D, Heyl JM, Hamzavi I. Dermatologic manifestations of urticarial vasculitis. Medscape Reference: Drugs, Diseases, and Procedures. http://emedicine.medscape.com/article/1085087-overview. Accessed June 26, 2012.

10. Jedele KB, Michels VV. Familial dermographism. *Am J Med Genet.* 1991;39(2):201-203.

11. Grattan EH, Charlesworth EN. Urticaria. In: Holgate ST, Church MK, eds. *Allergy.* New York, NY: Gower Medical Publishing; 1993:93-104.

12. Soter NA. Acute and chronic urticaria and angioedema. *J Am Acad Dermatol.* 1991;25:146-154.

13. Armenaka M, Lehach J, Rosenstreich DL. Successful management of chronic urticaria. *Clin Rev Allergy.* 1992;10:371-390.

14. White MV. The role of histamine in allergic disease. *J Allergy Clin Immunol.* 1990;86(4 pt 2):599-605.

15. Lessof MH. Food, food additives and urticaria. *Clin Exper Allergy.* 1991;21(suppl 1):316-320.

16. Sattler J, Hafner D, Klotter H, Lorenz W, Wagner PK. Food-induced histaminosis as an epidemiological problem: plasma histamine elevation and haemodynamic alterations after oral histamine administration and blockade of diamine oxidase (DAO). *Agents Actions.* 1988;23(3/4):361-365.

17. Murdoch DD, Lessof MH, Pollock I, Young E. Effects of food additives on leuko-cyte histamine release in normal and urticaria subjects. *J Roy Coll Phys London.* 1987;21(4):251-256.

18. Guin JD. The evaluation of patients with urticaria. *Dermatol Clin.* 1985;3(1):29-49.

19. Warin RP, Smith RJ. Challenge test battery in chronic urticaria. *Br J Dermatol.* 1976;94(4):401-406.

20. Ehlers I, Niggemann B, Binder C, Zuberbier T. Role of nonallergic hypersensitivity reactions in children with chronic urticaria. *Allergy.* 1998;53(11):1074-1077.

21. Magerl M, Pisarevskaja D, Scheufele R, Zuberbier T, Maurer M. Effects of a pseudo-allergen-free diet on chronic spontaneous urticaria: a prospective trial. *Allergy.* 2010;65(1):78-83.

22. Verschave A, Stevens E, Degreef H. Pseudo-allergen-free diet in chronic urticaria. *Dermatologica.* 1983;167(5):256-259.

23. Joneja JMV, Carmona Silva C. Outcome of a histamine-restricted diet based on chart audit. *J Nutr Environ Med.* 2001;11(4):249-262.

24. Bunselmeyer B, Laubach HJ, Schiller M, Stanke M, Luger TA, Brehler R. Incremental build-up food challenge—a new diagnostic approach to evaluate pseudoallergic reactions in chronic urticaria: a pilot study: stepwise food challenge in chronic urticaria. *Clin Exp Allergy.* 2009;39(1):116-126.

CHAPTER **37**

Asthma and Diet

Food allergy involves an immunologically mediated response to specific foods that results in the release of inflammatory mediators. It is the action of these mediators on the tissues of various organ systems that results in the symptoms of allergy. When these mediators act on tissues in the respiratory tract, symptoms of allergic rhino-conjunctivitis or hay fever result; mediators acting in the lungs may result in asthma.

Inhalation of Food Particles

In addition to ingestion, the allergenic food can impact the lung via inhalation of food particles released when the food is cooked or otherwise dispersed in an aerosol. An example of the latter is baker's asthma that results from inhalation of wheat particles in aerosolized flour.[1] Allergy to aerosolized allergens in cooked foods has been reported in highly allergic individuals who have been exposed to their allergenic foods, such as fish, shellfish, and eggs, in an enclosed area, such as a restaurant, during cooking.[2] Most of the examples of aerosolized food allergens triggering asthma are reported in adults in specific occupations that expose them regularly to the allergens.[3] In contrast, most of the foods that are associated with asthma in children trigger the response when they are eaten, not inhaled.

Ingestion of Food Allergens and Asthma

In 1992, one of the earliest studies that linked asthma and food allergy was published.[4] In 279 children with asthma, 168 experienced wheezing in double-blind placebo-controlled food challenges with foods. The foods that triggered wheezing in this study, in order of frequency, were peanut, milk, egg, tree nuts, soy, wheat, legumes (beans), and turkey. In all cases, the wheezing occurred within 2 hours of the children eating the test foods. All of the selected children were known to be allergic to the foods and had other symptoms that indicated their allergic status.

Another study of asthma triggered by foods[5] identified the culprit food, in order of prevalence, as egg, milk, peanut, wheat, soy, and fish. In another study,[6] peanut and milk allergies were both associated with an increased number of hospitalizations for acute asthma. Milk allergy was associated with increased use of systemic steroids for control of asthma in the children.[6]

In most cases of food-associated asthma in children, asthma symptoms rarely occur alone; other symptoms of allergy are triggered when the food is ingested.[7] Food-induced anaphylaxis is the most dramatic example of multiple organ systems being involved as a response to food allergy in asthmatics.

The relationship between food allergy and asthma is most obvious in children, rather than adults, and was highest in the youngest of the children studied.[8] In a group of babies allergic to milk, with a mean age of 10 months, 29% of 27 infants had lung responses typical of asthma on challenge with milk.[8]

Sulfite Sensitivity and Asthma

Sensitivity to sulfites is common in people with asthma. Of these people, individuals who are steroid dependent are considered most at risk for sulfite sensitivity.[9] Although the incidence of adverse reactions to sulfites is estimated to be as high as 1% of the U.S. population, sulfite sensitivity in people without asthma is considered rare. (For more details about sulfite sensitivity, see Chapter 21.)

Anaphylaxis and Asthma

Studies examining food allergy deaths suggest that those who die as a result of food allergy usually have coexistent asthma. The increasing prevalence of severe food allergies and awareness of its risk in those with asthma demands a rigorous approach to the diagnosis and management of coexistent food allergy and asthma, especially in young people who appear to be at highest risk from death from severe food allergy.[10]

Patients with underlying asthma are more likely to experience a fatal or near-fatal food reaction. Food reactions tend to be more severe or life threatening when they involve the respiratory tract. The presence of a food allergy is a risk factor for the future development of asthma, particularly for children with sensitization to egg protein.[7]

Asthma, Leukotrienes, and Inhibition of the Cyclooxygenase Pathway

Many asthmatics are sensitive to aspirin and some nonsteroidal anti-inflammatory drugs (NSAIDs). This sensitivity is due to the ability of aspirin (as acetyl salicylic acid [ASA]) to inhibit the cyclooxygenase pathway of arachidonic acid metabolism.

As a result of this inhibitory effect, the lipoxygenase pathway from arachidonic acid enhances the production of leukotrienes, leading to an increase in these mediators (see Chapter 26 for details and pictorial representation of this mechanism). Leukotrienes are largely responsible for the bronchoconstriction that causes asthma. Therefore, anything that will enhance leukotriene production is likely to exacerbate asthma.

Food additives such as azo dyes, particularly tartrazine; preservatives such as benzoates and sulfites; and naturally occurring salicylates have all been implicated in inhibiting the cyclooxygenase pathway and thus increasing the production of leukotrienes. These additives therefore may all have an adverse effect on a person with asthma who is sensitive to them.

In addition to their role in increasing leukotriene production, food additives such as preservatives and food colors have been shown in animal studies to suppress the Th1 pathway of immune response[11] (see Chapter 1 for details). This could shift the Th1/Th2 type immune balance toward the Th2 response of IgE-mediated allergy. The same studies also implicated antioxidant supplements such as vitamins C and E in suppressing the Th1 response and thus potentially contributing to asthma. These additives should be taken into account when investigating the possible role of foods in the symptoms of asthma, especially acute attacks where the effects may be immediately apparent after ingestion.

Prevention of Asthma in the Food-Allergic Child

Research studies indicate that there is no benefit from the delayed introduction of highly allergenic foods in young infants as a measure to prevent food allergy in the young child. On the contrary, research from 2010 indicates that introducing potentially allergenic foods such as oats at an early age may be associated with a reduced risk of persistent asthma.[12]

By the age of 5 to 7 years, most food allergies may be outgrown, but asthma may persist well into adulthood. The numbers of children with asthma and hay fever are typically the same whether or not the diet has been restricted because of food allergy management in infancy.[13] Inhalant allergies tend to be the most important triggers in older children with respiratory allergy. Foods probably contribute very little to these conditions, except in aggravating the situation when inflammatory mediators are released in the food-induced allergy.

Management of Food-Associated Asthma

Food allergy contributes to asthma in only a small number of people. There are so many other asthma triggers (eg, inhaled dust mites, mold spores, animal dander, pollens, etc) that can also contribute to the condition that it is very unlikely that removing the allergenic foods will result in control of asthma entirely. It is most probable that food allergy is making the asthma worse rather than being solely responsible for triggering the symptoms.

Nevertheless, it is possible to get some idea of whether foods are triggering wheezing or asthma by challenging suspect foods individually and monitoring symptom development after a period of avoiding the food (see Chapter 6 for details). Changes in the response of the airways after food challenge can be monitored using peak flow meters (spirometry). A decrease in airflow indicates an adverse response to the food. However, no food or food additive should be avoided unless it has been demonstrated to trigger or exacerbate a person's asthma.

Management of the food allergy that is associated with asthma is no different from managing food allergy that causes other symptoms. The foods must be avoided as long as the individual shows symptoms when the food is eaten. Persons with asthma, parents, and caregivers of the child with asthma must become familiar with terms on product labels and other sources where the food may be present. However, it is important to realize that avoidance of any food or additive will not cure asthma.

After long-term avoidance of the food, many children outgrow their food allergies as they become older, so periodic challenge with the offending food should be undertaken to determine whether a child is still allergic to it. Skin and blood tests tend to remain positive long after the symptoms have resolved, so direct challenge with the food is usually necessary. Once the food causes no problem, it should be eaten regularly to maintain tolerance.

Because of the increased risk of anaphylaxis in an asthmatic individual, it is becoming increasingly apparent that early and accurate determination of the foods responsible for food allergy, especially in a child with asthma, is crucial. Blood tests for allergen-specific IgE, followed by carefully monitored elimination and challenge, are essential to identify the foods and additives to which the asthma sufferer may be sensitive. Sulfites, benzoates, azo dyes, and other additives, and naturally occurring forms of these such as benzoates and salicylates, which may inhibit the cyclooxygenase pathway of arachidonic acid metabolism (see earlier discussion), should be considered during this process.

References

1. Baur X, Degens PO, Sander I. Bakers asthma: still among the most frequent occupational respiratory disorders. *J Allergy Clin Immunol.* 1998;102(6 pt 1):984-997.
2. Cartier A. The role of inhalant food allergens in occupational asthma. *Curr Allergy Asthma Rep.* 2010;10(5):349-356.
3. Nordman H, Karjalainen A, Keskinen H. Incidence of occupational asthma: a comparison by reporting systems. *Am J Ind Med.* 1999;(suppl 1):130-133.
4. Bock SA. Respiratory reactions induced by food challenges in children with pulmonary disease. *Pediatr Allergy Immunol.* 1992;3:188-194.
5. Sicherer SH, Sampson HA. The role of food allergy in childhood asthma. *Immunol Allergy Clin North Am.* 1998;18(1):49-60.
6. Simpson AB, Glutting J, Yousef E. Food allergy and asthma morbidity in children. *Pediatr Pulmonol.* 2007;42(6):489-495.

7. Beausoleil JL, Fiedler J, Spergel JM. Food intolerance and childhood asthma: what is the link? *Paediatr Drugs.* 2007;9(3):157-163.

8. Hill DJ, Firer MA, Shelton MJ, et al. Manifestations of milk allergy in infancy: clinical and immunological findings. *J Pediatr.* 1986;109:270-276.

9. Vally H, Misso NL, Madan V. Clinical effects of sulphite additives. *Clin Exp Allergy.* 2009;39(11):1643-1651.

10. Gillman A, Douglass JA. What do asthmatics have to fear from food and additive allergy? *Clin Exp Allergy.* 2010;40(9):1295-1302.

11. Zaknun D, Schroecksnadel S, Kurz K, Fuchs D. Potential role of antioxidant food supplements, preservatives and colorants in the pathogenesis of allergy and asthma. *Int Arch Allergy Immunol.* 2011;157(2):113-124.

12. Virtanen SM, Kaila M, Pekkanen J, et al. Early introduction of oats associated with decreased risk of persistent asthma and early introduction of fish with decreased risk of allergic rhinitis. *Br J Nutr.* 2010;103(2):266-273.

13. Zeiger R, Heller S. The development and prediction of atopy in high-risk children: follow-up at seven years in a prospective randomized study of combined maternal and infant food allergen avoidance. *J Allergy Clin Immunol.* 1995;95:1179-1190.

CHAPTER **38**

Migraine and Diet

An estimated 5% to 30% of the population has experienced migraine headaches. They affect women about three times more frequently than men and are an inherited condition in 60% to 80% of cases.

Many authorities have attempted to define migraine; one of the more succinct is: "Recurrent attacks of headache, widely varied in intensity, frequency, and duration. The attacks are commonly unilateral in onset; are usually associated with anorexia and, sometimes, with nausea and vomiting; in some cases are preceded by, or associated with, conspicuous sensory, motor, and mood disturbances; and are often familial."[1]

The causes of migraine are still unknown, and many theories have been propounded to account for their etiology. Probably several different mechanisms are involved.[1]

Factors That May Precipitate Migraine Headache

Several factors may trigger a migraine headache. These include stress, bright lights, loud sounds, physical exertion, inhalation of chemicals such as petroleum derivatives, fasting, menstruation, use of oral contraceptives, and foods. An adverse reaction to foods or food additives may play a part in causing migraine headaches in some people. Research indicates:[2]

- About a third of people with frequent migraines will experience significant reduction in headache frequency on an elimination diet.
- A small percentage (less than 10%) will become headache free.
- In general, the number of provoking foods is small.
- Skin tests are not helpful in determining which foods to eliminate from the diet.

Food Allergies and Migraine

Skin tests are of little value in identifying foods that trigger or exacerbate migraine headaches because the hypersensitivity reaction that skin testing is designed to detect (ie, IgE-mediated hypersensitivity) is not an important or frequent cause of migraine in adults. A 2010 study[3] suggested that the immune complexes associated with foods in migraine sufferers were of the IgG type, rather than IgE, indicating that immunologically mediated reactions other than IgE-mediated atopy may be involved in the etiology of food-induced migraine. However, the value of IgG in the diagnosis of adverse reactions to foods is presently controversial (see Chapter 5 for details).

Food allergy may be an important migraine trigger in atopic (allergic) children. A 1983 study[4] indicated that food allergens provoked migraine in these children: 78 of 88 children were free from migraine when the offending food(s) were removed from their diet. Monro et al[5] found that 66% to 80% of migraine patients in their 1980 study were allergic (food-specific IgE RAST positive) to foods that precipitated a migraine on challenge. A 2010 study reported that individuals with IgG against specific foods achieved relief of their migraine symptoms by eliminating the foods from their diet and that the migraine seemed to be triggered when the food was consumed.[3]

Foods Implicated in Triggering Migraines

Many foods have been implicated in triggering migraines. One study reported the frequency with which specific foods appeared to trigger migraine on challenge:[5]

- Milk (43%)
- Chocolate (29%)
- Hot dog (14%)
- Cheese (14%)
- Fish (10%)
- Wine (9%)
- Coffee (9%)
- Garlic (5%)
- Eggs (5%)

The role of specific triggering factors in these foods has been explained on the basis of an immunologically mediated (IgE- and non-IgE-mediated) allergic reaction[6] or a physiological response to chemicals in the foods. For example, in the previous list:

- Milk, fish, egg, and garlic may be acting as allergens that release inflammatory mediators in a hypersensitivity reaction.
- Chocolate, cheese, and wine contain biogenic amines such as histamine, tyramine, octopamine, and phenylethylamine.

▪ Hot dog contains nitrites.
▪ Coffee contains caffeine, a methylxanthine.

Other foods reported to be frequently involved in precipitating a migraine headache include:[1]

▪ Tea
▪ Beans
▪ Beef
▪ Citrus fruits
▪ Corn
▪ Tomato
▪ Nuts
▪ Shellfish
▪ Pork
▪ Fried foods

It is clear from the variety and types of foods and food additives that are reportedly involved in the etiology of migraine that the triggers are as diverse in their range and actions as the food components that cause allergy and other food intolerance reactions. Unfortunately, as in the diagnosis of food allergy and intolerances, there is no single laboratory test that will indicate the foods and additives responsible. The detection of food triggers for migraine headaches requires the same approach as that suggested for determining other food sensitivities—namely, elimination and challenge. The difference in this case is that only one symptom needs to be monitored.

The current thinking[7] regarding the role of diet in the management of migraine has been expressed thus: "Food as a sole cause of migraine is uncommon, but many patients experience significant relief with dietary manipulation. Therefore, this avenue should be pursued in patients continuing to suffer from frequent migraine headaches."

The types of foods, food components, and food additives that are most frequently reported to trigger migraine headaches in sensitive individuals include food allergens, biogenic amines, other pharmacologically active chemicals, nitrates, nitrites, alcohol, and food additives.

Food Allergens

When IgE-mediated hypersensitivity is a cause of migraine, almost without exception other signs of allergy are also evident as symptoms in the respiratory tract, skin, or digestive tract. Some studies have suggested that an IgG-mediated reaction might be involved in triggering migraine.[8] There are no well-controlled studies to substantiate this, although tests for food-specific IgG are becoming widely used in looking for food culprits for the condition. In most cases, food-specific IgG is a normal response to foods that are most commonly consumed. Elimination and challenge of the suspect foods is always the best way to determine which foods precipitate a reaction. The most commonly reported food allergens as migraine triggers include:

- Egg
- Milk and milk products
- Wheat
- Specific legumes, especially peanuts, soy, black-eyed peas, and pinto beans
- Corn
- Pork

Less common allergens include:

- Shellfish
- Nuts
- Finfish
- Tomato
- Beef
- Citrus fruits

Biogenic Amines

Biogenic amines[9,10] contribute to migraine by inducing a change in blood vessels, either by narrowing (vasoconstriction) or widening (vasodilation) them. The biogenic amines most frequently implicated in triggering migraine headaches include histamine, tyramine, octopamine, phenylethylamine, and putrescine.

Histamine

Dietary sources of histamine include:

- Fish and shellfish
- Fermented cheeses
- Fermented soy products, soy sauce
- Fermented beverages: wine (red and white), beer, lager, ale, and similar beverages
- Dry pork and beef sausages (pepperoni, salami, bologna, etc)
- Tomato
- Spinach
- Eggplant
- Egg white
- Strawberry
- Chocolate
- Sauerkraut

Tyramine

Dietary sources of tyramine include the following:

- Aged cheeses
- Processed and fermented sausages
- Sour cream
- Wine (red and white)
- Pickled herring
- Smoked and pickled fish (eg, smoked salmon)
- Sauerkraut
- Broad bean (fava) pods
- Banana
- Vinegar and foods containing vinegar such as pickles, relishes, prepared mustard, salad dressings
- Avocado
- Peanut
- Chicken liver
- Yeast extract

Phenylethylamine

Dietary sources of phenylethylamine include chocolate, aged cheeses, and red wine.

Other Pharmacologically Active Chemicals

Several pharmacologically active (druglike) chemicals also affect the *vasculature* (blood vessels) and other smooth muscles in the body and have been implicated as migraine triggers in a number of studies. Such chemicals include methylxanthines, such as caffeine, theobromine, theophylline, and aminophylline.[1]

Caffeine is the major source of dietary methylxanthine and can be found in foods, beverages, and nonprescription supplements such as coffee, cocoa, tea, cola drinks, chocolate (except white chocolate), weight-control aids (such as diet pills), and caffeine tablets.

Nitrites and Nitrates

The mechanism of action of nitrates and nitrites[11] in triggering migraine headaches is not completely understood. There appears to be two effects involved in different individuals:[12] headaches, which arise immediately on consuming nitrate-rich foods and are connected to vasodilation caused by nitric oxide (NO) release, and migraines, which are triggered by other actions such as the release of calcitonin gene-related peptide or glutamate or changes in ion channel function mediated by cyclic guanosine monophosphate or S-nitrosylation.[12] Further information on sensitivity to nitrates and nitrites can be found in Chapter 28.

Nitrates and nitrites are used in foods as preservatives and coloring agents. Foods most commonly containing nitrates and nitrites include:

- Cured meats such as hot dogs, salami, bologna, pepperoni, luncheon meats, ham, and bacon
- Smoked meats and fish such as smoked salmon, smoked bacon
- Aged cheeses

Alcohol

There is some evidence that chemicals in alcohol,[13] such as biogenic amines and sulfites, are more important triggers for migraine than the alcohol itself.[10]

Food Additives

Food additives are chemicals that fall into a number of the preceding categories of compounds. The additives most frequently associated with migraine headaches include:

- Artificial colors, especially azo dyes such as tartrazine, which act as histamine-releasing agents (see Chapter 27)
- Preservatives, especially sulfites and benzoates, which act as histamine-releasing agents (see Chapters 21 and 25)
- Monosodium glutamate (MSG; see Chapter 30)
- Some spices and herbs such as cinnamon, cayenne, curry spices, nutmeg, and thyme, which are associated with histamine release, probably due to the presence of natural benzoates
- Artificial sweeteners, especially aspartame

Aspartame

Aspartame is an artificial sweetener marketed under a variety of brand names. It is a white, odorless, crystalline powder and consists of two amino acids, L-aspartic acid and L-phenylalanine. It is 180 times as sweet as sugar. The Food and Drug Administration (FDA) first allowed its use in dry foods in July 1981 and then in July 1983 approved its use in carbonated beverages.[14] It is found in many diet products and some medications and supplements. Studies on the effect of aspartame in triggering migraine headaches indicate that a subset of people who have migraines experience more headaches while consuming aspartame.[15] In one study, 8.2% of 171 patients reported aspartame as a trigger of their migraine headaches.[16,17]

Determining the Culprit Foods in Migraines

Because many people believe that certain foods, food components, or additives trigger their migraine headaches, and because no laboratory tests can determine foods responsible for the adverse reaction in migraine, it is worthwhile to conduct a careful elimination and challenge to determine whether the suspect foods are indeed associated with their migraines. Unnecessary avoidance of foods can lead to nutritional deficiency and can place social and financial burdens on the individual and their families, especially if the migraineur is a child.

The most efficient way to determine whether foods are contributing to a person's symptoms is to conduct the elimination and challenge process as described in Chapters 5, 6, and 7, using the following process:

- A food and symptoms record should be kept for a sufficient period of time to cover at least three migraine episodes; this may take several weeks if the episodes are infrequent. Analysis of the food and symptoms record may reveal specific food triggers if the reaction is due to immediate food allergy; however, this is not a common finding. Further analysis might indicate a dose-related response to food intolerance triggers, such as histamine, tyramine, or food additives. This is often difficult to determine from the record but may be suspected if an unusual number of foods containing the component are consumed within a day or so of the migraine's onset.
- The elimination diet will be formulated based on the preceding analysis; however, a simpler and quicker method is for the person to follow a few foods elimination diet (see Chapter 6) for 14 days for an adult or 7 days for a child.
- Following the elimination diet, sequential incremental dose challenge (SIDC; see Chapter 7) should be conducted over 4 days for each food or food component. This will reveal both immediate-type reactions to the foods and the delayed response that will occur with dose-dependent triggers, such as biogenic amines, as they build up to a level that exceeds the person's limit of tolerance.

Biogenic Amines as Triggers of Migraine and Other Headaches

The most frequently suspected triggers of migraines and other types of headaches are the biogenic amines, specifically histamine and tyramine, and sometimes octopamine, phenylethylamine, and putrescine. It is often worthwhile for the individual to undertake a time-limited trial on a biogenic amine–restricted diet prior to attempting the more drastic few foods elimination diet to rule out biogenic amines as a trigger for their symptoms.

References

1. Weber RW, Vaughan TR. Food and migraine headache. In: Anderson JA, ed. *Food Allergy*. Immunology and Allergy Clinics of North America. Vol. 11. Philadelphia, PA: WB Saunders; 1991:831-841.
2. Weber RW. Neurologic reactions to foods and food additives. In: Metcalfe DD, Sampson HA, Simon RA, eds. *Food Allergy: Adverse Reactions to Foods and Food Additives*. 4th ed. Boston, MA: Blackwell Publishing; 2008:531-542.

3. Alpay K, Ertaş M, Orhan EK, Üstay DK, Lieners C, Baykan B. Diet restriction in migraine, based on IgG against foods: a clinical double-blind, randomised, cross-over trial. *Cephalalgia*. 2010;30(7):829-837.

4. Egger J, Wilson J, Carter CM, Turner MW, Soothill JF. Is migraine food allergy? A double-blind trial of oligoantigenic diet treatment. *Lancet*. 1983;2:865-868.

5. Monro J, Carini C, Brostoff J, Zilkha K. Food allergy in migraine: study of dietary exclusion and RAST. *Lancet*. 1980;2(8184):1-4.

6. Pradalier A, Launay JM. Immunological aspects of migraine. *Biomed Pharmacother*. 1996;50(2):64-70.

7. Weber RW, Vaughan TR. Neurological reactions to foods and food additives. In: Metcalfe DD, Sampson HA, Simon RA, eds. *Food Allergy: Adverse Reactions to Foods and Food Additives*. 2nd ed. Boston, MA: Blackwell Scientific; 1997:499-507.

8. Arroyave Hernández CM, Echevarría Pinto M, Hernández Montiel HL. Food allergy mediated by IgG antibodies associated with migraine in adults. *Rev Alerg Mex*. 2007;54(5):162-168.

9. Millichap JG, Yee MM. The diet factor in pediatric and adolescent migraine. *Pediatr Neurol*. 2003;28(1):9-15.

10. Perkin HE, Hartje J. Diet and migraine; a review of the literature. *J Am Diet Assoc*. 1983;83:459-463.

11. Henderson WR, Raskin NH. "Hot dog" headache: individual susceptibility to nitrite. *Lancet*. 1972;2:1162-1163.

12. Bagdy G, Riba P, Kecskeméti V, Chase D, Juhász G. Headache-type adverse effects of NO donors: vasodilation and beyond. *Br J Pharmacol*. 2010;160(1):20-35. www.ncbi.nlm.nih.gov/pmc/articles/PMC2860203/pdf/bph0160-0020.pdf. Accessed January 27, 2012.

13. Diamond S, Freitag FG, Solomon GD, Millstein E. Migraine headache—working for the best outcome. *Postgrad Med*. 1987;81(8):174-183.

14. Garriga MM, Metcalfe DD. Aspartame intolerance. *Ann Allergy*. 1988;61(6 pt 2):63-69.

15. Van den Eeden SK, Koepsell TD, Longstreth WT Jr, van Belle G, Daling JR, McKnight B. Aspartame ingestion and headaches: a randomized crossover trial. *Neurology*. 1994;44(10):1787-1793.

16. Lipton RB, Newman LC, Cohen JS, Solomon S. Aspartame as a dietary trigger of headache. *Headache*. 1989;29:90-92.

17. Newman LC, Lipton RB. Migraine MLT-down: an unusual presentation of migraine in patients with aspartame-triggered headaches. *Headache*. 2001;41(9):899-901.

CHAPTER 39

Eosinophilic Gastrointestinal Diseases

As a result of the expanded definition of food allergy to encompass any immunological response to food components that results in symptoms when the food is consumed,[1] several conditions are now included under the term *food allergy* that previously were excluded from this field of practice. Included in this group of conditions are those in the digestive tract in which infiltration of *eosinophils* is diagnostic. Collectively, these diseases are known as *eosinophilic gastrointestinal diseases* (EGID).

About Eosinophils

Eosinophils are *granulocytes*, white blood cells that contain granules that store inflammatory mediators (see Chapter 1 for more details). Eosinophils are almost always present where there is an inflammatory condition; for example, the inflammation associated with asthma in the lungs and hay fever in the upper respiratory tract. They are frequently seen in IgE-mediated allergy in which *chemotaxins* (chemicals that draw additional immune cells to a reaction site) attract eosinophils to augment the allergic response. However, not all inflammatory reactions are mediated by IgE. In the case of the eosinophilic digestive diseases, there is little evidence of IgE; therefore, tests for IgE-mediated allergy are usually negative. Research studies are indicating that a key event in eosinophilic gastrointestinal diseases is the attraction of the eosinophils to the reaction site, mediated by the chemotaxin *eotaxin*.[2]

Eosinophils are found in abundance in the intestinal canal in diseases such as IgE-mediated food allergy, inflammatory bowel disease, infections caused by viruses, parasites such as helminths and nematodes, collagen vascular disease, malignancies, and drug sensitivities, among others.[3] In the diagnosis of EGID, these conditions need to be excluded before the diagnosis can be confirmed.

Eosinophilic Esophagitis

Currently, the most frequently diagnosed EGID is eosinophilic esophagitis (EE; sometimes abbreviated EoE).[4] Before 1995, this condition, which affects mainly children (rarely babies) and young adults, was thought to be associated with gastro-esophageal reflux disease (GERD). More recent research has identified an allergic component to the disease in which eosinophils are present in significant numbers. Because most studies suggest that an immunological response to foods can be an important precipitating event, many allergists consider EE to be a distinct type of food allergy.

The reported incidence of EE is 6 in 100,000.[5] The condition is more common in whites, and males compared with females.[6] EE is a chronic disease. The vast majority of individuals do not outgrow it. In a 12-year study of adults, no patients had remission,[5] and in a 14-year study of children, 2% had remission of disease.[7]

In eosinophilic esophagitis, there is a great deal of eosinophil buildup in the esophagus, the muscular canal that connects the mouth to the stomach. Eosinophils are rarely seen in this location in healthy people. Eosinophils, being granulocytes, like other granulocytes such as mast cells and basophils, contain inflammatory chemicals (mediators). The inflammatory mediators are released from the eosinophils and act on local tissues in the esophagus, causing an inflammation.

EE differs from the type of food allergy that typically results in symptoms such as hives, angioedema, vomiting, diarrhea, abdominal pain and bloating, and, in severe cases, anaphylaxis. These conditions are triggered by IgE antibodies produced against a specific food, which cause the release of inflammatory mediators from mast cells. In EE, food-specific IgE is not usually evident, and it is eosinophils rather than mast cells that release the inflammatory mediators.

Symptoms of EE

EE occurs in toddlers, older children, and adults but rarely in babies. The symptoms of EE tend to differ somewhat in different age groups:[8] (a) young children experience failure to thrive or classic gastroesophageal reflux symptoms; (b) school-aged children have abdominal pain or vomiting; and (c) older adolescents and adults experience food impaction and dysphagia (difficulty in swallowing).

The symptoms most frequently associated with EE and considered to be typical of the disease[9] include:

▪ Vomiting
▪ Regurgitation of food
▪ Difficulty in swallowing: foods are said to be sticking on the way down
▪ Choking on food
▪ Heartburn and chest pain
▪ Water brash (regurgitation of a watery fluid not containing food material)
▪ Poor eating
▪ Failure to thrive (poor or no weight gain, or weight loss)

Although the symptoms resemble gastroesophageal reflux disease (GERD), the reflux of EE does not respond to the medications used to suppress the gastric acid and control regurgitation (antireflux therapy) in GERD. In fact, emerging data suggest that use of acid-suppressing medications may predispose these individuals to the development of EE.[10]

Diagnosis of EE

Currently, there is no diagnostic test or laboratory marker to diagnose or predict the course of the disease. Diagnosis is made by suspicious history, a 2-month trial of antireflux medications (up to 2 mg/kg/day of proton pump inhibitor [PPI]) without benefit, and esophageal biopsy.[11]

The diagnosis of EE relies on the appearance of eosinophils in endoscopic biopsy. For diagnosis, pathology must reveal 15 eosinophils or more per high-powered field (HPF) in one or more specimens in the absence of other causes (eg, drug allergy, infections, inflammatory bowel disease, and eosinophilic gastroenteritis).[8] In a third of patients, the appearance of the esophagus itself may be normal. A higher-than-normal level of eosinophils in a blood sample taken at the same time will also suggest the diagnosis.

Other evidence to confirm an EE diagnosis include finding that the usual antireflux medications are of no benefit but that elimination diets are often helpful, suggesting an underlying food allergy or intolerance as a triggering event. Medications to reduce inflammation, typically corticosteroids such as prednisone, are effective in treating the symptoms of EE.

Potential Causes of EE

Although IgE-mediated food allergy does not seem to be a primary contributing factor in EE, some foods have been frequently associated with the condition, and therefore in a sense this can be considered to be a variant of food allergy. The foods most frequently reported to trigger EE tend to be the same ones that are involved in most cases of IgE-mediated food allergy:[12,13]

▓ Egg
▓ Cow's milk
▓ Soy
▓ Wheat
▓ Corn
▓ Peanuts
▓ Tree nuts
▓ Shellfish
▓ Fish
▓ Beef
▓ Rye

Even though EE itself is not caused by IgE-mediated allergy, as many as 80% of patients with EE reportedly have symptoms of allergy, such as hay fever or asthma.[14] Because the immunological response in asthma and hay fever typically leads to a large number of eosinophils in the respiratory tract, it has been suggested that the close proximity of the upper GI tract tissues to the inflamed tissues of the upper respiratory tract might result in the eosinophils associated with asthma and hay fever to infiltrate the esophageal tissues and cause EE. This theory remains to be proven.

Some people with EE find that their symptoms appear only during the season in which they are exposed to their allergenic pollen. This observation would seem to reinforce the respiratory allergy/EE connection, because active allergy to the pollen will result in large numbers of eosinophils in the upper airways and lungs.

Not all EE is related to allergy. Around a quarter of individuals with EE have no evidence of allergy. Some have underlying conditions that can cause similar inflammation in the digestive tract. These people will not respond to diet manipulation but may respond to medication.

A puzzling observation is that some people do feel better when certain foods are removed from their diet, but when examined, evidence of inflammation in the esophagus remains. This suggests that in these cases, although foods contribute to the symptoms, they actually only aggravate the situation and are probably not the cause.

If EE is left untreated, the inflammation may start to damage the esophagus, resulting in narrowing of the canal (stricture) and increase in the fibrous tissue surrounding it (fibrosis). Therefore, it is essential that anyone with the type of symptoms listed earlier should be examined, diagnosed, and treated.

Management of EE

Treatment of EE consists of swallowed corticosteroids to suppress the eosinophilia and elimination of food antigens by excluding the most common allergens, or an elemental diet.[15] For details of this procedure, see "Dietary Management of EGID" later in this chapter.

Eosinophilic Gastroenteritis (EG)

Eosinophilic gastroenteritis also involves infiltration of eosinophils into digestive tract tissues—in this case into the stomach and small intestine. The condition is less common than EE and often more difficult to diagnose.[16] The actual incidence of EG is unknown but currently it is considered to be a rare disease,[16] although researchers think that the condition has been underdiagnosed because of the difficulty in its diagnosis. Most patients with EG are between 20 and 50 years of age.[16]

Symptoms of EG

Typical symptoms include:[17]

- Abdominal pain
- Nausea
- Vomiting
- Diarrhea
- Occult blood in the stool
- Abdominal bloating
- Protein wasting enteropathy
- Malnutrition, weight loss, and wasting due to malabsorption of nutrients

Diagnosis

Endoscopic biopsy showing increased eosinophils in gastric and intestinal tissues, after all other causes for the pathology have been ruled out, is usually the basis for definitive diagnosis.[16]

Cause of EG

The cause of EG is presently unknown, but because of the presence of large numbers of eosinophils, it is assumed that there is an allergic component to the condition. Most patients with EG are atopic and exhibit allergic diseases such as asthma, atopic dermatitis (eczema), food, and inhalant allergy. The presence of these IgE-mediated allergies heightens suspicion of EG as a cause of otherwise undiagnosed gastrointestinal symptoms.[18]

Management of EG

As with other immunologically mediated conditions, oral steroids are often used to control the symptoms.[14] Food allergy or intolerance is frequently either part of the etiology or an exacerbating factor in EG, so elimination and challenge to identify the culprit foods is an important part of managing the condition.

The foods most frequently reported[19] to be associated with EG include those that often trigger IgE-mediated food allergy. Cow's milk, eggs, peanuts, tree nuts, shellfish, fish, soy, wheat, and beef have all been implicated as triggers of the condition. An initial trial on removing these from the diet is often worthwhile before embarking on the more restricted few-foods elimination diet, followed by challenge, which is the best way to identify any foods contributing to the condition. (See "Dietary Management of EGID" later in this chapter for details.)

Eosinophilic Colitis (EC)

Eosinophilic colitis is distinguished by the presence of eosinophil infiltration into the colon. EC is exceptionally rare, with only a few cases being reported since 1979.[20]

Diagnosis is difficult, so the true incidence of the condition is unclear. The precise cause of EC is presently unknown. In a few cases, especially in infants, IgE-mediated food allergy with eosinophilic involvement has been identified as the cause.[20]

The condition mainly affects infants and young adults and both sexes equally.[21] The EC that develops in infancy tends to spontaneously resolve, often within days. After a few years, the children can even tolerate the implicated foods, particularly in cases where IgE-mediated food allergy is involved. For young adults with EC, the condition tends to become chronic with periods of activity and periods of apparent remission.[20]

Symptoms of EC

Symptoms of EC may appear similar to those of eosinophilic gastroenteritis (EG) and include diarrhea, malabsorption, weight loss and wasting. In more severe cases, intestinal obstruction, *intussusception* (a prolapse of one part of the intestine into the lumen of an adjacent part, which may result in an obstruction), and perforation may occur.[22]

Diagnosis of EC

Biopsy shows eosinophils in various regions of the colon; however, a small number of eosinophils can be seen regularly in normal biopsies of the colon, and at present there is no consensus as to the number of eosinophils that can be considered diagnostic of EC. Changes in the bowel wall in radiographs may provide a better indication of the condition.[22]

Management of EC

As in all cases of eosinophilic digestive diseases, because the condition is undeniably associated with local inflammation, a food component is strongly suspected as a triggering factor either in its etiology or as an exacerbating factor.

Dietary Management of EGID

Because IgE-mediated food allergy does not cause EGIDs (although in some cases eosinophilia occurs as a consequence of IgE-mediated food allergy), skin tests and blood tests for allergen-specific IgE are of very limited value in identifying foods that may be involved. However, all strategies for management of EGID involve food exclusion to determine the extent to which food is contributing to the problem. The most important question is, which foods should be avoided? And how do we know which ones are actually associated with the condition?[23]

The foods most frequently associated with EGID (listed earlier in this chapter) should be removed from the diet for a defined period of time to see whether symptoms improve. While avoiding these foods, nutritionally equivalent replacements should be included in the diet, especially if the person is a child. The diet provided in Chapter 19 can be used as a guideline for avoiding the most commonly reported food triggers of EGID. If symptoms still persist, a trial on the few foods elimination diet (see Chapter 6) can be implemented for a short period of time (7 to 10 days for a child; 10 to 14 days for an adult). If food elimination does not solve the problem, a time-limited trial on an elemental formula is an effective way to determine whether foods are contributing to the condition.

When symptom relief is achieved using any of these strategies, each food should then be reintroduced separately, in increasingly large quantities, while symptoms are monitored (see Chapter 7 for details of this process). This will provide a good idea of whether that food is causing a problem. If the food makes no difference, it can then be incorporated into the regular diet. If symptoms are triggered, or if existing symptoms are made worse, the food should be permanently removed from the diet. In the future, if symptoms improve, the foods should be reintroduced one at a time and reactions carefully monitored. It is possible for the condition to resolve, especially in a child as he or she matures. If the foods still make things worse, they will need to be avoided for the long term, by implementing a maintenance diet to provide all restricted nutrients from alternative sources (see Chapter 8 for details).

References

1. Johansson SGO, Hourihane JOB, Bousquet J, et al. A revised nomenclature for allergy. An EAACI position statement from the EAACI nomenclature task force. *Allergy.* 2001;56:813-824.
2. Khan S, Orenstein SR. Eosinophilic gastroenteritis. *Gastroenterol Clin North Am.* 2008; 37(2):333-348.
3. Laxa BU, Bouchard A, De Petris G, Heigh R, Heppell J. Eosinophilic enteritis confined to an ileostomy site. *Case Rep Gastroenterol.* 2011;5(2):422-427.
4. Liacouras CA, Ruchelli E. Eosinophilic esophagitis. *Curr Opin Pediatr.* 2004;16(5): 560-566.
5. Staumann A, Spichtin HP, Grize M, Bucher KA, Beglinger C, Simon HU. Natural history of primary eosinophilic esophagitis: a follow-up of 30 adult patients up to 11.5 years. *Gastroenterology.* 2003;125:1660-1669.
6. Heltzer ML, Franciosi JP, Shuker M, Liacouras CA, Spergel JM. Demographic information of patients with eosinophilic esophagitis. *J Allergy Clin Immunol.* 2007;119:S111.
7. Spergel JM, Brown-Whitehorn TF, Beausoleil JL, et al. 14 years of eosinophilic esophagitis: clinical features and prognosis. *J Pediatr Gastroenterol Nutr.* 2009;48(1):30-36.
8. Brown-Whitehorn TF, Spergel JM. The link between allergies and eosinophilic esophagitis: implications for management strategies. *Expert Rev Clin Immunol.* 2010;6(1):101-109.
9. Liacouras CA. Eosinophilic esophagitis in children and adults. *J Pediatr Gastroenterol Nutr.* 2003;37(suppl 1):S23-S28.
10. Merwat SN, Spechler SJ. Might the use of acid-suppressive medications predispose to the development of eosinophilic esophagitis? *Am J Gastroenterol.* 2009;104:1897-1902.

11. Furuta GT, Liacouras CA, Collins MH, et al. Eosinophilic esophagitis in children and adults: a systematic review and consensus recommendations for diagnosis and treatment. *Gastroenterology.* 2007;133(4):1342-1363.

12. Kagalwalla AF, Sentongo TA, Ritz S, et al. Effect of six-food elimination diet on clinical and histologic outcomes in eosinophilic esophagitis. *Clin Gastroenterol Hepatol.* 2006;4:1097-1102.

13. Franciosi JP, Liacouras CA. Eosinophilic esophagitis. *Immunol Allergy Clin North Am.* 2009;29(1):19-27.

14. Shifflet A, Forouhar F, Wu GY. Eosinophilic digestive diseases: eosinophilic esophagitis, gastroenteritis, and colitis. *J Formos Med Assoc.* 2009;108(11):834-843.

15. Arora AA, Weiler CR, Katzka DA. Eosinophilic esophagitis: allergic contribution, testing, and management. *Curr Gastroenterol Rep.* 2012;14(3):206-215.

16. Powell N, Walker MM, Talley NJ. Gastrointestinal eosinophils in health, disease and functional disorders. *Nat Rev Gastroenterol Hepatol.* 2010;7(3):146-156.

17. Kalantar SJ, Marks R, Lambert JR, Badov D, Talley NJ. Dyspepsia due to eosinophilic gastroenteritis. *Dig Dis Sci.* 1997;42:2327-2332.

18. Jyonouchi S, Brown-Whitehorn T, Spergel JM. Association of eosinophilic gastrointestinal disorders with other atopic disorders. *Immunol Allergy Clin North Am.* 2009;29:85-97.

19. Bischoff SC. Food allergy and eosinophilic gastroenteritis and colitis. *Curr Opin Allergy Clin Immunol.* 2010;10(3):238-245.

20. Alfadda AA, Storr MA, Shaffer EA. Eosinophilic colitis: epidemiology, clinical features, and current management. *Therap Adv Gastroenterol.* 2011;4(5):301-309.

21. Rothenberg ME. Eosinophilic gastrointestinal disorders (EGID). *J Allergy Clin Immunol.* 2004;113:11-28.

22. Velchuru VR, Khan MA, Hellquist HB, Studley JG. Eosinophilic colitis. *J Gastrointest Surg.* 2007;11:1373-1375.

23. González-Cervera J, Angueira T, Rodriguez-Domínguez B, Arias A, Yagüe-Compadre JL, Lucendo AJ. Successful food elimination therapy in adult eosinophilic esophagitis: not all patients are the same. *Clin Gastroenterol.* Epub ahead of print 2012 Feb 13.

CHAPTER 40

Food Protein–Induced Enteropathies

In recent years, there has been increasing recognition of a group of non-IgE-mediated food-related gastrointestinal problems associated with delayed or chronic reactions.[1] The conditions include food protein–induced enterocolitis syndrome (FPIES) and food protein proctocolitis (FPIP). These digestive disorders tend to appear in the first months of life. They are progressive and generally self-limiting, typically resolving at about 2 years of age.

The most commonly implicated food is milk, but fish, egg, rice, and several other foods have been reported. Reactions can be triggered by any protein introduced into the infant diet. The symptoms disappear after removing the causal protein from the diet.

In a 2011 study,[2] the incidence of FPIES triggered by cow's milk was reported to be 0.34% in the first year of life compared with 0.5% for IgE-mediated cow's milk allergy. FPIES typically presents before 6 months of age in formula-fed infants. A few cases of FPIES in breastfed infants have recently been reported.[2]

Characteristics of FPIES

FPIES is triggered by foods but is not mediated by IgE. The symptoms in infants typically include:[3]

- Profuse vomiting
- Diarrhea, which can progress to dehydration and shock in severe cases
- Increased intestinal permeability
- Malabsorption
- Dysmotility (changes in the speed at which food passes through the digestive tract)
- Abdominal pain
- Failure to thrive (typically weight gain less than 10 g/d)
- In severe episodes, the child may be hypothermic (body temperature less than 36°C)[2]

Because FPIES is not mediated by IgE, tests for IgE-mediated allergy (eg, skin tests and blood tests for allergen-specific IgE) are typically negative.

Most reports of FPIES indicate that the condition develops in response to food proteins as a result of digestive tract and immunological immaturity. Symptoms develop in the infant after exposure to certain proteins in foods; early reports indicated that cow's milk and soy proteins, usually given in infant formulas, were the most frequent causes of the reaction. More recent research claims that rice is the most common food causing FPIES.[3] Milk- and soy-associated FPIES usually starts within the first year of life; most frequently within the first 6 or 7 months.[4] When solid foods are introduced, other foods may cause the condition.

Diagnosis of FPIES

There are currently no diagnostic tests for FPIES. The clinical picture of development of acute symptoms immediately after consuming the offending foods (often milk- or soy-based infant formula), together with the absence of positive tests for food allergy, will usually alert the clinician to the possibility that FPIES is the cause of the problem.

Foods Associated with FPIES

Foods that have been identified as triggers of FPIES in individual cases include:[5]

- Cow's milk
- Soy
- Grains such as oats, barley, and rice
- Legumes (peas, peanuts, lentils)
- Vegetables (sweet potato, squash)
- Poultry (chicken, turkey)
- Egg

Removing the culprit foods usually leads to immediate recovery from the symptoms. After the offending foods have been avoided for a period of time, eating the food may cause a recurrence in which the symptoms are mild, and instead of an immediate reaction, the symptom onset is 2 or more hours after ingestion.[3]

Cause of FPIES

The immune system reaction in FPIES appears to involve T helper cells that release the cytokine TNF-α, which is typical of a Th1 response.[6] This is in contrast to allergy, in which a Th2 response releases the cytokines that result in the production of IgE (see Chapter 1 for an explanation of Th1 and Th2 responses). In addition, a low level of TGF-β, which is the cytokine most frequently involved in developing tolerance to foods, suggests that a lack of immunological tolerance results in the immune system treating the food as if it were a threat to the body's health and survival.[3] The subsequent release of inflammatory mediators in response to the entry of the offending food into the body results in the "defensive" symptoms of vomiting and diarrhea.

Breastfeeding and FPIES

Most reports of FPIES indicate that exclusive breastfeeding is protective in potential cases of FPIES.[3] None of the infants who later developed FPIES after the introduction of solids had symptoms while being exclusively breastfed. Authors of these studies suggest that babies who had FPIES while being breastfed, but who had occasionally been given an infant formula, were sensitized to the proteins in the formula during a period of immunological susceptibility.

Management of FPIES

Like food allergy, the management of FPIES involves avoiding the food that triggers the child's symptoms. In most cases, a reaction to milk- and soy-based formula with severe vomiting and diarrhea, without other signs of allergy such as skin reactions, is suggestive of the diagnosis.

Elimination and challenge with the suspect foods will usually confirm the syndrome. In most cases, delayed introduction of solid foods is advised because of the possibility that until the child's immune system has matured, a similar reaction to proteins in other foods may elicit the same response.

There is a long way to go before we understand all of the different immunological and physiological mechanisms responsible for FPIES and therefore how best to manage the condition. Until we have more well-conducted research studies, the directive is to avoid the foods that clearly trigger FPIES (usually milk- and soy-based formulas) in the early months, and delay the introduction of solids until after 6 or 7 months of age.[3] The introduction of solids should be undertaken with caution. The protocols in Chapter 44 should be followed so that any adverse response to potential triggers of FPIES can be detected on first exposure to them.

Exclusive breastfeeding is the best preventive to the early development of FPIES. When the infant has already developed FPIES, the mother should remove any milk and soy from her diet. When the baby is formula-fed, an extensively hydrolyzed formula (EHF) such as Similac Alimentum (Abbott Nutrition), Enfamil Nutramigen (Mead Johnson), and Enfamil Pregestimil (Mead Johnson) may be tolerated. If EHF is not tolerated, an elemental formula such as EleCare (Abbott Nutrition) or Neocate (Nutricia) should be tried.[1]

Most babies outgrow FPIES by the age of 2 or 3 years, when their immune and digestive systems have matured.[3] If a child has exhibited the symptoms of FPIES, and the offending foods have been avoided, reintroduction of the foods is usually undertaken under medical supervision at about the age of 2 years or later.[4]

Food Protein–Induced Proctitis/Proctocolitis

Many parents are understandably concerned when their apparently healthy baby has visible flecks of blood, often mixed with mucus, in the stool. Food protein–induced proctitis or proctocolitis (FPIP) is often the cause.[7] The condition typically appears in the first few months of life, on average at the age of 2 months. The absence of other symptoms, such as vomiting, diarrhea, and failure to thrive, usually rules out other causes such as food allergy and food protein enteropathies. Usually the blood loss is very slight, and anemia from it is rare. A diagnosis is usually made after other conditions that could account for the blood, such as anal fissure and infection, have been ruled out.

Cow's milk proteins and soy proteins are the most common triggers of food-protein proctitis. Many babies develop the symptoms during breastfeeding in response to milk and soy in the mother's diet.[8]

Causes and Management of FPIP

The cause of FPIP is unknown but does not involve IgE, so all tests for allergy are usually negative. In most cases, avoiding the offending food leads to a resolution of the problem.

When the baby is breastfed, elimination of milk and soy from the mother's diet is usually enough to resolve the infant's symptoms. Occasionally egg can cause the symptoms, in which case, the mother must avoid all sources of egg in her diet as well.

When the baby is formula-fed, an EHF will often lead to recovery. However, a few babies do develop symptoms on this type of formula, in which case an elemental formula such as Neocate (Nutricia) or EleCare (Abbott Nutrition) is usually the answer. Bleeding will usually disappear within 72 hours of eliminating the protein responsible for the reaction.

In most cases, the disorder will resolve by the age of 1 or 2 years.[7] After this age, the offending foods may be reintroduced gradually, with careful monitoring for the reappearance of blood in the baby's stool.

References

1. Boné J, Claver A, Guallar I, Plaza AM. Allergic proctocolitis, food-induced enterocolitis: immune mechanisms, diagnosis and treatment. *Allergol Immunopathol (Madr)*. 2009;37(1):36-42.
2. Leonard SA, Nowak-Węgrzyn A. Food protein-induced enterocolitis syndrome: an update on natural history and review of management. *Ann Allergy Asthma Immunol*. 2011;107(2):95-101.
3. Nowak-Wegrzyn A, Muraro A. Food protein-induced enterocolitis syndrome. *Curr Opin Allergy Clin Immunol*. 2009;9(4):371-377.
4. Nowak-Wegrzyn A, Sampson HA, Wood RA, Sicherer SH. Food protein-induced enterocolitis syndrome caused by solid food proteins. *Pediatrics*. 2003;111:829-835.

5. Levy Y, Danon YL. Food protein-induced enterocolitis syndrome—not only to cow's milk and soy. *Pediatr Allergy Immunol.* 2003;14(4):325-329.
6. Chung HL, Hwang JB, Park JJ, Kim SG. Expression of transforming growth factor β1, transforming growth factor type I and II receptors, and TNF-α in the mucosa of the small intestine in infants with food protein-induced enterocolitis syndrome. *J Allergy Clin Immunol.* 2002;109:150-154.
7. Sicherer SH. Clinical aspects of gastrointestinal food allergy in childhood. *Pediatrics.* 2003;111(6):1609-1616.
8. Anveden HL, Finkel Y, Sandstedt B, Karpe B. Proctocolitis in exclusively breast-fed infants. *Eur J Pediatr.* 1996;155:464-467.

CHAPTER 41

Celiac Disease (Gluten-Sensitive Enteropathy)

Celiac disease or gluten-sensitive enteropathy (previously referred to as *celiac sprue*) is another disease that is caused by an adverse reaction to specific foods, mediated by the immune system, but that is not an IgE-mediated hypersensitivity reaction. Although not considered to be an allergic condition according to the traditional meaning of the term, celiac disease sits uneasily under an expanded definition of allergy that includes immunologically mediated reactions to food components. The topic is included here for completeness.

Celiac disease is a genetically inherited condition that affects the small intestine.[1] Gluten in certain cereal grains (wheat, rye, and barley) triggers an immune response involving IgA antibodies[2] that results in damage to the brush border cells in the epithelium lining the intestines. These cells have numerous projections, called *villi* (singular *villus*) that serve to increase the total surface area over which food can be absorbed into circulation. In celiac disease, the brush border cells are "attacked" by components of the immune system. As a result, the villi are damaged, and under the microscope appear flattened and distorted. This is the most important diagnostic indicator that a person has celiac disease.

Because the villi are damaged, absorption of food across the epithelial lining of the intestine is impeded. The affected person cannot absorb nutrients efficiently and loses weight or fails to gain weight appropriately. In addition, unabsorbed food materials pass into the colon, where they are fermented by the microorganisms that colonize the area. The result is the gas, bloating, and diarrhea typical of some forms of the disease.

Although celiac disease can be diagnosed at any age, it appears most commonly in either early childhood (between 9 and 24 months) or in the third or fourth decade of life. About the same number of girls and boys have the disease, which is different from adults, where twice as many women as men are diagnosed with the condition.

Recent reports indicate that celiac disease is much more common than previously thought. Antibody assays have shown the prevalence of celiac disease to be nearly 1 in 100 in many populations.[2] Part of the reason for the increase in incidence is probably due to a greater awareness of the condition among doctors, the availability of more precise serological tests for detection of the disease,[3] and the fact that many more symptoms than had previously been recognized are now included under the diagnosis.

Symptoms of Celiac Disease

The symptoms of celiac disease[4] most commonly begin in children younger than 1 year, although the condition can manifest at any age, sometimes well into adulthood.

Previously, celiac disease was thought to be characterized by the "classical" symptoms of gastrointestinal malabsorption syndrome, which included:

- Diarrhea
- Stool that contains unabsorbed fat, which floats on the water in a lavatory (steatorrhea)
- Weight loss
- Fatigue
- Anemia
- Vomiting
- Poor appetite

In infants and young children, the following may be additional signs of celiac disease:

- Chronic diarrhea
- Weight loss
- Failure to gain weight (failure to thrive)
- Short stature for age
- Iron deficiency anemia
- Protuberant abdomen

These symptoms are now known to be associated with severe celiac disease. Most patients are now recognized to have milder symptoms, such as abdominal discomfort, bloating, indigestion, or nongastrointestinal symptoms such as fatigue and anemia, or sometimes no symptoms at all.[5]

Mechanism of Celiac Disease

Our understanding of the key steps underlying the intestinal inflammatory response to celiac disease has increased dramatically in recent years. The first stage in the immunological reaction sequence that ultimately leads to damage of the brush border cells is the release of a specific molecule that is present in certain types of gluten. Specifically:

▪ Alpha-gliadins in wheat
▪ Hordeins in barley
▪ Secalins in rye

This molecule is present in wheat, rye, and barley glutens, but not in gluten from any other grains. It is also a different molecule from the ones that are responsible for triggering IgE-mediated allergy to these grains. The "celiac molecule" is freed from the complete protein by an enzyme called transglutaminase that is present in the digestive tract.

The celiac molecules are recognized by the immune system. Together with a specific type of "self-antigen" called HLA-DQ2 and/or HLA-DQ8 on antigen presenting cells, which are present in most people who inherit the tendency to develop celiac disease,[6] gluten-specific T cells are activated. This enhances cytotoxicity of intraepithelial lymphocytes against the intestinal epithelium, which results in the cell damage characteristic of the disease.[6] In addition, research suggests that this interaction leads to an increase in permeability of the digestive tract lining (leaky gut) by weakening the tight junctions between epithelial cells.[6]

Celiac disease is an example of tissue damage that results in malabsorption of nutrients rather than a net increase in permeability of the mucosal tissue. However, these two mechanisms are not mutually exclusive. Inflammation causes tissue damage, and in the case of celiac disease, the absorptive villous cells are damaged, significantly reducing their capacity to transport nutrients. However, access to antigens through the damaged epithelium is increased. This means that food molecules and other materials that would normally be excluded can pass more readily through the more "porous" epithelium. This may explain the frequency in which other immunologically mediated conditions accompany the condition.

Diagnosis of Celiac Disease

Celiac disease is now diagnosed by highly sensitive immunological tests that identify antibodies in blood that are produced against various antigens that arise as a result of the events leading to tissue damage in the disease. When these tests are positive, microscopic examination of samples taken from the lining of the intestine by biopsy is necessary to confirm the diagnosis.

Testing for celiac-related antibodies in children younger than 5 years old may not be reliable. However, since celiac disease is hereditary, family members, particularly first-degree relatives—meaning parents, siblings, or children of people who have been diagnosed—may wish to be tested for the disease. About 5% to 15% of an affected person's first-degree relatives will also have the disease. About 3% to 8% of people with type 1 diabetes will have biopsy-confirmed celiac disease, and 5% to 10% of people with Down syndrome will be diagnosed with celiac disease.[7]

Previously, IgA antibodies against gliadin, reticulin (a connective tissue component that is released when tissue damage occurs), and an antiendomysial antibody formed against transglutaminase in blood were measured in active cases of celiac disease; these antibodies disappear when a gluten-free diet is followed. Nowadays, newer tests that detect the presence of IgA antibodies against transglutaminase have proved to be more reliable than any of the older methods.[5] The presence of these antibodies in blood is an indication that celiac disease may be the cause of a person's symptoms.

However, the diagnosis cannot be made on the presence of these antibodies alone because of the false-positive and false-negative reactions associated with the tests:

▪ False-negative reactions can result from an IgA deficiency that is sometimes associated with the condition.
▪ False-positive reactions may occur in inflammatory bowel disease such as Crohn's disease, and in communities where other causes of enteropathy are common.[8]

Positive immunological tests are almost always followed by examination of the cells lining the digestive tract, taken by endoscopic biopsy. If the tests and symptoms suggest celiac disease, a small bowel biopsy should be performed. During the biopsy, a tiny piece of tissue from the small intestine will be removed to check for damage to the villi. To obtain the tissue sample, a long, thin tube called an *endoscope* is inserted through the mouth and stomach into the small intestine. The sample is obtained by using instruments passed through the endoscope. Abnormalities in the appearance of the villi of the brush border cells will confirm the diagnosis.

The symptoms of celiac disease quickly resolve when all sources of the gluten responsible for the disease are removed from the diet. Strict avoidance of wheat, rye, and barley leads to recovery of the intestinal villi, which return to their normal shape, and the IgA antibodies associated with celiac disease disappear from blood. This means that if a person has been on a gluten-free diet for about a month before the test, all evidence of the disease will be absent. Therefore, in order for the tests to be valid, gluten needs to be eaten for at least 2 weeks (preferably at least 4 weeks) prior so that evidence of the disease can be detected. This may cause some temporary digestive tract distress but is nevertheless necessary in order for an accurate diagnosis to be made.

An accurate diagnosis is essential because celiac disease is a lifelong condition. Gluten must be avoided in order for the person to remain symptom-free and to avoid the complications of the condition that can arise as a consequence of inadequately controlled celiac disease. Such complications may include:[9]

▪ Osteoporosis, from chronic malabsorption of essential nutrients
▪ Iron-deficiency anemia
▪ The troublesome skin condition *dermatitis herpetiformis*
▪ Several neurological and endocrine diseases

- Persistent chronic hypertransaminasemia of unknown origin
- Various types of cancer
- Some autoimmune disorders

However, if all the tests for celiac disease are negative, there is no reason for the individual to be subjected to the often cumbersome and tedious dietary restrictions of a gluten-free diet.

Management of Celiac Disease

The acute symptoms in the gastrointestinal tract resolve when all sources of gluten are removed from the diet. This means complete avoidance of wheat, rye, and barley, and any foods that contain these ingredients or their derivatives.

For most people, following this diet will stop symptoms, heal existing intestinal damage, and prevent further damage. Improvements begin within days of starting the diet. The small intestine is usually completely healed in 3 to 6 months in children and younger adults and within 2 years for older adults.

Adherence to the dietary restrictions will be lifelong, because tissue damage and the resulting symptoms recur rapidly when gluten is reintroduced. Damage can be detected in microscope preparations of epithelial tissue within a few hours of eating gluten. It is important that celiac disease should be detected early because of the risk of developing the more severe and permanent conditions, especially malignancies, associated with it.

Celiac Disease and Oats

In the past, oats were excluded from the diet in celiac disease. Oat avenin was thought to trigger an IgA response similar to that against wheat, rye, and barley glutens. However, in 1995, studies[10] demonstrated that after 6 to 12 months, persons with celiac disease who had avoided wheat, rye, and barley but had continued to consume oats had no signs of the disease. Subsequent studies have confirmed these results.[11] Nevertheless, concerns about persons with celiac disease eating oats have continued in some cases. Oats may be contaminated with gluten-containing grains, especially when the oats are imported, or if oats are processed and packaged in a facility that also processes wheat, rye, and barley. A 2011 report from Canada[12] indicated that the commercial oat supply in Canada is heavily contaminated with gluten from other grains. Approximately 88% of 133 oat samples were contaminated above 20 mg per kilogram, and there were no differences among the oat types tested. It is likely that similar contamination occurs in oats in the United States. It is possible that contamination occurred in the field, in the transport of the grain, in the storage of the grain, and in the milling and packaging facilities.[12]

In general, however, pediatricians and registered dietitians have encouraged the consumption of labeled gluten-free oats to make the gluten-free diet more liberal, and hence encourage compliance in children and adults alike. Nevertheless, a few patients have reportedly shown both clinical and immunological responses to a pure oat product; signs and symptoms of the disease should be carefully monitored in anyone on a gluten-free diet who is consuming oats.[13,14]

When the symptoms resolve, labeled gluten-free oats and oat products can be introduced into the diet in increasing doses. If symptoms remain quiescent, labeled gluten-free oats can be eaten regularly, but continue to carefully monitor symptoms and remove the oats at the earliest sign of digestive tract disturbances.

Celiac Disease and Corn

A 2012 Italian study[15] suggests the possibility that prolamins in corn, specifically zeins, contain amino acid sequences that resemble the wheat gluten peptides involved in celiac disease. IgA from some celiac patients with HLA-DQ2 or DQ8 haplotypes (the gene sequences associated with celiac disease) recognized (that is, formed an immunological complex with) two of the corn zeins tested. The authors suggest that these findings may be of clinical importance, especially in cases of refractory celiac disease that does not respond to a gluten-free diet. If the validity of these preliminary findings is proven by subsequent research, then the inclusion of corn, which is often used in the formulation and preparation of gluten-free foods, will need to be reevaluated in some cases of celiac disease.

References

1. Schuppan D, Junker Y, Barisani D. Celiac disease: from pathogenesis to novel therapies. *Gastroenterology*. 2009;137(6):1912-1933.
2. Leffler DA, Schuppan D. Update on serologic testing in celiac disease. *Am J Gastroenterol*. 2010;105(12):2520-2524.
3. Van Heel DA, West J. Recent advances in celiac disease. *Gut*. 2006;55:1037-1046.
4. Ensari A. Gluten-sensitive enteropathy (celiac disease): controversies in diagnosis and classification. *Arch Pathol Lab Med*. 2010;134(6):826-836.
5. American Gastroenterological Association medical position statement: celiac sprue. *Gastroenterology*. 2001;120:1522-1525.
6. Tjon JM, van Bergen J, Koning F. Celiac disease: how complicated can it get? *Immunogenetics*. 2010;62(10):641-651.
7. Cerqueira RM, Rocha CM, Fernandes CD, Correia MR. Celiac disease in Portuguese children and adults with Down syndrome. *Eur J Gastroenterol Hepatol*. 2010;22(7): 868-871.
8. Calabuig M, Torregosa R, Polo P, et al. Serological markers and celiac disease: a new diagnostic approach? *J Pediatr Gastroenterol Nutr*. 1990;10(4):435-442.
9. Rodrigo L. Celiac disease. *World J Gastroenterol*. 2006;12(41):6585-6593.
10. Janatuinen EK, Pikkarainen PH, Kemppainen TA, et al. A comparison of diets with and without oats in adults with celiac disease. *N Engl J Med*. 1995;333:1033-1037.
11. Hogberg L, Laurin P, Falth-Magnusson K, et al. Oats to children with newly diagnosed coeliac disease: a randomised double blind study. *Gut*. 2004;53:649-654.

12. Koerner TB, Cléroux C, Poirier C, Cantin I, Alimkulov A, Elamparo H. Gluten contamination in the Canadian commercial oat supply. *Food Addit Contam Part A Chem Anal Control Expo Risk Assess*. 2011;28(6):705-710.

13. Lundin KE, Nilsen EM, Scott HG, et al. Oats induced villous atrophy in coeliac disease. *Gut*. 2003;52:1649-1652.

14. Rashid M, Butzer D, Burrows V, et al. Consumption of pure oats by individuals with celiac disease: a position statement by the Canadian Celiac Association. *Can J Gastroenterol*. 2007;21(10):649-651.

15. Cabrera-Chávez F, Iametti S, Miriani M, de la Barca AM, Mamone G, Bonomi F. Maize prolamins resistant to peptic-tryptic digestion maintain immune-recognition by IgA from some celiac disease patients. *Plant Foods Hum Nutr*. 2012;67(1):24-30.

PART VI

Pediatric Food Allergy

CHAPTER 42

Food Allergy in Infancy and Early Childhood

The prevalence of food allergy is highest in infants and toddlers, and pediatric food allergy is of increasing concern worldwide. Cow's milk allergy has been estimated to occur in 2.5% of infants, and up to 8% of children under 3 years of age in North America are estimated to have allergy to a limited number of foods, mainly cow's milk, egg, soy, peanut, wheat, fish, shellfish, and tree nuts.[1] Using diagnostic food challenges, the incidence of peanut allergy in young children in North America (United States[2] and Canada[3]) has been estimated to be 1.5% of the population. The estimated incidence of food allergy differs somewhat in other countries. For example, reports in 2009 from Japan indicate that food allergies affect 12.8% of infants, 5.1% of 3-year-olds, and 1.3% to 2.6% of school-age children.[4]

The incidence of food allergy in children differs widely between the numbers reported by parents compared to those determined by oral food challenges. Two large population-based studies found that, although 40% to 60% of parents believed their child's symptoms were related to food consumption, only 30% to 40% reported symptoms that would support a diagnosis of food allergy, and merely 4% to 8% of the children were confirmed to be food allergic as a result of oral food challenges.[5,6] However, the actual numbers of children suffering from food allergies is difficult to ascertain, due in part to the lack of definitive diagnostic tests. All laboratory tests need to be confirmed by elimination and challenge to confirm food allergy and to determine the identity of the foods responsible.[4] Because such procedures are time-consuming and expensive to perform, many childhood food allergies may be misdiagnosed.

The greater numbers of children with food allergies compared with adults is largely due to the differences in the immune response of infants and children compared to that of adults. As the child's immune system matures, he or she starts to outgrow early food allergies. This change reflects the way in which a person's body processes and handles foreign food materials at different life stages. Thus, a good place to start the discussion on pediatric food allergy is to look at the immune system itself and how it changes with age.

The Immune System of the Developing Baby: Importance in Childhood Food Allergy

The Production of Antibodies in the Fetus, Baby, and Child

Each of the different types of antibody is produced at different times during development of the fetus and child, and each has a specific role to play in defense against pathogens and other agents that could harm the developing baby.[7,8] Compiled from a variety of sources cited in the reference list, Figure 42.1 depicts the way in which antibodies develop from fetal life through 9 years of age.

FIGURE 42.1

Comparative levels of antibodies in the fetus and child from conception to 9 years of age. Levels of antibodies are shown as a percentage of the adult level (designated 100%) of each antibody, rather than as actual values of the antibodies, which may be expressed in milligrams per deciliter (mg/dL) or other units of measurement, such as international units (IU), units (U), or kilounits (kU) per liter. For example, the adult level of IgM is about 100 mg/dL, whereas the adult level of IgG is about 1,300 mg/dL. Data are from multiple sources cited in the reference list.

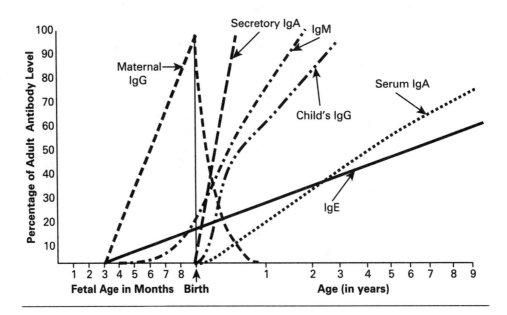

IgG

IgG is the only antibody that can cross the placenta from mother to fetus. All of the other antibodies that can be detected in the fetus or newborn are actually made by the immune system of the fetus while in the womb.

When the mother has been exposed to a specific microorganism such as a bacterium or virus, her immune system makes antibodies of the IgG class to protect her from further infection or invasion by that same microorganism. The IgG antibodies then cross the placenta to become part of the blood circulation of her unborn child and will protect it from the same microorganism while it is in the womb and during the first few months of life. In most cases, this system is extremely efficient in protecting the fetus from infections to which the mother is exposed.

The IgG in the fetus and newborn is solely of maternal origin. After birth, maternal IgG declines quite rapidly, and by about 9 months has disappeared altogether. Production of IgG by the baby begins at birth and increases quickly; by the age of 12 months, the baby is producing a level of IgG about 60% of that of an adult.

IgE

The earliest of the antibodies of nonmaternal origin detectable in the fetus is IgE. Antibodies of this class are made by the immune system of the fetus as early as 11 weeks' gestation. Because IgE is the antibody whose *protective* role (in contrast to its role in allergy) is defending the body from parasites such as intestinal helminths and nematodes, babies with high levels of IgE at birth are most effectively protected from these parasites. Under the "natural conditions" of what we now consider to be the developing countries where parasite infestations are endemic, such babies are the survivors. However, a baby similarly protected by a high IgE level in our sanitized Western world is most unlikely to encounter intestinal parasites at birth and consequently is the one most likely to develop allergies.

The level of IgE in the baby and child varies widely between different individuals. The level often depends on the allergic status of the child—the more allergens to which he or she is sensitized, the higher the level of IgE. And conversely, the higher the IgE level, the more likely the infant is to becoming sensitized to allergens in food and in his or her environment. However, the specific relationship between IgE level and clinical symptoms (atopy) is currently unknown. Some children with low levels of IgE may develop symptoms of allergy, while others with high levels of IgE may not show any signs of allergy. Factors in addition to IgE, as yet incompletely understood, are important in the process.

The expert panel (EP) guidelines[9] on the diagnosis and management of food allergy in the United States recommends that the routine use of measuring total serum IgE should not be used to make a diagnosis of food allergy. The guidelines state, "Although an elevated total serum IgE level is frequently found in atopic individuals and some investigators suggest that it may be useful when interpreting allergen-specific IgE levels, the EP could find no studies to support such a claim. In addition, the sensitivity and specificity of this test compared with the outcome of oral food challenges is insufficient to warrant routine use in evaluating FA." For more details about this topic, see Chapter 5.

IgM

IgM in the fetus and newborn are entirely of fetal origin. Production of IgM may start as early as 22 weeks' gestation and reach 10% of the adult level at birth. Thereafter, the level of IgM rises rapidly and typically reaches 75% of the adult level at 12 months of age. However, if the fetus becomes infected by a virus in utero, the fetal immune system can produce a higher level of IgM in an attempt to protect the unborn baby. A few viruses do infect the fetus directly; for example, the HIV virus that is responsible for AIDS and the rubella virus that causes German measles. When such viruses gain access to the fetus, the level of IgM in the fetus and newborn would then be much higher than shown in Figure 42.1.

IgA

The newborn baby is born without any IgA. However, IgA is produced rapidly by the baby's immune system, starting at birth, and secretory IgA (sIgA) may reach the adult level as early as 6 months of age. The lack of sIgA at birth, however, means that the baby is vulnerable to invasion by infective microorganisms or other foreign material through orifices that are normally protected by a coating of mucus. The digestive tract is especially vulnerable, because at every feeding, foreign material enters through the mouth. Fortunately, this lack of sIgA is adequately supplied to the newborn in the form of maternal sIgA in mother's colostrum and continues in her mature milk. Ninety percent of the antibody in the mother's colostrum and breastmilk is sIgA, which will protect all of the mucous membrane–lined cavities[a] until the baby is making sufficient sIgA of his or her own. Thus, every effort should be made to provide the newborn with colostrum as soon after birth as possible, and certainly before any other material, such as an infant formula, is given to the baby by mouth. Ideally, breastfeeding should commence within half an hour of birth, and exclusive breastfeeding should continue until solid foods are introduced at 4 to 6 months of age; for the infant with allergies, 6 months is preferable and recommended. Refer to Chapter 1 for a discussion of the role and relevance of these antibodies in the immune response in allergy.

Symptoms of Food Allergy in Babies and Children

In most cases, the first sign of allergy, or atopy, in a baby is an allergic reaction to foods. In the exclusively breastfed baby, this is usually a response to components of the mother's diet, which pass into her breastmilk. Symptoms frequently start in the digestive tract and skin and may be followed by symptoms in the upper respiratory tract and in the lungs.[10,11] Respiratory tract symptoms in the first year are frequently

---

[a] Mucous membranes line all of the organs that have external orifices. These include the digestive tract from the mouth to the anus; the respiratory tract, including the mouth, nasal passages, inner ear canals, upper respiratory tract, and lungs; and the urogenital tract.

triggered by food allergy, but as early food allergies are outgrown, allergy to airborne allergens may continue the symptoms, often into adulthood.

The most important question that parents ask is, "How do I know if my child has food allergies?" With older children who are eating solid foods, this is often apparent when symptoms develop in minutes, and usually within 2 hours, after he or she eats a specific food. With exclusively breastfed infants, it is more difficult to spot because the culprit food may come from the mother's diet and her baby may show symptoms several hours (typically 2 to 8 hours) after she has eaten the meal that contains the allergen. Most importantly, though, any other causes for the baby's or child's symptoms must be ruled out before food allergy is considered.

Allergy Symptoms in the Major Organ Systems

Digestive Tract

The first signs of a problem may appear in the digestive tract soon after birth, with persistent colicky pain, frequent spitting up or projectile vomiting after a feeding, and abnormally liquid or frothy stool, which sometimes continue for several weeks. Of course, not all food-allergic babies start with these symptoms, but these early symptoms may be signs that an adverse reaction to foods might be the problem if no other cause is found.

In older children, food allergy might appear as nausea and vomiting, frequent stomachaches, bloating, and diarrhea. Although not usually considered to be a common symptom of food allergy, chronic constipation that does not respond to laxatives is being increasingly recognized as a possible symptom of food allergy in children.[12] Further studies need to be carried out to obtain firmer evidence for the role of allergy in constipation and clarify the pathogenic mechanisms involved.

Skin

Allergic skin reactions may also start early—eczema (atopic dermatitis) can appear soon after birth—or in some unusual cases, the baby may have signs of eczema at birth. In the early stages, eczema may be present on the baby's cheeks, upper surfaces of the feet, legs, hands, and arms. Later the eczematous patches are more commonly found in the creases in the elbow and behind the knees, behind the ears and where the ear meets the face, and sometimes in the ear itself. A baby with eczema often has dry, flaky skin, which is easily irritated. Further details about eczema and food allergy can be found in Chapter 35.

Hives (urticaria) and facial reddening and swelling (angioedema) may also be indicators of an allergic reaction to foods in a baby and young child, which may appear and disappear with apparently very little association with specific foods. However, careful observation often does provide some indication of frequent triggers in the diet of either the baby or the mother. Persistent rashes that have no other cause (such as infection) may also be associated with early food allergy. See Chapter 36 for more details about urticaria and food allergy.

Respiratory Tract

Symptoms of nasal stuffiness; congestion; runny nose; itchy, irritated eyes; cough; and the wheeze associated with asthma are unusual as symptoms of food allergy in young babies. These types of symptoms are more commonly associated with airborne allergens such as pollens from trees, grasses, and weeds; dust mites; mold spores; and animal dander. Respiratory allergies to airborne allergens usually start to appear after about the age of 18 months to 2 years; such allergies are uncommon in infants.

Respiratory symptoms in babies under the age of about 18 months may be associated with foods, but symptoms in the respiratory tract in this age group rarely occur alone; there is usually some sign of reactions in other organ systems, such as the digestive tract (often as prolonged or unusually severe colic) or skin reactions such as eczema.

Anaphylaxis in the Young Infant

The whole-body involvement of an anaphylactic reaction is rare in babies and very young children. Most life-threatening anaphylactic reactions tend to occur in the teens and early twenties. Occasional reports of anaphylactic reactions to foods in early childhood indicate that the food most frequently responsible for this most extreme food allergy is cow's milk.[13]

Anaphylaxis is a life-threatening allergic reaction[14] that affects several different parts of the body. It may affect the skin: flushing, itching, or hives; the airway: swelling of the throat, difficulty in talking or breathing; the digestive tract: nausea, vomiting, or diarrhea; the ability of the heart to pump blood: low blood pressure, increased pulse rate, and may proceed to unconsciousness and shock.

Symptoms usually appear rapidly, sometimes within minutes of exposure to the allergen and can be life-threatening. Immediate medical attention is necessary when anaphylaxis occurs. Standard emergency treatment often includes an injection of epinephrine (adrenaline) to open up the airway and help reverse the reaction. Transportation to the nearest hospital is essential. The subject of anaphylactic reactions to foods is discussed in more detail in Chapter 4.

Common Symptoms of Allergy in Relation to Age

Figure 42.2 provides a visual summary of the comparative occurrence of the various allergy symptoms with age.[15] Food allergy is the earliest of the allergic responses to become apparent, with skin reactions such as eczema closely following a similar pattern for approximately 12 to 18 months. After this time, the incidence of food allergy tends to decline as children start to outgrow their early allergy, especially to foods such as egg and milk. The incidence of eczema does not follow the same curve, because environmental factors begin to play a role in eczema as airborne allergens (eg, dust and dust mites, mold spores, animal dander, and pollens) gain access through the abraded skin of eczema and elicit an IgE-mediated allergy.[16] This

FIGURE 42.2

Age relationship between food allergy and atopic symptoms. Reprinted with permission from Werfel T, Knapp A. Atopic dermatitis and allergic contact dermatitis. In: Holgate ST, Church MK, Lichtenstein LM, eds. *Allergy*. 2nd ed. Maryland Heights, MO: Elsevier/Mosby; 2001:110. Copyright Elsevier, 2001.

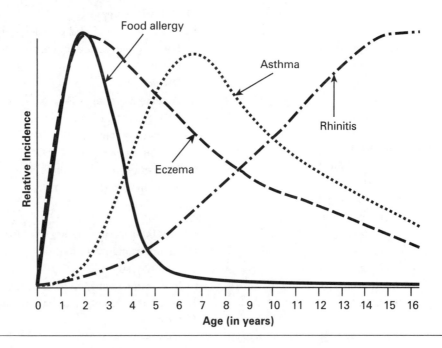

reaction continues the atopic dermatitis that may have earlier been a result of an allergic response to food.

Asthma may begin early, but the incidence in the first 2 years tends to be low. It reaches a peak at about 7 years and then declines, especially at puberty. However, asthma may continue to be a lifelong problem in many atopic individuals.

Upper respiratory tract allergy may be associated with food allergy in the early stages of life, but allergy to airborne allergens resulting in hay fever symptoms tends to rise in incidence significantly at about 7 years of age, reaching a peak at about 14 to 15 years. Typically, hay fever continues into adulthood and is often a lifelong condition.

As most allergies to foods are outgrown, the symptoms in the major organ systems may continue in response to allergens in the air and environment. However, a few food allergies do persist into adulthood in some people; these tend to be allergies to the most highly allergenic foods (peanuts, tree nuts, fish, shellfish, and, less frequently, egg, wheat, and other grains) and may be responsible for a severe or anaphylactic reaction.

The major effects of food allergy occur in the first 2 years, and then rapidly decline as the child begins to grow out of the early food allergies. As environmental and airborne allergies start to make their appearance at about 2 years of

---

BOX 42.1   Symptoms That May Indicate Food Allergy in the Baby and Young Child

Gastrointestinal tract
- Persistent colic
- Abdominal distress
- Frequent spitting up
- Nausea
- Vomiting
- Diarrhea
- Constipation

Respiratory tract
- Nasal stuffiness
- Sneezing
- Nose rubbing
- Noisy breathing
- Persistent cough
- Wheezing
- Asthma
- Itchy, runny, reddened, eyes
- Frequent earaches

Skin
- Urticaria (hives)
- Facial reddening and swelling (angioedema)
- Swelling and reddening around the mouth
- Eczema
- Dry itchy skin
- Persistent diaper rash
- Redness around anus
- Redness on cheeks
- Reddened ears
- Rash of unknown origin
- Scratching and rubbing

Other
- Feeding problems (baby may forcibly reject food)
- Failure to gain weight (failure to thrive)
- Weight loss
- In extreme cases, involvement of all body systems in anaphylaxis, which can be life-threatening

---

age, there is an overlap of allergies. This sometimes results in a combined effect of both food allergies and environmental allergies between about 2 and 4 years of age. IgE antibodies to airborne allergens, and the inflammatory mediators released in response, will add on top of the mediators of food allergy; as a result, the child's symptoms may appear more frequently and seem more severe. This may change over the next year or so as the child outgrows his or her early allergies to foods. See Box 42.1 for a summary of the more common symptoms of allergy in babies and young children.

Infant Colic and Allergy

Up to one-third of infants under the age of 4 months experience some degree of colic. *Colic* is defined as a condition affecting healthy, well-fed infants, consisting of irritability and excessive, inconsolable crying (usually in the evening) that lasts for at least 3 hours a day and occurs more than 3 days a week. Although the cause of colic is still unknown, it seems to be self-limiting and in most cases resolves by the age of 4 months.[17]

A number of causes for colic have been postulated, none of which fit every situation. Most often, food allergy or intolerance has been suggested, and a variety of dietary strategies have been advised, which sometimes help. The most frequently suggested cause has been milk allergy, and elimination of milk and milk products from the diet of breastfeeding mothers has proven to be beneficial in many cases. For the formula-fed infant, some studies have shown that switching from a cow's-milk-based formula to one that is based on soy has relieved the distress of several colicky infants.[18]

Transient lactose intolerance has also been investigated as a cause. In one study, treating infant food with lactase reduced the symptoms in a significant number of cases.[19] (The subject of lactose intolerance in the breastfed baby is discussed in Chapter 11.)

In other cases, feeding a hydrolyzed whey-based formula or a casein-based formula that has been extensively hydrolyzed seems to reduce the symptoms in many colicky babies.[20] Other studies indicate that an overload of sugar—for example, in apple juice—may have contributed to the problem. Fructose intolerance (see Chapter 24) may be a factor in causing colic-like symptoms in some infants.

From the many studies on dietary triggers for infant colic, it would appear that food allergy or intolerance may be a contributing factor. However, it is probable that infant colic has multiple causes, and no single dietary strategy is likely to improve the situation in all cases.

References

1. Bock SA, Atkins FM. Patterns of food hypersensitivity during sixteen years of double-blind, placebo-controlled food challenges. *J Pediatr*. 1990;117:561-567.
2. Grundy J, Matthews S, Bateman B, Dean T, Arshad SH. Rising prevalence of allergy to peanut in children: data from 2 sequential cohorts. *J Allergy Clin Immunol*. 2002; 110:784-789.
3. Kagan RS, Joseph L, Dufresns C, et al. Prevalence of peanut allergy in primary school children in Montreal, Canada. *J Allergy Clin Immunol*. 2003;112:1223-1228.
4. Ito K, Urisu A. Diagnosis of food allergy based on oral food challenge test. *Allergol Int*. 2009;58:467-474.
5. Bock SA. Prospective appraisal of complaints of adverse reactions to foods in children during the first 3 years of life. *Pediatrics*. 1987;79:683-688.
6. Roehr CC, Edenharter G, Reimann S, et al. Food allergy and non-allergic food hypersensitivity in children and adolescents. *Clin Exper Allergy*. 2004;34:1534-1541.
7. Holt PG, Jones CA. The development of the immune system during pregnancy and early life. Allergy Review Series VI: the immunology of fetuses and infants. *Allergy*. 2000;55:688-697.
8. Kesarwala HH, Fischer TJ. Introduction to the immune system. In: Lawlor GJ, Fischer TJ. *Manual of Allergy and Immunology: Diagnosis and Therapy*. 2nd ed. Boston, MA: Little, Brown and Company; 1988:1-14.
9. Boyce JA, Assa'ad A, Burks AW, et al. Guidelines for the diagnosis and management of food allergy in the United States: report of the NIAID-sponsored expert panel. *J Allergy Clin Immunol*. 2010;126(6):S1-S58. (Guideline 6.)

10. Vieira MC, Morais MB, Spolidoro JVN, et al. A survey on clinical presentation and nutritional status of infants with suspected cow's milk allergy. *BMC Pediatr*. 2010;10:25-31.
11. Sampson HA. Food allergy part 1. Immunopathogenesis and clinical disorders. *J Allergy Clin Immunol*. 1999;103(5):717-728.
12. Carroccio A, Iocono G. Review article: chronic constipation and food hypersensitivity—an intriguing relationship. *Aliment Pharmacol Ther*. 2006;24(9):1295-1304.
13. Pumphrey RS. Lessons for management of anaphylaxis from a study of fatal reactions. *Clin Exper Allergy*. 2000;30:1144-1150.
14. Sampson HA, Munoz-Furlong A, Campbell RL, et al. Second Symposium on the Definition and Management of Anaphylaxis: Summary Report—Second National Institute of Allergy and Infectious Disease/Food Allergy and Anaphylaxis Network Symposium. *Ann Emerg Med*. 2006;47(4):373-380.
15. Werfel T, Knapp A. Atopic dermatitis and allergic contact dermatitis. In: Holgate ST, Church MK, Lichtenstein LM, eds. *Allergy*. 2nd ed. Maryland Heights, MO: Elsevier/Mosby; 2001:110.
16. Strid J, Strobel S. Skin barrier dysfunction and systemic sensitization to allergens through the skin. *Curr Drug Targets Inflamm Allergy*. 2005;4(5):531-541.
17. Cohen-Silver J, Ratnapalan S. Management of infantile colic: a review. *Clin Pediatr (Phila)*. 2009;48(1):14-17.
18. Hill DJ, Hosking CS. Infantile colic and food hypersensitivity. *J Pediatr Gastroenterol Nutr*. 2000;30(1):S67-S76.
19. Kanabar D, Randhawa M, Clayton P. Improvement of symptoms in infant colic following reduction of lactose load with lactase. *J Human Nutr Diet*. 2001;14(5):359-363.
20. Jakobsson I, Lothe L, Ley D, Borschel MW. Effectiveness of casein hydrolysate feedings in infants with colic. *Acta Paediatric*. 2000;89(1):18-21.

CHAPTER **43**

Prevention and Management of Food Allergy in Babies and Children

O ne of the most significant changes in pediatric food allergy management in recent years has been in strategies to prevent food allergy in early infancy. Previously the idea prevailed that if foods are withheld from the infant until the immune and digestive systems are more mature, allergic sensitization would be prevented or significantly reduced. Frequently the advice regarding the introduction of the most highly allergenic foods was the later the better. It was hoped that this would prevent allergy to food and to inhalant and contact allergies in later life. We now know that this is not the best advice. In fact, new research seems to indicate the opposite—that *exposure* to allergens in early life may actually tolerize the infant's immune system and prevent allergic sensitization to food.

Examples of Changes in Approach to Management of Food Allergies

Fish Allergy

Previously it was thought that fish, being a highly allergenic food, should be avoided until the child is at least a year; some authorities suggested not introducing fish until even later if the child is considered to be at high risk for allergy.[1] However, recent research has provided evidence that children are less likely to develop allergy to fish if the mother consumes fish two or three times a week during pregnancy[2] (if the mother is not allergic to fish, of course). Another paper provided evidence that regular fish consumption during the first year of life was associated with a reduced risk for allergic disease by 4 years of age,[3] and a further study indicated that early introduction of fish (before 9 months of age) reduces the risk of eczema in children.[4]

Adverse Reactions to Wheat

Even more revolutionary is evidence that it is possible that adverse reactions to certain foods might be prevented by introducing those foods to the baby during a specific "window of opportunity" that lasts only a few months when the baby's immune system is most likely to become tolerant. Timing of the introduction of grains, especially wheat, seems to strongly affect the baby's immunological response to the food.[5] This is applicable not only to food allergy but also to other conditions such as celiac disease that are triggered by food.[6] These studies suggest that wheat should be introduced after age 3 months but before age 7 months to promote tolerance to it.

Peanut Allergy

Repeatedly, reports indicate that the incidence of peanut allergy in children has increased dramatically in recent years. A 2007 study[7] reported that the incidence of peanut allergy in children younger than 5 years of age had doubled in the years from 2002 to 2007, and the current incidence of peanut allergy in the U.S. population is reported to be 1%.[8] Despite strong advice from pediatric groups and governmental guidelines recommending avoidance of peanuts during pregnancy, lactation, and infancy in the United Kingdom, Australia, and North America, peanut allergy continues to increase in these countries.

A 2008 article shed light on this apparent anomaly.[9] This study of peanut allergy in Jewish children in primary school (elementary school) in two populations—in Israel and the United Kingdom—showed the prevalence of peanut allergy in the United Kingdom to be 10 times higher than that in Israel (1.85% in the United Kingdom compared to 0.17% in Israel). The difference could not be accounted for by differences in atopy, social class, genetic background, or peanut allergenicity. The difference was in the age of exposure to peanut: Israeli infants 8 to 14 months of age consume peanut in high quantities (median monthly consumption 7.1 g), whereas infants in the United Kingdom strictly avoid peanuts.

Late Introduction of Allergenic Foods and Development of Food and Inhalant Allergies

A 2009 study from Finland[10] examined the effects of maternal diet during pregnancy and lactation and the infant's diet during infancy and childhood on the development of type 1 diabetes, allergic diseases, and asthma. The study suggested that late introduction of solid foods was associated with increased risk of allergic sensitization to food and inhalant allergens. In light of this research, the directives for feeding in the early stages of life have changed significantly.[11] Whereas previously the directive was to avoid highly allergenic foods until the immune system was sufficiently mature to process them, the current directives recommend exposing the developing infant to food antigens in an environment that provides the optimum opportunity for development of tolerance. However, what the optimum environment is remains to be determined.[12]

It is possible that optimal specific introduction stages do exist for different foods, but research has a long way to go before we can confidently advise parents on when to introduce specific foods to their allergic babies. At the moment, we must rely on consensus documents and practice guidelines (see "Introducing Solid Foods" later in this chapter), which are based on extensive reviews of studies published in reputable, peer-reviewed medical and scientific journals, and wait for more good studies.

Early Allergy Predictors

Allergic diseases result from a strong relationship between genetic and environmental factors. Sensitization to food allergens occurs mainly in the first year of life, and cow's milk allergy is often the first food allergy to appear in susceptible infants. The incidence of allergy in children of allergic parents is significantly greater than in children of parents without allergies; it is estimated that genetic factors account for 50% to 70% of asthma and allergy.[13] However, many children who develop atopic diseases during the first years of life come from families without any history of allergy.

It is important to understand that inheriting the potential to develop allergy is actually an inheritance of the Th2 response to allergens, not inheritance of a specific allergy. In other words, the baby's immune system is primed at birth to respond to certain harmless proteins as if they posed a threat to the body, but it is not programmed to respond to any allergen in particular. For example, even if both parents are allergic to peanuts, the baby does not inherit peanut allergy; he or she inherits an increased likelihood of responding to an allergen. The development of peanut allergy in the baby would require sensitization to the peanut allergen under conditions appropriate to that sensitization. The baby is just as likely to develop allergy to milk, or soy, or even some obscure tropical fruit—or none at all (although some foods are more likely than others to leads to allergy; see Chapter 2). It depends on the baby's exposure to the allergen and the response of his or her immune system at the time of exposure.

Many authorities have tried to provide parameters to identify those babies who are most likely to develop early allergies, based on their inherited allergic potential. As these babies are identified, it is hoped that strategies can be implemented to reduce their sensitization to allergens during the period in which they are most likely to become allergic.

Various definitions of high-risk infants have been used. The prevailing definition, published as a joint statement of the European Society of Pediatric Allergology and Clinical Immunology (ESPACI) and the European Society for Pediatric Gastroenterology, Hepatology and Nutrition (ESPGHAN)[14] and the American Academy of Pediatrics (AAP)[15] defines high-risk infants as those with at least one first-degree relative (parent or sibling) with documented allergic disease. Most authorities rely on this definition as the basis of their assessment of the at-risk-for-allergy pediatric population.

The bottom line is that there are no objective scientific tests to determine exactly which baby will develop allergy. The best we can do is to make an informed guess, based on family history of allergy.

Food Allergy and Other Allergic Diseases

For many years it was assumed that if the early onset of allergy could be prevented or delayed, the child might avoid what allergists like to call the "allergic march"—the progression from food allergy to inhalant-triggered respiratory allergy and asthma, which usually have their onset at a later age. It was assumed that the early expression of allergy in the form of allergic reaction to foods "primed" the immune system to take the Th2 route, and once started, the Th2 response would progress to respiratory allergy and asthma. However, newer research has demonstrated that this is not necessarily the case. Prevention of food allergy in early infancy prevents or reduces *food* allergy. However, the direct effect of food allergy in the development of allergy to airborne and environmental allergens has yet to be identified by scientific studies. Nevertheless, it is important to prevent, reduce, or relieve food allergy as early as possible because of the central role of allergy to foods in many allergic diseases (particularly eczema), its contribution to asthma and allergic rhinitis, and the real danger of life-threatening anaphylactic reactions.

This brings us to an important concept in understanding food allergy: An allergy to food is not a "stand-alone" disease. The mediators released in an allergic reaction affect many tissues and organ systems, resulting in a variety of symptoms. Therefore, a reaction to a food may cause a flare-up of eczema; trigger an asthma attack or make existing asthma worse; increase the severity of hay fever, especially in the pollen season; or cause digestive tract upset; or all of the above at the same time. Of course, each of these conditions may have a "primary allergy trigger" apart from food, such as airborne pollens, dust mites, mold spores, animal dander, or contact allergens that cause a skin reaction when they come into contact with the sensitized skin or mucous membranes. This means that in most cases, mediators released in a food allergy can impact any vulnerable area of the body, depending on the individual's sensitivity; therefore, successfully managing a child's food allergy will avoid the direct effects of food sensitivity and will relieve or reduce the impact of other allergies at the same time.

So, how can we make a difference in the baby's risk of developing allergy? How early in life can we implement strategies to promote tolerance and avoid sensitization of the baby to allergens?

Does Atopic Disease Start in Fetal Life?

During pregnancy, immune responses in the uterus are skewed to the Th2 type rather than the Th1, because the fetus must be protected from rejection by the mother's system. Obviously, the fetus, having inheritance from both father and mother, has a different cellular composition from its mother. Therefore the developing baby might be at risk of rejection by the mother's immune system, which is designed to reject anything "foreign" within her body. This rejection would be a Th1 response (see Chapter 1 for a detailed discussion of Th1 and Th2 immune responses). To avoid this rejection, the fetal environment develops a predominantly Th2 milieu, which suppresses the mother's protection/rejection response. This effectively bathes the fetus in Th2-type cytokines that keep it safe in its environment.

Since the fetus is enveloped by Th2-type cytokines in the womb, it is logical to question whether allergic sensitization to foods in the mother's diet might gain access to the developing baby's system and thereby start allergic sensitization even before birth. In fact, allergens have been detected in amniotic fluid, indicating that allergens to which the mother has been exposed can cross the placenta.[16] However, there is no real evidence to suggest that the fetal immune system is primed to respond to these allergens.[17] In fact, some authorities suggest that exposure to food antigens in utero may promote fetal tolerance[2]—that is, the immune system is "educated" to recognize the food as "foreign but safe" and not to mount a defensive action against it when the food is encountered at any time in the future. So, in utero exposure to food molecules may mark the beginning of our ability to consume food with impunity.

At birth, all newborns have low levels of INF-γ and produce the cytokines associated with the Th2 response, especially IL-4, and newborns of both atopic and nonatopic inheritance have a predominantly Th2 response to antigens. As the baby matures, there is a switch from the Th2 to the "protective" Th1 response, except in atopic babies, where the Th2 response continues to predominate and sets the stage for allergen sensitization and allergy.[18] So here the important question is, why do all neonates not have allergy? New research is indicating that the answer may lie with the mother's immune system, which plays a significant role in the expression of allergy in her baby.[19]

The only antibody that crosses the placenta from mother to fetus is IgG. As has been mentioned previously in the discussion on antibodies (see Chapter 1), there are four subtypes of IgG, designated IgG1, IgG2, IgG3, and IgG4. IgG4 is frequently associated with IgE in allergy. The nonatopic mother produces abundant IgG1 and IgG3, which cross the placenta to protect her fetus in utero. Because food proteins can cross the placenta, it is thought that fetal exposure to these antigens in the uterus, protected by the mother's IgG1 and IgG3, may promote fetal tolerance to these foods, and this continues into the neonatal period. In contrast, the allergic mother tends to produce IgE and IgG4; IgG4 is very poor at crossing the placenta, and the mother's IgE-to-IgG ratio is thought to have the greatest consequences for the offspring.[19] In allergic mothers, there is likely to be insufficient IgG1 and IgG3 to downregulate (reduce the level of) fetal IgE, and thus at birth her baby may be primed to become sensitized to allergens and to develop allergic symptoms very early.

Although there is no evidence that the fetus of the allergic mother can mount an IgE-mediated response to specific allergens in utero, the potential to produce allergen-specific IgE predominates at birth. The only defense against this at present is to reduce the allergic mother's exposure to her own allergens throughout pregnancy in an attempt to decrease her production of IgE and IgG4 and hopefully enhance production of the protective IgG1 and IgG3. The mother should avoid foods to which she is allergic at all times and obtain complete balanced nutrition from alternate sources. No evidence suggests that maternal avoidance of any foods other than her own allergens during pregnancy will improve the allergic status of her baby. A 1988 report[20] indicated that excluding highly allergenic foods from the mother's diet from week 28 to the end of pregnancy did not affect the atopic status of the infant in any way.

Several studies suggest that women tend to have a weaker immune response to allergens with each successive pregnancy, which might explain why children born later tend to suffer less from eczema, hay fever, and asthma than their older siblings. In addition, firstborn children generally have a higher level of IgE in their blood (measured in cord blood at birth) than children born subsequently. The authors of these studies suggest that the mother's immune response influences the baby's immune system, which subsequently affects the child's sensitivity to allergens later.[21]

The Newborn Baby: Conditions That Predispose to Allergy

Immaturity of the Infant's Immune System

At birth, the major elements of the immune system are in place but do not function at a level that provides adequate protection against all infections. The level of antibodies (except maternal IgG) is a fraction of that of the adult, and secretory IgA (sIgA), the "first-line defense" of all mucous membranes, is absent at birth. Babies at risk of developing atopic disease are commonly described as having impaired function/delayed maturation of various immunologic processes, including cytokine production.[4]

Permeability of the Digestive Tract

The infant's intestine is highly permeable to the absorption of large molecules during the first 3 years of life, especially during the first 6 months and up to 1 year. The larger food molecules (10,000 to 70,000 daltons in molecular size) trigger the Th2 response and the production of food-specific IgE. Therefore, during the period that the digestive tract is most permeable, sensitization to food allergens occurs, and food allergy is most likely to develop.

Consequently, the newborn is at risk for developing food allergies as a result of a predominance of the Th2 response, the lack of protective secretory IgA at mucosal surfaces, and a hyperpermeable digestive epithelium. The offspring of the allergic mother has the additional risk factors associated with an increased potential to mount an IgE-mediated response as a result of lacking the maternal IgG1 and IgG3 that would normally downregulate the production of Th2 cytokines.

In an important study of 1,749 newborns in Odense, Denmark, 39 (2.2%) were identified as being sensitized to cow's milk proteins soon after birth. Of these, 9 infants developed symptoms of cow's milk allergy before 3 months of age, in spite of being exclusively breastfed. Review of records from the newborn nursery revealed that all 9 of these infants had been exposed to cow's milk formula in amounts corresponding to approximately 0.4 to 3 g of beta-lactoglobulin (BLG) during the first 3 days of life. Similar proteins were detected in their mother's breastmilk to which the allergic infants reacted with the development of symptoms. The authors conclude that early inadvertent and occasional exposure to cow's milk proteins may initiate sensitization in predisposed neonates; subsequent exposure to minute amounts of bovine milk proteins in human milk may then act as booster doses, eliciting allergic reactions.[22]

Breastfeeding and Allergy

Breastmilk provides the ideal nutritional, immunological, and physiological nourishment for all newborns. Components of human milk enhance the baby's natural defenses and promote maturation of the immune system.[23] Ninety percent of antibodies in human colostrum and milk are secretory IgA, which provide the baby with protection at mucosal surfaces until the infant is producing adequate quantities of its own sIgA at about 6 months of age.[24] However, the effect of breastfeeding on the development of allergic diseases in the breastfed infant remains controversial.

As discussed by Arshad,[25] several studies report that breastfeeding is protective against allergy with a definite improvement in infant eczema and associated gastrointestinal complaints and a reduced risk of asthma in the first 24 months, when the baby is exclusively breastfed and mother eliminates highly allergenic foods from her diet. A 2010 report indicates that IgG immune complexes found in breastmilk are potent inducers of tolerance to aerosolized antigens to which the mother was sensitized, providing antigen-specific protection from asthma in their babies.[26]

However, other studies seem to indicate that breastfeeding has no effect on the infant's symptoms of allergy, or worse, may be associated with an increased prevalence of atopic eczema.[27,28] One of the reasons for this apparent contradiction may be explained by data that indicates that the breastmilk of atopic mothers differs immunologically from that of mothers without allergies.[29,30]

Atopic mothers tend to have a higher level of the cytokines and chemokines associated with allergy in their breastmilk and have a lower level of the cytokine known as *transforming growth factor-beta-1* (TGF-β1) that promotes tolerance to food components in the intestinal immune response. A normal level of TGF-β1 in the mother's colostrum and breastmilk is likely to facilitate tolerance to food encountered by the infant in the breastmilk and later to formulas and solids.[31] Evidence seems to suggest that breastfeeding is protective against allergies when the mother is not atopic,[32] but that babies of allergic mothers may be at risk of developing allergies, especially to foods, during breastfeeding.

In view of the large amount of evidence regarding the role of breastmilk in promoting the well-being of all babies, and based on careful analysis of all research data on the topic, ESPACI and ESPGHAN strongly recommend exclusive breastfeeding for 4 to 6 months, and the AAP[15,33] recommends breastfeeding for at least 4 months, with introduction of complementary foods no earlier than age 4 to 6 months as the hallmark for allergy prevention.[15,34]

Prevention of Food Allergic Sensitization During the First 6 Months

From the results of epidemiological studies, it is thought that initial sensitization to food allergens in the exclusively breastfed baby occurs predominantly from external sources, such as a single feeding of infant formula or perhaps by accident. Thereafter, the baby's immune system responds to the allergen in the mother's milk. The question of whether allergens from the mother's diet appearing in her breast-milk can act as the initial sensitizing dose for development of food allergy in the breastfed baby has often been investigated, but the answer is still not clear.[35] However, current evidence in general supports the concept that restricting the mother's diet during pregnancy and lactation has no beneficial effect in preventing allergy in her baby.

The current directives from position papers and consensus documents from many countries now recognize that restricting the maternal diet during pregnancy and lactation is contraindicated in allergy prevention:

■ The AAP states[15] that antigen avoidance during lactation does not prevent atopic disease, with the caveat that more data are needed to substantiate this conclusion.
■ The European Academy of Allergology and Clinical Immunology states that "no conclusive evidence for protective effect of maternal exclusion diet during pregnancy or lactation has been documented."[14]
■ The Australasian Society of Clinical Immunology and Allergy states that "dietary restrictions in pregnancy are not recommended" and "maternal dietary restrictions during breast feeding are not recommended."[36]

In summary, professional groups do not recommend the elimination of any specific foods from the maternal diet during breastfeeding except for the mother's own allergens unless the baby has been diagnosed with allergy to one or more foods, in which case the baby's allergenic food should be avoided by its mother as long as she is breastfeeding.

Formula Feeding

It is not always possible for a baby to be breastfed, and when the infant is at risk for or has developed allergies, making the best choice of formula is important. Most authorities suggest that if a baby has no signs or symptoms of cow's milk allergy, a conventional cow's milk–based formula is safe for infant feeding. However, for babies who are at high risk for allergy, emerging evidence suggests that hydrolyzed infant formulas provide a measure of protection against the development of atopic disease[37] compared to conventional milk–based formulas. Hydrolysis of cow's milk breaks the protein into smaller, potentially less allergenic proteins. A Cochrane review states that "in high risk infants who are unable to be breast-fed, there is limited evidence that prolonged feeding with a hydrolysed formula compared to a cow's milk formula reduces infant and childhood allergy and infant cow's milk allergy."[37]

A 2003 study in Germany compared conventional cow's milk formula (CMF) with extensively hydrolyzed casein formula (EHF), an extensively hydrolyzed whey formula, and a partially hydrolyzed whey formula (PHF) in their role in preventing allergic disease in the first year of life. The results showed that the incidence of allergy was significantly reduced in the babies fed the extensively hydrolyzed formulas compared to CMF, and the incidence of eczema was significantly reduced in babies fed EHF or PHF in comparison to those fed CMF.[38] A follow-up study in 2007 reported that a significant reduction in the incidence of atopic dermatitis (eczema) was achieved with the extensively hydrolysed casein formula and with the partially hydrolysed whey formula, but that none of the formulas reduced the incidence of asthma.[39] Further results from the study published in 2008 confirmed that hydrolyzed infant formulas had a long-term allergy-preventive effect on the development of atopic eczema until 6 years of age.[40]

Based on the evidence from a variety of studies, the AAP concluded in 2008 that "in studies of infants at high risk of developing atopic disease who are not breast-fed exclusively for 4 to 6 months or are formula fed, there is modest evidence that atopic dermatitis may be delayed or prevented by the use of extensively hydrolyzed or partially hydrolyzed formulas, compared with cow's milk formula, in early childhood."[15] The AAP further stated that "extensively hydrolyzed formulas may be more effective than partially hydrolyzed in the prevention of atopic disease."[15]

However, the authors of a 2011 research study stated that "despite current dietary guidelines, we found no evidence to support recommending the use of pHWF [partially hydrolysed whey formula] at weaning for the prevention of allergic disease in high-risk infants."[41] Their conclusion was based on a study of 620 infants with a family history of allergic disease who were recruited at birth to receive a conventional cow's milk formula, a partially hydrolyzed whey formula, or a soy formula. Follow-up was conducted at 2 years and at 6 or 7 years of age. There was no evidence that infants allocated to the pHWF or the soy formula were at a lower risk of allergic manifestations in infancy compared with conventional formula. There was also no evidence of reduced risk of skin prick test reactivity or childhood allergic disease.

Pediatric groups worldwide agree that there is no evidence for the use of soy-based infant formula for the purpose of allergy prevention.[15,33,36] In summary, if a baby at high risk for allergy cannot be exclusively breastfed to 4 to 6 months of age, the preferred method of feeding in prevention of atopic disease is an extensively hydrolyzed formula (see Box 43.1 for hydrolyzed infant formulas available in the United States).

BOX 43.1   Hydrolyzed Infant Formulas Available in the United States

- Extensively hydrolyzed casein (cow milk protein; EHF):
  - Enfamil Nutramigen (Mead Johnson)
  - Enfamil Pregestimil (Mead Johnson)
  - Similac Alimentum Advance (Abbott)
- Partially hydrolyzed whey (cow milk protein; PHF): Good Start Supreme (Nestlé USA)
- Partially hydrolyzed whey and casein (cow milk protein; PHF): Enfamil Gentlease Lipil (Mead Johnson)
- Free amino acid based (elemental formula):
  - Neocate (Nutricia North America)
  - EleCare (Abbott Nutrition)

Introducing Solid Foods

The question of when to introduce foods into the diet of the allergic or potentially allergic infant and which foods to introduce has been largely a matter of following previous practices rather than using evidence-based or consensus-based guidelines. In fact, there is no standard schedule for weaning infants, whether healthy or at risk for allergies. In July 2006, the Adverse Reactions to Foods Committee of the American College of Allergy, Asthma and Immunology[42] published the first consensus document on the introduction of solid foods for the food-allergic infant. They recommended delaying the introduction of the most common allergens in solid foods to the allergic infant until after 6 months of age. Until this age, the authors suggest that the infant's immature digestive tract and immune system may increase the risk of sensitization and development of allergy.

Furthermore, it was recommended that the most highly allergenic foods should not be introduced until after 1 year of age or later. Specific times of introduction were suggested as follows: cow's milk at 12 months; egg at 24 months; and peanut, tree nut, and fish at 3 years. However, more recent research has demonstrated that these recommendations were neither supported by evidence-based research nor were they effective in practice. Newer position papers reflect this change in approach. The AAP position paper published in 2008 states that the evidence "does not allow one to conclude that there is a strong relationship between the timing of the introduction of complementary foods and development of atopic disease."[15]

The current directive is that solid foods should be introduced to the potentially allergic infant no later than 6 months of age, ideally following 4 to 6 months of exclusive breastfeeding. Some studies suggest that foods, especially gluten-containing grains, should be introduced while breastfeeding for optimum tolerance development.[43] The optimal sequence of introducing foods is presently unknown. Current research indicates that there may be a "window of opportunity" when the child's immune system is most likely to tolerate the food, and if this is missed, there may be an increased likelihood of sensitization. Future research will undoubtedly reveal the ideal times for introduction of specific foods.

Method of Introducing Solid Foods

According to the guidelines of all pediatric societies and consensus committees, solid foods should be introduced individually and gradually, starting at about 4 to 6 months of age. Each food should be introduced, ideally over a 4-day period, with careful monitoring of the baby for the development of signs of allergy. No mixed foods should be given until each food in the mixture has been given to the baby and is tolerated.

The following sequential incremental dose method of introducing solid foods to the allergic baby has been used by this book's author for many years with great success.[44] This protocol introduces graded quantities of individual foods, starting with very small amounts, and allows monitoring of the baby's response as each food is tested:

- Before introducing a new food to infants who are at high risk for allergy, especially if they have demonstrated any type of allergic reaction previously, apply the food to the baby's cheek and wait 20 minutes to see whether a reddened area appears at the site of application. This "early warning sign" indicates the release of histamine, which presages a probable allergic response to the food.
- If a reddened area does not appear, apply a little of the food to the outer border of the baby's lower lip (not inside the mouth). If there is no response to this, such as reddening, swelling, blistering, or irritation (sometimes indicated by baby rubbing the area), place a tiny amount of the food on the baby's tongue and monitor for a reaction.
- If the above signs are all negative, feed the infant a small amount (½ teaspoon or less) of the food. The baby should be carefully observed for any reactions for the next 4 hours.
- If no adverse signs appear, the infant can be fed more (usually ½ to 1 teaspoon) of the food. Again monitor the baby for 4 hours.
- If no adverse reactions occur, 1 to 2 teaspoons of the food can then be given. This is three incremental doses on day 1.
- The next 24 hours (day 2) should be a monitoring time for delayed reactions, which may be apparent in several ways, including disturbed sleep patterns, irritability, and overt allergic symptoms. Delayed reactions, especially to cow's milk proteins, are not uncommon.
- If no adverse reactions are observed, more of the same food can be introduced on the third day, in three doses as previously described, using slightly greater quantities than on the first, ending with feeding the baby as much of the food as he or she wants.
- The fourth day is a second monitoring day in which none of the test food is eaten, and the baby is observed for any signs that would indicate a delayed reaction.

- If the baby is free from any signs of allergy after the 4-day introduction period, the food may be assumed safe and included in the regular diet.
- Each new food should be introduced separately.
- As each food is tolerated, it can be incorporated regularly into the baby's diet.
- If there is an obvious adverse reaction at any stage, stop that food immediately. Wait until all signs of the reaction have resolved, and wait another 24 to 48 hours before trying a new food.

Sequence of Introducing Solids

There is no particular order in which the different categories of foods should be introduced. However, if the baby has been exclusively breastfed, it is a good idea to introduce meats early because a food source of iron is important from 6 months of age onward. The Recommended Dietary Intake for iron for babies ages 6 to 11 months is 11 mg/d. Once babies start ingesting solid food, the iron in breastmilk is not as easily absorbed. The belief that babies cannot digest red meats has become entrenched in popular thought, but it lacks scientific evidence. Many registered dietitians and pediatricians advocate the use of iron-enriched baby cereals for early infant feeding. However, the best source of iron is heme iron, which is derived from animal sources and is abundant in red meat. Heme iron is readily absorbed and it enhances the uptake of nonheme iron from plant sources, which is generally more poorly absorbed. A welcome change in policy regarding the early introduction of meat is reflected in the 2012 joint statement of Health Canada, Canadian Paediatric Society, Dietitians of Canada, and breastfeeding committee for Canada,[45] which recommends that a baby's first complementary foods should be meat, meat alternatives (meat, poultry, fish), and iron-fortified cereal.

Before "hypoallergenic" formulas based on extensively hydrolyzed casein were available, babies who were allergic to milk were fed a meat-based infant formula from birth.[46] Every hospital had its own meat-based formula that was made up whenever a newborn was unable to breastfeed and could not tolerate cow's milk–based formula. In most cases, babies on this formula did extremely well.[47] Meats can be readily prepared for early introduction to babies by cooking ground meats well in water, then puréeing the meat into a soft paste and diluting with water as required.

In Western countries, it has become traditional to introduce grains as the first solid food, probably because it seems easier to cook cereals into a soft purée suitable for early infant feeding. Grains should be introduced as the pure grain before manufactured baby cereals containing the grain are tried. Some baby cereals contain ingredients other than the grain. If the cereal is a baby's first exposure to the grain and an allergic reaction occurs, it is not possible to tell whether the baby is reacting to the grain or the additional ingredients, unless each has been introduced separately. In all cases, it is important that the baby's first introduction to a specific food be the individual food in a cooked and puréed form.

Oral Tolerance and Allergy Prevention

Current research suggests that delaying exposure to foods until after the first year or even later may bypass the stage at which oral tolerance may be most effectively achieved. Furthermore, advising avoidance of any food by the breastfeeding mother, apart from her own and her baby's known allergens, may preclude the infant's development of tolerance to them. It is well known that continuous exposure to small quantities of antigen is an effective way of "informing" the immune system that the material is safe. As discussed earlier, this may be the way that the immune system of the fetus in utero is first primed to become tolerant of the molecules of food found in the amniotic fluid in the womb. The next stage of achieving tolerance to food may be exposure to the small quantities of food molecules that find their way into the breastmilk from a mother's diet. By excluding these foods, the mother may in fact deny her baby the tolerizing potential of the foods that he or she will eat later.

On the other hand, we know that an excessive quantity of allergen can cause an immunological response as a result of "allergen overload." Although there is mainly anecdotal evidence to support it, the consumption of large quantities of single foods, especially if the food is highly allergenic (eg, peanut), is thought to possibly promote sensitization of the breastfeeding baby, or even the fetus in utero. A 2010 study[48] of peanut sensitization in 503 infants, ages 3 to 15 months, who were allergic to egg or milk indicated that 27.8% (140 out of 503) had peanut IgE levels greater than 5 kU_A/L (a measure of allergen-specific IgE in kilounits per liter of blood sample); this indicates sensitization, even though none of the children had a previous diagnosis of peanut allergy. The mothers of these infants had consumed peanut during pregnancy, and the sensitization appeared to be dose-related. The higher the level of peanut consumption by the mother during pregnancy, the greater the likelihood of the baby having peanut-specific IgE. Further studies on this observation need to be conducted in order for a dose-related effect to be confirmed. However, at this time, mothers are advised to avoid "bingeing" on any food during pregnancy and lactation and to eat all foods, except their own and their baby's allergens, in moderate quantities.

Prognosis for Infant Food Allergy

Many children outgrow their early allergies to foods spontaneously. Consider, for example, the following allergies:

■ Cow's milk allergy: Most children with early cow's milk allergy outgrow their allergy by 3 years of age. In a 1990 study, 56% of the infants with cow's milk allergy outgrew their allergy at 1 year, 77% at 2 years, and 87% by 3 years of age.[49] In contrast, a 2007 study[50] reported that 19% of its participants with cow's milk allergy developed tolerance by age 4 years, 42% by 8 years, 64% by 12 years, and 79% by 16 years. Those children with the highest level of cow's milk–specific IgE were least likely to outgrow their cow's milk allergy. Furthermore, children with asthma, atopic rhinoconjunctivitis (hay fever), and atopic dermatitis (eczema) are reported to be less likely to outgrow their early cow's milk allergy, suggesting that it is the most highly allergic individuals who are most at risk for persistent food allergies.[51]

■ Egg allergy: It has been reported that 80% of infants with egg allergy are able to consume egg by 5 years of age.[52] Other more recent reports using predicted resolution of egg allergy are more pessimistic: 4% of egg-allergic children were predicted to outgrow their allergy by 4 years, 12% by 6 years, 37% by 10 years, and 68% by 16 years of age.[53] The persistence of egg allergy was related to the presence of asthma and allergic rhinitis (hay fever) and higher levels of egg-specific IgE. Nevertheless, the consensus from published studies concludes that most patients with egg allergy are likely to develop tolerance to egg by late childhood, with the exception of patients with an egg IgE greater than 50 kU_A/L in which egg allergy is likely to persist into adulthood.

■ Peanut allergy: Recent reports suggest that at least 21% of peanut-allergic children will outgrow their peanut allergy over time (median age 6 years).[54] Traditionally, allergy to peanut was considered to be lifelong. Those children with lower peanut-specific IgE (less than 5 kU_A/L at time of challenge) and lower rates of asthma and allergic rhinitis were reported to be more likely than those with high levels to outgrow their peanut allergy. An earlier report from the United Kingdom indicated that 9.8% of their peanut-allergic patients outgrew their peanut allergy[55] in childhood.

■ Tree nut allergy: Allergy to tree nuts is another condition that traditionally has been considered to be rarely outgrown. However, a study of 278 people allergic to tree nuts reported that 9% outgrew their tree nut allergy, including some who had previous severe reactions.[56] The authors suggested that patients aged 4 years or older with tree nut-specific IgE levels of 5 kU_A/L or less should be considered for challenge of tree nuts under medical supervision to determine whether they still remain allergic.

Children who have outgrown their early allergy to foods should be identified so that the previously allergenic food can be included in their diet. This is important for several reasons:

■ The diet becomes easier to formulate and maintain.
■ The vigilance previously exerted to avoid the culprit food can be relaxed, which reduces the stress associated with maintaining restricted diets, especially those that contain foods that may be considered life-threatening.
■ Including the now-tolerated food in the diet on a regular basis reduces the likelihood of recurrence of the allergy, because maintenance of tolerance reduces this risk.[57]

Oral Tolerance in the Management of Established Food Allergy

In some cases, desensitization or tolerance to a food allergen can be achieved even if the child has not spontaneously outgrown the allergy. This is a relatively new concept, as previous directives for food allergy management emphasized strict avoidance of the culprit allergen. Now specific desensitization protocols are being developed that expose the allergic child to the offending allergen by the oral route in a safe environment in order to induce tolerance to it.

Several studies have reported achievement of tolerance to cow's milk by starting with minute quantities of milk and increasing the dosage over time, a process termed *specific oral tolerance induction* (SOTI). Examples include:

- One study reported that starting with 1 drop of milk and increasing to 120 mL over a period of 136 days, 13 out of 16 children achieved tolerance to 120 mL milk in 3 to 12 months.[58]
- Starting with an initial dose of 0.05 ml cow's milk, reaching 1 mL on the first day and increasing the dosage weekly until a dose of 200 to 250 mL of milk taken once a day was tolerated, 16 of 18 patients 4 years and older achieved tolerance after a median length of 14 weeks (range 11 to 17 weeks). Thirteen of the children continued to tolerate 200 to 250 mL per day of milk after more than a year.[59]
- Another study[60] reported achievement of tolerance to cow's milk in 7 of 10 children with established milk allergy, starting with one drop of milk and increasing weekly over a period of 4 months until a dose of 200 mL was tolerated.

A similar tolerance to foods other than milk has been achieved, such as to egg[61,62] and peanut.[63,64] Undoubtedly, successful SOTI to other allergenic foods will be achieved over time.

Notable Aspects of SOTI

Oral tolerance to allergenic foods has a number of important features and considerations:

- Even though a child still may not be able to consume the allergenic food ad lib, successful SOTI does provide an important measure of safety in that the threshold dose required to trigger an allergic reaction has been raised considerably. Consequently, exposure to a minute quantity of the allergen may no longer pose the threat of a life-threatening reaction. This reduces the stress and vigilance required on the part of the child and the family, which has a significant positive impact on their quality of life.

■ However, there is always a risk for an anaphylactic reaction to the food, so great care is required in exposing a highly allergic child to their food allergen except in a carefully controlled environment in a medical facility until tolerance has been achieved.

■ After tolerance is achieved, it is important for the child to consume the food regularly in order to maintain tolerance to it; there is evidence of an increased risk for recurrence of the allergy if the food continues to be avoided after tolerance has been achieved.

■ Although this type of management of food allergy in children shows great promise, clinicians recommend caution. Careful avoidance of the allergenic food is still considered to be the mainstay of food allergy management until more basic and clinical trials on SOTI and other methods of tolerance induction have been conducted.[65,66]

Hygiene Theory in Allergy Prevention

Before concluding the subject of allergy prevention, we should look at what has become known as the "hygiene hypothesis." Research indicates that when the Th1 pathway of immunological protection against potentially disease-causing bacteria and viruses is triggered, there is a corresponding downregulation, or reduction, in the Th2 pathway that would lead to allergy. It therefore seemed logical to assume that if babies and children were exposed early to a wide range of microorganisms, the Th1 pathway would predominate, and the incidence of allergy would be reduced. This theory appeared to be validated by observations that children in third world countries, those living in lower socioeconomic conditions, and those living on farms had a lower incidence of allergy compared to babies and children living in the highly sanitized homes in urban centers of the developed world.

Further evidence for the idea that early exposure to microorganisms might reduce allergenic sensitization has come from a study on allergic children and their pets. A team of researchers compared 184 children who were exposed to two or more dogs or cats in their first year of life with 220 who didn't have pets. To their surprise, the scientists found that children raised with pets were 45% less likely to test positive for allergies than those without pets.[67]

A 2006 study showed that children drinking unpasteurized milk (which would contain many more microorganisms than pasteurized milk) had fewer eczema symptoms and a generally lower incidence of overall allergies than children who never drank unpasteurized milk.[68] Unpasteurized milk consumption was associated with a 59% reduction in total IgE levels and higher production of whole blood IFN-γ compared to levels in children drinking only pasteurized milk, indicating that the former had less allergy than the latter group. A further study reported similar results, indicating that consumption of (unpasteurized) farm milk may offer protection against asthma and allergy.[69] Of course, this is not to suggest that drinking unpasteurized milk should be advised for all children, because the risks from exposure to a disease-causing pathogen are too great, but these types of studies do suggest that the hygiene hypothesis is probably valid in its basic assumption that exposure to micro-organisms early in life may reduce or prevent allergen sensitization and development of allergy by promoting Th1-type immune development.

These observations suggest that exposing babies and children to appropriate "safe" microorganisms in early life may reduce the incidence of allergy. This is currently being attempted by feeding probiotic foods, a topic that is discussed in some detail in Chapter 47.

Summary of Dietary Guidelines for Babies at High Risk for Allergy[70]

In infants, a high risk for allergy is defined as having one first-degree relative (parent or sibling) with a diagnosed allergy.

Maternal Diet During Pregnancy

There should be no dietary restriction during pregnancy except the mother must avoid her own allergenic foods. It is essential that the mother obtain complete balanced nutrition appropriate for pregnancy and eat as wide a range of foods as possible. The allergic mother must ensure that she is consuming equivalent nutrients in the alternative foods she is eating as substitutes for her allergens.

Breastfeeding and Introduction of Complementary Foods

The mother should not restrict her own diet while breastfeeding other than avoiding her own allergenic foods *and* any foods to which her baby has been diagnosed as allergic. Exclusive breastfeeding should be continued for 4 to 6 months.

For the breastfed baby, the introduction of solid foods or infant formula (complementary foods) should be delayed until at least the age of 4 to 6 months. There is no benefit in delaying the introduction of solid foods beyond 6 months of age.

The first complementary food should be iron-rich, preferably meat.

There is no convincing scientific evidence that avoidance or delayed introduction of potentially allergenic foods reduces allergies.

Early (younger than 4 months) or late (older than 7 months) introduction of gluten should be avoided. Gluten should be introduced gradually while the infant is still breastfed.

Formula Feeding

If breastfeeding is not possible, hydrolyzed infant formula can be used as a measure to prevent food allergy. Extensively hydrolyzed formulas are more effective than partially hydrolyzed formulas in allergy prevention. Soy-based formulas and formulas based on milks other than cow's milk (eg, goat's milk) are not recommended for reducing the risk of food allergy.

If the child is allergic to cow's milk, extensively hydrolyzed casein-based formulas or amino acid–based formulas should be used if breastfeeding is not possible. If the baby is not allergic to cow's milk, a normal cow's milk formula can be introduced as complementary food at the age of 4 to 6 months.

References

1. Fiocchi A, Assa'ad A, Bahna S. Food allergy and the introduction of solid foods to infants: a consensus document. *Ann Allergy Asthma Immunol*. 2006;97(1):10-21.
2. Calvani M, Alessandri C, Sopo SM, et al. Consumption of fish, butter and margarine during pregnancy and development of allergic sensitizations in the offspring: role of maternal atopy. *Ped Allergy Immunol*. 2006;17(2):94-102.
3. Kull I, Bergstrom A, Lilja G, Pershagen G, Wickman M. Fish consumption during the first year of life and development of allergic diseases during childhood. *Allergy*. 2006;61(8):1009-1015.
4. Alm B, Aberg N, Erdes L, et al. Early introduction of fish decreases the risk of eczema in infants. *Arch Dis Child*. 2009;94:11-15.
5. Poole JA, Barriga K, Leung DY, et al. Timing of initial exposure to cereal grains and the risk of wheat allergy. *Pediatrics*. 2006;117(6):2175-2182.
6. Norris JM, Barriga K, Hoffenberg EJ, et al. Risk of celiac disease autoimmunity and timing of gluten introduction in the diet of infants at increased risk of disease. *JAMA*. 2005;293:2343-2351.
7. Hourihane JO, Aiken R, Briggs R, et al. The impact of government advice to pregnant mothers regarding peanut avoidance on the prevalence of peanut allergy in United Kingdom children at school entry. *J Allergy Clin Immunol*. 2007;119(5):1197-1202.
8. Sicherer SH, Munoz-Furlong A, Godbold JH, Sampson HA. US prevalence of self-reported peanut, tree nut, and sesame seed allergy: 11-year follow-up. *J Allergy Clin Immunol*. 2010;125(6):1322-1326.
9. Du Toit G, Katz Y, Sasieni P, et al. Early consumption of peanuts in infancy is associated with a low prevalence of peanut allergy. *J Allergy Clin Immunol*. 2008;122(5):984-991.
10. Nwaru BI, Erkkola M, Ahonen S, et al. Age at the introduction of solid foods during the first year and allergic sensitization at age 5 years. *Pediatrics*. 2009;125(1):47-56.
11. Sicherer SH, Burks AW. Maternal and infant diets for prevention of allergic diseases: understanding menu changes in 2008. *J Allergy Clin Immunol*. 2008;122:29-33.
12. Jennings S, Prescott SL. Early dietary exposures and feeding practices: role in pathogenesis and prevention of allergic disease? *Postgrad Med J*. 2010;86:94-99.
13. Moat MF, Cookson WOCM. Gene identification in asthma and allergy. *Int Arch Allergy Immunol*. 1998:116:247-252.
14. Host A, Koletzko B, Dreborg S, et al. Dietary products used in infants for treatment and prevention of food allergy. Joint statement of the European Society of Paediatric Allergology and Clinical Immunology (ESPACI) Committee of Hypoallergenic Formulas and the European Society for Paediatric Gastroenterology, Hepatology and Nutrition (ESPGHAN) Committee on Nutrition. *Arch Dis Child*. 1999;8:80-84.
15. Greer FR, Sicherer SH, Burks AW, and the Committee on Nutrition and Section on Allergy and Immunology Effects of Early Nutritional Interventions on the Development of Atopic Disease in Infants and Children: the role of maternal dietary restriction, breastfeeding, timing of introduction of complementary foods, and hydrolyzed formulas. *Pediatrics*. 2008;121(1):183-191.

16. Szepfalusi Z, Loibichler C, Pichler J, Reisenberger K, Ebner C, Urbanek R. Direct evidence for transplacental allergen transfer. *Pediatr Res.* 2000;48(3):404-407.

17. Prescott S. Early origins of allergic disease: a review of processes and influences during early immune development. *Curr Opin Allergy Clin Immunol.* 2003;3(2):125-132.

18. Prescott S, Macaubas C, Smallcombe T, Holt B, Sly P, Holt P. Development of allergen-specific T-cell memory in atopic and normal children. *Lancet.* 1999;353:196-200.

19. Jones CA, Holloway JA, Warner JO. Does atopic disease start in foetal life? *Allergy.* 2000;55:2-10.

20. Kjellman N-IM. Allergy prevention: does maternal food intake during pregnancy or lactation influence the development of atopic disease during infancy? In: Hanson LA, ed. *Biology of Human Milk.* Nestle Nutrition Workshop series 15. New York, NY: Vevey/Raven Press; 1988: 197-203.

21. Karmaus W, Archad SH, Sadeghnejad A, Twiselton R. Does maternal immunoglobulin E decrease with increasing order of live offspring? Investigation into maternal immune tolerance. *Clin Exp Allergy.* 2004;34(6):853-859.

22. Host A, Husby S, Osterballe O. A prospective study of cow's milk allergy in exclusively breast-fed infants. Incidence, pathogenetic role of early inadvertent exposure to cow's milk formula, and characterization of bovine milk protein in human milk. *Acta Paediatr Scand.* 1988;77(5):663-670.

23. Goldman AS. The immune system of human milk: antimicrobial, anti-inflammatory and immunomodulating properties. *Pediatr Inf Dis J.* 1993;12:664-671.

24. Joneja JMV. Breast milk: a vital defense against infection. *Can Fam Physician.* 1992;38: 1849-1855.

25. Arshad SH. Primary prevention of asthma and allergy. *J Allergy Clin Immunol.* 2005; 116(1):3-14.

26. Mosconi E, Rekima A, Seitz-Polski B, et al. Breast milk immune complexes are potent inducers of oral tolerance in neonates and prevent asthma development. *Mucosal Immunol.* 2010 May 19. [Epub ahead of print.]

27. Miyake Y, Yura A, Iki M. Breastfeeding and the prevalence of symptoms of allergic disorders in Japanese adolescents. *Clin Exp Allergy.* 2003;33:312-316.

28. Miyake Y, Tanaka K, Sasaki S, et al. Breastfeeding and atopic eczema in Japanese infants: the Osaka Maternal and Child Health Study. *Pediatr Allergy Immunol.* 2009;20(3):234-241.

29. Wright AL, Sherrill D, Holberg CJ, Halonen M, Martinez FD. Breast-feeding, maternal IgE, and total serum IgE in childhood. *J Allergy Clin Immunol.* 1999;104:589-594.

30. Bottcher MF, Jenmalm MC, Bjorksten B, Garofalo RP. Chemoattractant factors in breast milk from allergic and non-allergic mothers. *Pediatr Res.* 2000;47:592-597.

31. Saarinen KM, Vaarala O, Klemetti P, Savilahti E. Transforming growth factor-β1 in mothers' colostrums and immune responses to cow's milk proteins in infants with cow's milk allergy. *J Allergy Clin Immunol.* 1999;104(5):1093-1098.

32. Jarvinen KM, Suomalainen H. Development of cow's milk allergy in breast-fed infants. *Clin Exper Allergy.* 2001;31:978-987.

33. American Academy of Pediatrics, Committee on Nutrition. Hypoallergenic infant formulas. *Pediatrics.* 2000;106:346-349.

34. Zeiger RS. Food allergen avoidance in the prevention of food allergy in infants and children. *Pediatrics.* 2003;111:1662-1671.

35. Saarinen KM, Juntunen-Backman K, Jarvenpaa AL, et al. Supplementary feeding in maternity hospitals and the risk of cow's milk allergy: a prospective study of 6209 infants. *J Allergy Clin Immunol.* 1999;104:457-461.

36. Prescott SL, Tang MLK. The Australasian Society of Clinical Immunology and Allergy position statement summary of allergy prevention in children. *Med J Aust.* 2005;182(9): 464-467.

37. Osborn DA, Sinn JKH. Formulas containing hydrolysed protein for prevention of allergy and food intolerance in infants (review). *Cochrane Database Syst Rev.* 2006;(4): CD003664.

38. Von Berg A, Koletzkop S, Grubl A, et al. The effect of hydrolyzed cow's milk formula for allergy prevention in the first year of life: the German Infant Nutritional Intervention Study, a randomized double-blind trial. *J Allergy Clin Immunol.* 2003;111(3):533-540.

39. Von Berg A, Koletzko S, Filipiak-Pittroff B, et al. Certain hydrolyzed formulas reduce the incidence of atopic dermatitis but not that of asthma: three-year results of the German Infant Nutritional Intervention Study. *J Allergy Clin Immunol.* 2007;119(3):718-725.

40. Von Berg A, Filipiak-Pittroff B, Kramer U, et al. Preventive effect of hydrolyzed infant formulas persists until age 6 years: long-term results from the German Infant Nutritional Intervention Study (GINI). *J Allergy Clin Immunol.* 2008;121(6):1442-1447.

41. Lowe AJ, Hosking CS, Bennett CM, et al. Effect of a partially hydrolyzed whey infant formula at weaning on risk of allergic disease in high-risk children: a randomized controlled trial. *J Allergy Clin Immunol.* 2011;128(2):360-365.

42. Fiocchi A, Assa'ad A, Bahna S. Food allergy and the introduction of solid foods to infants: a consensus document. *Ann Allergy Asthma Immunol.* 2006;97(1):10-21.

43. Ivarsson A, Hernell O, Stenlund H, Persson LA. Breast-feeding protects against celiac disease. *Am J Clin Nutr.* 2002;75:914-921.

44. Joneja, JMV. *Dealing with Food Allergies in Babies and Children.* Boulder, CO: Bull Publishing; 2007.

45. Health Canada. Draft: Nutrition for Healthy Term Infants. Recommendations from birth to six months. A joint statement of Health Canada, Canadian Paediatric Society, Dietitians of Canada, and Breastfeeding Committee for Canada. April 2012. http://hc-sc.gc.ca/fn-an/consult/infant-nourrisson2/recommendations/index-eng.php. Accessed July 11, 2012.

46. Weisselberg B, Dayal Y, Thompson JF, Doyle MS, Senior B, Grand RJ. A lamb-meat based formula for infants allergic to casein hydrolysate formulas. *Clin Pediatr (Phila).* 1996;35(10):491-495.

47. Cantani A. A home-made meat-based formula for feeding atopic babies: a study in 51 children. *Eur Rev Pharmacol Sci.* 2006;10(2):61-68.

48. Sicherer SH, Wood RA, Stablein D, et al. Maternal consumption of peanut during pregnancy is associated with peanut sensitization in atopic infants. *J Allergy Clin Immunol.* 2010;126(6):1191-1197.

49. Host A, Halken S. A prospective study of cow milk allergy in Danish infants during the first 3 years of life. Clinical course in relation to clinical and immunological type of hypersensitivity reaction. *Allergy.* 1990;45(8):587-596.

50. Skripak JM, Matsui EC, Mudd K, Wood R. The natural history of IgE-mediated cow's milk allergy. *J Allergy Clin Immunol.* 2007;120(5):1172-1177.

51. Saarinen KM, Pelkonen AS, Makela MJ, Savilahti E. Clinical course and prognosis of cow's milk allergy are dependent on milk-specific IgE status. *J Allergy Clin Immunol.* 2005;116(4):869-875.

52. Sampson HA, McCaskill CC. Food hypersensitivity in atopic dermatitis: evaluation of 113 patients. *J Pediatr.* 1986;107:669-675.

53. Savage JH, Matsui EC, Skrpak JM, Wood RA. The natural history of egg allergy. *J Allergy Clin Immunol.* 2007;120(6):1413-1417.

54. Skolnick HS, Conover-Walker MK, Koerner CB, Sampson HA, Burks W, Wood RA. The natural history of peanut allergy. *J Allergy Clin Immunol.* 2001;107:367-374.

55. Hourihane JO, Roberts SA, Warner JO. Resolution of peanut allergy: case control study. *BMJ.* 1998;306:1271-1275.

56. Fleischer DM, Conover-Walker MK, Matsui EC, Wood RA. The natural history of tree nut allergy. *J Allergy Clin Immunol.* 2005;116:1087-1093.

57. Fleischer DM, Conover-Walker MK, Christie L, Burks AW, Wood RA. Peanut allergy: recurrence and its management. *J Allergy Clin Immunol.* 2004;114(5):1195-1201.

58. Patriarca G, Nucera E, Roncallo C, Pollastrini E, Bartolozzi F, De Paquale. Oral desensitizing treatment in food allergy: clinical and immunological results. *Aliment Pharmacol Ther.* 2003;17:458-465.

59. Zapatero L, Alonson E, Fuentes V, Martinez MI. Oral desensitization in children with cow's milk allergy. *J Investig Allergol Clin Immunol.* 2008;18(5):389-396.

60. Caminiti L, Passalacqua G, Barberi S, et al. A new protocol for specific oral tolerance induction in children with IgE-mediated cow's milk allergy. *Allergy Asthma Proc.* 2009; 30(4):443-448.

61. Morisset M, Moneret-Vautrin DA, Guenard L, et al. Oral desensitization in children with milk and egg allergies obtains recovery in a significant proportion of cases. A randomized study in 60 children with cow's milk allergy and 90 children with egg allergy. *Eur Ann Allergy Clin Immunol.* 2007;39(1):12-19.

62. Itoh N, Itagaki Y, Kurihara K. Rush specific oral tolerance induction in school-age children with severe egg allergy: one year follow-up. *Allergol Int.* 2010;59(1):43-51.

63. Blumchen K, Ulbricht H, Staden U, et al. Oral peanut immunotherapy in children with peanut anaphylaxis. *J Allergy Clin Immunol.* 2010;26(1):83-91.

64. Clark AT, Islam S, King Y, Deighton J, Anagnostou K, Ewan PW. Successful oral tolerance induction in severe peanut allergy. *Allergy.* 2009;64(8):1218-1220.

65. Prescott SL, Bouygue GR, Videky D, Fiocchi A. Avoidance or exposure to foods in prevention and treatment of food allergy? *Curr Opin Allergy Clin Immunol.* 2010;10(3):258-266.

66. Fisher HR, Toit GD, Lack G. Specific oral tolerance induction in food allergic children: is oral desensitization more effective than allergen avoidance? A meta-analysis of published RCTs. *Arch Dis Child.* 2010;96(3):259-264.

67. Ownby DR, Johnson CC, Peterson EL. Exposure to dogs and cats in the first year of life and risk of allergic sensitization at 6 to 7 years of age. *JAMA.* 2002;288:963-972.

68. Perkin MR, Strachan DP. Which aspects of the farming lifestyle explain the inverse association with childhood allergy? *J Allergy Clin Immunol.* 2006;117(6):1374-1381.

69. Waser M, Michels KB, Bieli C, et al. PARSIFAL study team. Inverse association of farm milk consumption with asthma and allergy in rural and suburban populations across Europe. *Clin Exp Allergy.* 2007;37(5):661-670.

70. Joneja JM. Infant food allergy: where are we now? *JPEN J Parenter Enteral Nutr.* 2012;36(1 suppl):49S-55S.

CHAPTER 44

Identifying a Child's Allergenic Foods

Unnecessary restriction of foods can be detrimental to a child's growth and development during the critical early months and years of his or her life. Thus, it is important to correctly identify the foods responsible for adverse reactions due to allergies and intolerances. Even if the foods are not a threat to the child's life, they do threaten his or her quality of life, which can be very important for a young person's emotional and psychological health.[1]

Unfortunately, there is no easy and direct way to identify the offending foods, especially in very young babies and children unable to communicate their distress. Tests for allergen-specific IgE are especially unreliable in babies younger than 6 months, and food-specific IgE for the diagnosis of food allergy is not definitive at any age (see Chapter 5 for details). Thus, determining the foods responsible for food allergy in a baby or young child is challenging. The best method for diagnosis is a careful medical examination and history, followed by elimination and challenge of the suspect foods.[2]

Identification of the offending foods in a baby or young child starts with analysis of dietary intake in conjunction with symptom development. The method for keeping a careful record of a child's intake of foods, beverages, supplements, and medications, and of the onset and duration of symptoms (ie, an exposure diary) is the same as for an adult (refer to Chapter 6). Information in the exposure diary should be recorded at the time of consumption, not in retrospect. Recalled dietary data (especially of ingredients in complex dishes) and symptoms is often inaccurate and of limited value in determining the potential food triggers in adverse reactions to foods.

Exposure Diary for a Breastfed Baby

When a baby is breastfed, it is important to record not only the baby's food and liquid intake, but also that of the breastfeeding mother. Food components from the mother's diet will be present in her breastmilk, so this will be a source of potential food allergens if the baby has already been sensitized to them. If the baby is exclusively breastfed without additional foods or formulas, the mother's dietary intake and the baby's symptoms should be recorded. If the baby is being breastfed but is also consuming some solids, the exposure diary should include:

■ The mother's dietary intake
■ The baby's times and duration of nursing
■ The baby's food and beverage intake
■ The baby's symptoms

The Elimination Diet

An appropriate elimination diet that excludes all of the suspected foods and liquids should be based on an analysis of the food and symptoms records and the following information:

■ The child's detailed medical history
■ Analysis of the exposure diaries for both baby and mother
■ Results of any allergy tests
■ Foods that parents and caregivers suspect may be a cause of the child's symptoms

Each of the following three types of elimination diet may have a place in the determination of the offending foods (see Chapter 6 for details of these elimination diets and their appropriate usage):

■ Selective elimination diets: one or a small number of foods are eliminated for a specified period of time—for example, milk-free diet, egg-free diet, wheat-free diet, or a combination of these (see Chapters 10 to 19).
■ Few foods elimination diets (sometimes referred to as oligoantigenic diets): only a few (usually less than 10) foods are allowed for a specified period of time.
■ Elemental diets: only an amino acid–based formula is allowed for the duration of the elimination phase; however, many clinicians favor an extensively hydrolyzed formula (EHF) rather than an elemental formula.

Elimination Diets for Breastfeeding Mothers

Molecules from the mother's diet pass into her breastmilk, so it is important for the breastfeeding mother of an allergic infant to avoid foods that may be triggers for her baby's food allergies. In determining the foods responsible for a nursing baby's symptoms, the mother consumes the elimination test diet. When it is time to initiate the challenge phase, the suspect foods can be introduced via the mother's milk, which is usually safer than giving them directly to the baby.

When just a few foods are suspected as potential triggers for the baby's food allergy, the mother will avoid the suspect foods while ensuring complete balanced nutrition by substituting the eliminated foods with those of equivalent nutrient value. Specific examples of selective elimination diets include diets free from the foods most frequently associated with infant allergies: milk (Chapter 10), egg (Chapter 12), peanut (Chapter 15), soy (Chapter 17), tree nuts (Chapter 16), seafood (Chapter 18), and wheat (Chapter 13). If several foods are suspected, the mother should follow a diet free from the top ten allergens (Chapter 19).

The elimination diet should be followed for 4 weeks and the baby's symptoms monitored for improvement. If many foods are suspected, or if the identity of the potential food allergens is difficult to determine, the mother should follow the few foods elimination diet (Chapter 6) for 10 to 14 days. This is usually a sufficient length of time for the baby's symptoms to improve.

It is usually unnecessary for mother to reduce her nutritional intake as far as an elemental diet, but very occasionally this has been a last-resort attempt to identify a highly allergic baby's food triggers. This should be undertaken only under close supervision by the mother's physician and registered dietitian.

Use of Formulas in Elimination Diets for Babies Who Are Not Breastfed and for Children

When allergy to multiple foods is suspected, and when either selective or few foods elimination diets have failed to resolve a child's symptoms, an extensively hydrolyzed casein-based formula used alone for a short period of time (about 7 days) should determine whether the child's symptoms are food related. An extensively hydrolyzed or elemental formula supplies calories and all essential macro- and micronutrients. Such diets are usually easy to administer in infancy but more difficult as the child becomes older. Unless the child has become used to the formula in infancy, they tend to dislike the unusual taste at first. Such formulas can be rendered more palatable by flavoring added by the manufacturer, but this adds the risk for adverse reactions to the chemicals in the flavoring compounds. Some children like the formula when fruit or fruit juice can be added—for example, blending peaches or pears into it. Elemental formulas are used only in rare cases where all other elimination diets have failed to resolve symptoms but the suspicion of an allergic etiology for the child's illness remains high.

Several extensively hydrolyzed casein and elemental formulas are available. None should be used without the knowledge and approval of the attending physician or health care professional. Hydrolyzed casein formulas for infants include Enfamil Nutramigen (Mead Johnson), Similac Alimentum (Abbott), and Enfamil Pregestimil (Mead Johnson). In cases where these are not tolerated, elemental formulas such as Neocate (Nutricia North America) or EleCare (Abbott) are available for infants.

Before a specific formula is chosen, a physician or registered dietitian should ascertain its suitability for the individual child. The number of daily calories supplied by the formula must be calculated for each child individually so that the required quantity of formula is consumed. In addition, the precise composition of each formula should be confirmed by application to the manufacturer, since sometimes the ingredients are changed without notice.

The Challenge Phase: Reintroduction of Foods

When the elimination test diet has been completed, the next step is reintroducing each component individually so that those responsible for symptoms can be clearly identified.[3] This is achieved by careful challenge with precise quantities of each food component[4] and careful monitoring of symptom development, looking for immediate reactions (within a 4-hour period) or delayed reactions (from 1 to 4 days) following ingestion.

Challenge of any food that poses a risk of anaphylaxis should be conducted only under medical supervision in a suitably equipped facility. Many allergists insist that challenge of the most highly allergenic foods in children (ie, egg, milk, peanuts, soy, tree nuts, all seafood, and wheat) should be carried out only under medical supervision, even when such foods have been eaten in the past with apparent impunity.

Details of the different methods of food challenges employed in the identification of offending foods in food allergies and intolerances are provided in Chapter 7. These methods can be followed for babies and children consuming solid foods, beverages, and infant formulas.

Challenge Phase for the Breastfeeding Mother and Infant

After avoiding the suspect foods for 4 weeks, the breastfeeding mother should determine which of the foods triggers symptoms in her infant. There is no advantage in consuming increasing doses of the food, as recommended for a direct challenge, since we have very little idea of the quantity that reaches the breastmilk in relation to the amount consumed. Therefore, the mother should consume a large quantity of the food or beverage (at least a serving, and as much more as she can tolerate), and monitor her baby's reactions for up to 8 hours following. In most cases, the baby will show symptoms from 2 to 6 hours after the mother has consumed a food. It is a good idea to repeat this procedure at least three times to confirm the results.

The following are suggested quantities of individual foods that the mother should consume to determine allergic reactivity in her baby:

- One cup or more of whole milk
- Three or more eggs (make them into an omelet if desired)
- One-half cup or more of peanuts or nuts of any individual type
- Two or more slices of whole wheat bread (toasted if preferred) to test for wheat allergy
- One-half cup of tofu (prepared to taste) to test soy allergy
- Three or more ounces of any fish
- Three or more ounces of beef or other meats

Challenge for an Older Child Eating Solid Foods

The selective or few foods elimination diet continues for all meals throughout the testing period. An initial screening challenge provides a measure of safety. Before offering the food for consumption, rub a little of the food on the child's cheek, and monitor for signs of a reaction, such as reddening or irritation, for about 20 minutes. If there is no reaction, place a small quantity of the food on the outer border of the child's lower lip and allow to stay in place for at least 2 minutes. Observe the area for the development of a local reaction for 30 minutes. Signs of a positive reaction are:

■ Swelling, reddening, or irritation at the site of application
■ Development of a rash of the cheek and/or chin
■ Rubbing of the site by a young child will indicate irritation
■ Rhinitis or conjunctivitis
■ A systemic reaction

If there is no sign of a reaction in any of the preceding tests, give the child a small quantity of the food three times on the test day at 4-hour intervals and carefully monitor him or her for the development of symptoms, as described in Chapter 7.

The Maintenance Diet

When the child's allergenic foods have been determined, the next step is to develop a maintenance diet for the long term. It must contain all of the nutrients that the child needs for growth and development during this critical stage of his or her life. But it must also contain foods that the child enjoys and those that are regarded as treats for times of celebrations such as birthdays and holidays. It is important that food allergy is not a central issue for the child and the family; it should be considered an issue that needs to be dealt with responsibly, but it should not be the focus of life.

If the child is old enough, he or she should be included in the process of diet design and should be recruited to help with recipe and meal preparation so that it becomes a pleasurable, not burdensome, process for everyone. The help of family members should be enlisted to make the meal planning a family affair to which everyone can contribute. Many grandparents love making special foods for their grandchildren and find it rewarding when they can come up with new and different recipes to delight the child and the whole family.

Maintenance Diets for Breastfeeding Mothers

When the breastfeeding mother has determined which foods cause symptoms in her baby, she will need to avoid them as long as she is breastfeeding. It is very important that she consumes a nutritionally complete, well-balanced diet to maintain her own health. Although her breastmilk will always be nutritionally complete for her baby's needs, if the mother is not consuming a nutritionally adequate diet, the deficient nutrients will be taken from her own body.

References

1. Sicherer SH, Noone SA, Munoz-Furlong A. The impact of childhood food allergy on quality of life. *Ann Allergy Asthma Immunol.* 2001;87(6):461-464.
2. Sampson HA. Food allergy part 2. Diagnosis and management. *J Allergy Clin Immunol.* 1999;103(6):981-989.
3. Ito K, Uriso A. Diagnosis of food allergy based on oral food challenge test. *Allergology Int.* 2009;58(4):467-474.
4. Sicherer SH. Food allergy: when and how to perform oral food challenges. *Pediatr Allergy Immunol.* 1999;10:226-234.

PART VII

Emerging Areas of Research in Adverse Reactions to Foods

CHAPTER 45

Hyperactivity and Diet

When parents and teachers have to cope every day with an unruly, disruptive, sometimes aggressive child in the home and classroom, and when every attempt at control has met with failure, the idea that the child's diet is the cause of the problem is often embraced with great enthusiasm, especially if the alternative is behavior-modifying drugs. In this chapter, we discuss several ways in which food may trigger behavior problems in children, and we cover what parents and caregivers might be able to do to help their child in this situation.

The Role of Diet in Behavioral Disorders

The idea of dietary components causing aberrant behavior is not new; it has been considered at various times since it was first suggested in the 1920s. Allergic reactions to wheat and corn as a cause of fatigue, irritability, and behavior problems was suggested in the 1940s.[1] Since then, numerous theories, some backed by well-conducted research studies, have been put forward to explain why food may be involved in triggering disruptive behavior in children. The most convincing of these suggest the following:

- Components of the food, either naturally occurring chemicals or man-made additives, act in a pharmacological manner on body systems and result in behavioral changes.
- Inflammatory mediators released in an allergic response to the food may be the pharmacological agents responsible for behavioral changes.
- Nutritional deficiencies may result in central nervous system dysfunction.
- Stress or anxiety may release neuropeptides in the digestive tract that can themselves trigger the release of inflammatory mediators and cause clinical symptoms.

Starting in the 1970s, many people became concerned about the widespread use of stimulant drugs, such as methylphenidate, to control children's hyperactive behavior. Some clinicians advanced claims that childhood hyperactivity was a perception created by intolerant teachers and parents and was caused by environmental factors rather than any neurological deficit. In response, components of a child's diet became the focus of attention as an alternative to drugs, and the psychological stigma attached to the caregivers of hyperactive children was repudiated.

In 1975, Dr. Benjamin Feingold published an article and then a book[2] promoting the theory that a toxic reaction to food additives was responsible for hyperactivity in children. He claimed that up to 70% of his hyperactive patients improved when food dyes, artificial flavors, and natural salicylates were eliminated from their diet. After the publication of Dr. Feingold's book in 1975, the "Feingold diet" became very popular as a nondrug treatment for childhood hyperactivity. Feingold Associations sprang up around the United States as sources of information and support for parents.

A number of research studies were conducted in an attempt to confirm or refute Feingold's theories. All of these studies can be criticized on the basis of differences in methodology, no clear consensus on diagnostic criteria, inadequate controls, and the diversity of the independent variables employed.[1] However, the consensus reached was that Feingold's claims were exaggerated and his findings were anecdotal and lacking in objective evidence. Finally, the idea that diet and food additives were the cause of "hyperkinesis" was strongly refuted in a 1983 statement from the National Advisory Committee on Hyperkinesis and Food Additives.[3] Nevertheless, all of the studies demonstrated that a few hyperactive children did benefit from an additive-free diet.

Attention Deficit Hyperactivity Disorder and Allergy

Children with problems in attention, impulse control, and overactivity are often diagnosed with attention deficit hyperactivity disorder (ADHD). However, the diagnosis and cause of the symptoms that constitute this disorder have been in dispute since the condition was first recognized. The disorder is currently considered to be divisible into several subcategories, including the inattentive type, the hyperactive impulsive type, and the combined type.[4] The debate continues regarding the degree to which the symptoms are due to a neurological deficit and how much can be attributed to aberrant environmental factors. Furthermore, no clear consensus exists that these are scientifically divisible conditions based on physiological differences.

The role of food allergy and intolerance of food additives in behavior and learning disorders (loosely designated ADHD) in children was the subject of several well-conducted research studies in the 1980s. In 1992, Robinson and Ferguson published a comprehensive review of research on the potential association between food allergy and intolerance to food additives on the one hand and pediatric learning and behavior disorders on the other.[5] An important point made by these reviewers is that "it must be recognized that adverse effects of foods on behavior may be either a manifestation of (probably pharmacologically based) food intolerance, or they may be psychologically based (eg, via suggestion or adverse conditioning)."

Subsequently, medical and scientific literature abounds with the results of studies on the role of food components in behavioral dysfunction in children. However, these experiments are often criticized on methodological grounds.[6] All of the studies that are designed to demonstrate a role for food components in children's behavior have two major handicaps:

■ The lack of clear diagnostic criteria for the behavioral conditions that are being studied
■ The absence of any definite tests that unequivocally demonstrate allergy to food or intolerance of food additives

Allergy tests such as skin prick and food-specific antibody tests (see Chapter 5 for details of these tests) are unhelpful in diagnosing food allergy and intolerance. The only way to demonstrate an adverse reaction to food components is elimination and challenge. Double-blind, placebo-controlled, cross-over food challenge is the standard method used to identify reactive foods to rule out as many confounding variables as possible.

Sugar and Hyperactivity

Following the decline in the belief that the Feingold diet was an effective management strategy for childhood hyperkinesis, the idea that refined sugar was an important etiological factor in the disorder became popular. "Reactive hypoglycemia" or "functional hypoglycemia" (FH) due to sugar in the diet has been blamed for many emotional problems, hyperactive behavior, and irritability. However, no studies have been reported that conclusively demonstrate low blood sugar levels and impaired insulin response in conditions other than diabetes. The scientific view regarding FH is that the condition is rare but "has become popular because it is a respectable metabolic illness rather than a symptom of psychological distress."[6]

The adverse effect of sugar in sensitive individuals may be mediated by mechanisms other than defective insulin control. A 1986 study on the response to sugar and aspartame in 39 children diagnosed with ADHD indicated that catecholamine control of sugar regulation may be impaired in children with ADHD.[7] The children with ADHD performed significantly worse on behavioral evaluation following a sucrose challenge compared with an aspartame challenge after a breakfast of carbohydrate, but the behavior improved in these children after a sucrose challenge following a protein breakfast. Normal children in the study were unaffected by the challenges after a carbohydrate, protein, or fasting breakfast condition. This research therefore suggests that children with ADHD require protein to offset the potential adverse effects of sugar.

Although an excess of sugar in the diet is often blamed for a range of behavioral problems, such as irritability, anxiety, violent behavior, and fatigue, in most cases sugar has the effect of making a person feel lethargic because it promotes the production of serotonin (the "sleep chemical") in the brain. When at midmorning, people reach for a cup of caffeinated coffee to keep them alert, they are exhibiting the effects of a high-sugar, high-starch breakfast such as toast or croissant and jam or breakfast cereals containing high levels of sugars and processed starches. Or they feel hungry and compound the problem with a snack of a muffin or doughnut to give them an "energy boost," which is inevitably followed by another rapid drop in alertness and energy as a result of the high-sugar and free starch content of the snack. A high-sugar, high-starch lunch is often followed by sleepiness in midafternoon. These same people wonder why they can't sleep well after an evening meal high in protein from foods such as meat or fish, which is going to promote alertness rather than sleep. Children are no different.

The idea that sugar causes hyperactivity in children probably arose because the foods that contain large amounts of sugar, such as soft drinks, candies, and other sweet manufactured foods, also contain artificial food colors and preservatives. Evidence now suggests that the latter (and not sugar) are responsible for the hyperactive behavior.[8] In addition, a diet high in commercial snack foods and drinks with a great deal of sugar and processed starches tends to lead to a lack of "whole foods," which may cause nutritional deficiencies, especially of essential vitamins and minerals.

Based on anecdotal evidence, phosphate and a variety of other ingredients have been suggested as a dietary component that could play a major role in hyperkinesis. This hypothesis was refuted by controlled studies,[1] but it is important to note that children on either a restricted sugar diet or a restricted phosphate diet would avoid many potentially allergenic foods and a variety of artificial colors and preservatives, and that might be the real reason for the apparent improvement in their behavior.

Nutritional Deficiencies as a Cause of Unacceptable Behavior

In 1986, the results of a 4-year dietary intervention program in 803 New York City schools involving 800,000 children were published. All school meals were virtually free from sucrose and all artificial food flavors, artificial food colors, and the preservatives butylated hydroxyanisole (BHA) and butylated hydroxytoluene (BHT). Academic achievement rather than behavior was chosen as a more objective measure of the performance outcome of this intervention. The average percentile rankings of the students in the study on the California Achievement Test (CAT) over the 4-year test period rose 15.7%, from 39.2% to 54.9%, with no changes in the school curricula or teaching staff.[9] The hypothesis was made that the improvements in academic achievement were due to diet, which treated marginal malnutrition.[10] Elimination of foods high in sucrose, artificial flavors, artificial colors, and preservatives removes many "junk foods" from a child's diet, giving place to more nutritionally dense foods and a more nutritionally adequate, balanced diet.

Food Additives as a Cause of Hyperactive Behavior

In a 2004 double-blind, placebo-controlled study of 277 three-year-old children on the Isle of Wight in England, all of the children, regardless of whether they would be considered abnormally hyperactive or not, demonstrated some degree of hyperactive behavior when they consumed artificial food dyes and benzoate preservatives. This study analyzed the effects of four artificial food colorings (sunset yellow, carmoisine, tartrazine, and ponceau 4R) and the preservative sodium benzoate on the participating children's behavior.[8]

According to parents' assessments of their children's behavior, a test drink containing 300 mL mixed fruit juices, 45 mg sodium benzoate, and 5 mg of each of the four food colorings triggered some level of hyperactivity in all participants. Even children who had no history of behavior problems became more active after consuming the additives. The effect of behavior was more striking on those children already diagnosed as hyperactive; their level of activity increased noticeably. Interestingly, the change in behavior was very obvious to the parents, even though they had no idea whether their child had been given the test drink or a placebo, but psychological tests administered by trained psychologists did not show any changes after either the test drink or placebo.

The authors suggest[8] that the increase in activity levels associated with the additives is likely to be "via a pharmacological effect which is best exemplified by the non-IgE-dependent histamine release." (For details about histamine sensitivity and the histamine-releasing properties of benzoates and azo dyes, refer to Chapter 31). The authors further state that "this suggests that benefit would accrue for all children if artificial food colours and benzoate preservatives were removed from their diet."

A follow-up study in 2007 included 153 three-year-olds and 144 eight- and 9-year-olds. In addition to the juice mix used in the original study, the follow-up study (a randomized, double-blind placebo-controlled trial) included a second test drink ("mix B") that contained 300 mL fruit juice mixed with 45 mg sodium benzoate and 5 mg each of the food colors sunset yellow, quinoline yellow, carmoisine, and allura red.[11] The behavior of the children was measured using a global hyperactivity aggregate (GHA) based on questionnaires completed by parents, teachers, and trained observers. Small but significant increases in GHA occurred with Mix A in both age groups, with the 3-year-olds showing a greater effect. Mix B was associated with a small significant increase in GHA in the 8- and 9-year-old participants but not in the 3-year-old subjects. The authors of the study[11] concluded that the results strongly support a relationship between food additives and behavior. However, they rightly point out that the additives increased activity levels but did not cause clinically defined ADHD.

After review of these studies, the British Committee on Toxicity concluded that the results could be clinically relevant for individual children, especially those who already show signs of hyperactivity. The British Food Standards Agency advised parents to consider eliminating the additives from the diet of children who exhibit hyperactive behavior. The British and the European Union parliament are seeking to ban the colors used in the test mixes (sometimes referred to as the *Southampton six*) based on the studies.

In conclusion, at the present stage in our knowledge, we can say that artificial colors and preservatives, specifically benzoates, in manufactured foods seem to have the potential to trigger hyperactive behavior in the greatest number of children, regardless of whether the child has food allergy or not. These additives should not be part of any child's regular diet.

Hyperactivity and Celiac Disease

Parents and caregivers have frequently observed that wheat and other gluten-containing grains seem to trigger hyperactivity in their children. Clinicians and researchers have observed that people with celiac disease often exhibit signs of psychological and behavioral disorders that improve significantly on a gluten-free diet.[12] Whether this response is related to wheat or gluten allergy, to an effect associated with celiac disease, or to a result of the malabsorption associated with celiac disease has been a topic of debate. A 2011 article[13] describes a 2004 to 2008 study done in South Tyrol, Italy, of 67 subjects, ages 7 to 42 years (mean, 11.4 years), who had ADHD. Ten of the subjects were diagnosed with celiac disease based on levels of antigliadin and antiendomysium antibodies (for the significance and details of these tests, see Chapter 41).

After initiation of a gluten-free diet, participants with celiac disease or their parents reported a significant improvement in their behavior and functioning compared to the period before celiac diagnosis and treatment. The authors conclude that "celiac disease is markedly overrepresented among patients presenting with ADHD." Future research could uncover the mechanisms responsible for these observations. In the meantime, as recommended by these researchers, celiac disease as a component of hyperactivity should be considered when attempting to identify a dietary trigger for hyperactivity at any age.

Management of Behavior Dysfunction That Results from Food Ingestion

When we look at the many different types of hyperactivity and related behavioral problems in children, which may or may not be attributable to a variety of biochemical or physiological triggers, it is difficult to advocate that diet, either as a cause (eg, a food allergy, a food additive, or a natural chemical in the food acting like a "drug") or as a deficiency (vitamin or mineral deficiencies), could be the major etiological factor in all of these phenomena. However, it is clear that some food components do trigger hyperactive behavior in some children. Of course, the question that every parent and caregiver of a child with abnormal behavior asks is, "Which child and what food components?" In response to this question, we can say with some degree of confidence:

■ A child suffering an allergic reaction will respond as any child would to an acute or chronic illness. He or she will feel miserable and appear irritable, restless, have difficulty sleeping, and may be unable to concentrate. The obverse of this will be that the child will experience fatigue and listlessness. The condition may result in prolonged absences from school, which will have a negative effect on scholastic achievement.

■ An allergic condition such as exercise-induced asthma may prevent a child from taking part in normal childhood activities, resulting in a feeling of being excluded from peers. Severe eczema can provoke revulsion in other children. Overanxious and overprotective parents may exacerbate the isolation felt by the allergic child, and the need for special diets can impede the normal socializing associated with food. All of these factors may promote an antisocial climate for the allergic child and possibly contribute to the child's problematic behavior.

■ Food allergy may be a direct physiological cause of behavior changes. The hypersensitivity reaction releases inflammatory chemicals that may have a direct effect on central nervous system functions. The *hypoxia* (decrease in oxygen reaching the brain) associated with even mild asthma has also been suggested as having significant effects on cerebral function, which might affect behavior.

■ Additives in foods, such as azo dyes (eg, tartrazine), preservatives (especially benzoates), and artificial flavors (such as glutamates), have a direct physiological effect on central nervous system functions. Histamine is a neurotransmitter, so excess histamine either from an allergic response or released by components of the diet such as azo dyes and benzoates can have a definite effect on a child's behavior.

■ Undiagnosed celiac disease may be a contributing factor.

However, when considering food allergy as a possible cause of a child's allergy, it is important to realize that hyperactivity is never the *only* symptom of allergy. If the child has allergies, he or she will have other symptoms, such as skin reactions (eg, eczema or hives), stomach problems (eg, diarrhea, stomachache), or a runny, stuffy nose and itchy watery eyes. Accurately identifying a child's food allergies and removing the culprit foods from the child's diet is of first importance. Equally important is that the allergic child should be provided with alternative foods that supply all his or her nutritional needs.

Additional Reasons for Behavioral Improvements with a Modified Diet

Several reasons have been proposed for the observation that a surprisingly large number of children with behavior issues improve significantly on a "hypoallergenic diet":

■ When food allergens are excluded from the diet, an allergic child's symptoms will disappear. They are then able to sleep, have more energy, and generally feel better, so their behavior will naturally improve.

- Effects of inflammatory mediators on behavior will be removed as a result of successful management of the allergy.
- When food additives are excluded from a child's diet, it is often the "junk food" and simple sugars that are removed. The resulting diet is often nutritionally much more adequate and balanced. The child's behavior is a response to a more nutritious diet.
- If artificial colors and preservatives affect a child's behavior, removing them from his or her diet will obviously result in a noticeable improvement in behavior.
- When a specifically formulated diet is prescribed, parents will take extra care in food preparation. The child feels "special" and commands more attention within the family. This change in status and family dynamics has a positive psychological effect on the child and behavior improves.

Most of these factors will likely have some effect on a child, especially an atopic child. A supervised, time-limited trial on an elimination diet and judicial reintroduction of foods with careful monitoring of a child's behavior is at present the most effective strategy for determining how diet affects a child's behavior.[14] Whatever the scientific basis may be, the opportunity to improve the quality of life for the child and family by dietary management is justified, as long as the diet does not pose any psychological, nutritional, or economic distress on an already stressed family situation. The best candidates for dietary intervention are children with poor eating habits and physical and behavioral symptoms.

References

1. Randolph TG. Allergy as a causative factor of fatigue, irritability, and behavior problems of children. *J Pediatr*. 1947;31:560-572.
2. Feingold BF. *Why Your Child Is Hyperactive*. New York, NY: Random House; 1975.
3. National Institutes of Health consensus development conference statement: defined diets and childhood hyperactivity. *Am J Clin Nutr*. 1983;37:161-165.
4. Barkley R. *Taking Charge of AD/HD: The Complete Authoritative Guide for Parents*. Rev ed. New York, NY: Guilford; 2000.
5. Robinson J, Ferguson A. Food sensitivity and the nervous system: hyperactivity, addiction and criminal behaviour. *Nutr Res Rev*. 1992;5:203-223.
6. Egger J. Psychoneurological aspects of food allergy. *Eur J Clin Nutr*. 1991;45(suppl 1): 35-45.
7. Connors CK, Caldwell J, Caldwell L, et al. Experimental studies of sugar and aspartame on autonomic, cortical and behavioral responses of children. In: *Proceedings of Interfaces in Psychology*. Lubbock, TX: Texas Tech Press; 1986.
8. Bateman B, Warner JO, Hutchinson E, et al. The effects of a double blind placebo controlled artificial food colourings and benzoate preservative challenge on hyperactivity in a general population sample of preschool children. *Arch Dis Child*. 2004;89:506-511.
9. Schauss AG. New York City public school dietary revisions 1979–1983. Positive effects on 800,000 students' academic achievement. *Int J Biosocial Res*. 1986;8(1):2-5.

10. Schauss AG. Nutrition, student achievement and behaviour: insights from new research. *Intermediate Teacher.* 1986;22(1):5-15.
11. McCann D, Barrett A, Cooper A, et al. Food additives and hyperactive behaviour in 3-year old and 8/9-year old children in the community: a randomised, double-blinded, placebo-controlled trial. *Lancet.* 2007;370(959B):1560-1567.
12. Bruzelius M, Liedholm LJ, Hellblom M. Celiac disease can be associated with severe neurological symptoms: analysis of gliadin antibodies should be considered in suspected cases. *Lakartidningen.* 2001;98(34):3538-3542.
13. Niederhofer H. Association of attention-deficit/hyperactivity disorder and celiac disease: a brief report. *Prim Care Companion CNS Disord.* 2011;13(3). www.ncbi.nlm.nih.gov/pmc/articles/PMC3184556/?tool=pubmed. Accessed July 11, 2012.
14. Pelsser LM, Frankena K, Toorman J, et al. Effects of a restricted elimination diet on the behaviour of children with attention-deficit hyperactivity disorder (INCA study): a randomised controlled trial. *Lancet.* 2011;377(9764):494-503.

CHAPTER **46**

Autism and Diet

Autism is a lifelong developmental disorder affecting as many as 1 in 500 children. Typically children with autism have difficulty with language, communication, and socialization. They have problems in learning and display a variety of atypical behaviors. The disorder is accompanied by mental retardation in three out of four cases. Asperger's syndrome (autism without retardation) is included in the range of different presentations of autism.[1]

The number of cases of autism has noticeably risen in recent years. It is unclear whether this is a result of an increasing awareness of autism spectrum disorders, a change in the way that autism is diagnosed so that cases that were not previously recognized as autism are now included under the diagnosis, or a real rise in the number of cases.

Diagnosis of Autism

The diagnosis of autism is usually determined when the child is 2 to 3 years old after extensive evaluation according to the criteria of the *Diagnostic Statistical Manual IV (DSM-IV)*.[2] Sometimes there is evidence of the condition soon after birth as the child does not meet the expected developmental milestones. In other cases the child loses newly acquired skills such as language, eye-to-eye contact, and sociability after a period of apparently normal development. The latter pattern is often referred to as *regressive autism* and occurs in about one-third of autistic children.[3]

Causes of Autism

There seem to be several different causes for autism, none of which are completely understood. Most authorities agree that there is a strong genetic factor in the condition, and it is not uncommon to see several children, usually boys, with the condition in the same family. However, the cause of the disorder for the great majority of autistic individuals has not been determined.

It is likely that there are different causes and different precipitating factors associated with the way that autism is experienced by different individuals. The term "autistic syndrome" is often used to describe a pattern of similar behaviors produced by a variety of triggers.[4]

Digestive Tract Disturbances in Autism

Children with autism seem to have a higher incidence of digestive tract symptoms than children without autism. Anecdotal reports by parents extending back more than 30 years described evidence that their autistic children had disturbed gastrointestinal (GI) tract function, citing symptoms such as abdominal pain, bloating, constipation, loose stools, and frequent diarrhea.[4] A survey of 500 parents of autistic children carried out in 2001 showed that almost one-half reported that their children had loose stools or frequent diarrhea.[5] Parents frequently reported an apparent intolerance to certain foods, especially wheat and cow's milk.

Several studies have demonstrated abnormal digestive tract function in autistic children. A *leaky gut* (increased permeability of the membrane lining the digestive tract, which allows food molecules that would normally be excluded to pass into circulation) was demonstrated in some studies (leaky gut is discussed in more detail later in this chapter). Others found evidence of low activity of intestinal carbohydrate digestive enzymes.[6] The results of these different studies taken together suggest that significant digestive tract pathophysiology may accompany autism, at least within a subpopulation of patients.[4]

However, other studies have refuted these claims. The authors of a UK study published in 2002 concluded that there was not a substantial association between gastrointestinal illness in children and the development of autism.[7] Nevertheless, the authors acknowledged that some children may have had subclinical GI symptoms that were overlooked and that severe GI disease may be associated with autism in certain individuals.

Sensitivity to Cow's Milk and Gluten in Autism

The frequent reports from parents that cow's milk and wheat seemed to increase their child's autistic symptoms prompted several studies on the possibility that components of these foods could be involved in triggering or exacerbating autistic symptoms in some children.

Two separate studies involving a large number of autistic patients reported that an improvement of social, cognitive, and communication skills occurred when they were placed on a diet free of gluten and cow's milk or a diet free of cow's milk alone.[8,9] A 2010 study of 72 children (ages 4 years to 10 years, 11 months) diagnosed with autism spectrum disorder (ASD) indicated that a gluten- and casein-free diet improved the test parameters of the treatment group compared with the placebo control group.[10]

The Possible Roles of Gluten and Casein in Autism

Two types of proteins have been reported to be involved in triggering or exacerbating certain types of autism, namely casein (in milk) and the gliadin fraction of gluten in wheat. Digestion of dietary casein and gluten in the small intestine by the action of pancreatic and intestinal peptidase enzymes leads to the production of short chain peptides, which are structurally similar to endorphins.[a] These products are called *exorphins* to reflect their dietary origin. Gliadomorphins are a family of exorphins released from the partial digestion of the wheat protein gliadin. Similarly, casomorphins are a family of exorphins released upon partial digestion of the milk protein casein. Casomorphins and gliadomorphins have been shown to affect the brain in experimental animals and may be psychosis-inducing agents.[4]

The Hyperpermeable Digestive tract (Leaky Gut) in Autism

In some autistic children the opioid peptides from the diet move through the lining of the digestive tract into blood and are carried to the brain as the blood circulates through the various organs in the body. This was found when it was discovered that the epithelium lining the digestive tract in some autistic children was more permeable than normal.[11] Thus, the "leaky gut hypothesis" was proposed (see Box 46.1).[4,12,13] It was suggested that because of the increased permeability, larger molecules than normal are able to pass through the lining of the digestive tract into circulation. Digestion products of natural foods such as casein and gluten-containing grains may thus be able to elicit immunological responses and interfere directly with the central nervous system.

A 2010 study[14] demonstrated that a significantly greater percentage of patients with autism and their close relatives had considerably higher scores on the intestinal permeability test (IPT)—36.7% and 21.2%, respectively—than the nonautistic population (4.8%). (Details of the lactulose/mannitol permeability test used in determining intestinal permeability are provided in Box 46.1.) The authors suggest that the increased IPT levels found in first-degree relatives indicates the possibility of an intestinal (tight-junction linked) hereditary factor in the families of subjects with autism. The study further reported a significant decrease in the IPT scores in autistic persons following a gluten- and casein-free diet.

---

[a] Endorphins are neuropeptides that bind to opioid receptors in the brain and affect pain perception.

BOX 46.1   A Closer Look: The Leaky Gut

The "leaky gut" and its relation to food-related reactions has been the subject of research and debate for some time. The term *leaky gut* was coined to describe food molecules passing more readily than normal through the lining of the digestive tract and into circulation. It has often been suggested that children with autism have this condition.

In early infancy, the digestive tract lining tends to be permeable to food molecules, possibly because components of the mother's breastmilk need to pass easily into the infant's circulation. Such components include active immune cells, hormones, and maturation factors that need to remain intact in order to exert their effects. After infancy, these molecules are not essential, and the digestive tract lining starts to "close up" in order to filter out materials that may be detrimental to the body. The gut lining becomes less permeable as the child ages, until at adulthood only the smaller molecular weight nutrients pass through after food has been broken down in the lumen of the digestive tract.

The digestive tract is lined by simple column-shaped (columnar) epithelial cells along its length. The epithelial cells are linked together by tight junction complexes. The epithelial cells as well as the tight junctional complexes are the principal barriers to the free movement into the blood of dietary foods and the products released during their break down (digestion) by digestive enzymes in the lumen of the intestine. This is called the *intestinal luminal barrier*.

Certain conditions can compromise the intestinal luminal barrier and cause the digestive lining to become less permeable. Inflammation in the digestive tract may damage the epithelial cells and allow food molecules through the nonintact epithelium. Infection, food allergy, and autoimmune disease are some of the insults that may cause inflammation and cell damage and cause the tight junctions to separate. This allows free movement of food molecules into circulation as they bypass the normal processing by the gut-associated lymphoid tissue (GALT). As a result, they encounter immune cells as "foreign material" and cause a variety of problems.

Identification of the Leaky Gut

A useful method of assessing the physical integrity of the luminal barrier is the sugar permeability test. This test measures the ability of small sugar molecules, taken by mouth, to gain entry into the blood and, eventually, to be excreted into the urine.[4]

The patient is given a measured quantity of two sugars to drink, dissolved in water.[12] Usually mannitol and lactulose are used:

- Mannitol is a monosaccharide sugar that is poorly absorbed by the human intestine, because it has no affinity for the glucose-galactose carrier protein molecules in the apical (luminal) brush border membrane of small intestinal cells (the enterocytes) that carry sugars across the membrane into circulation. The mannitol molecules pass through the luminal membrane by way of aqueous pores in the brush border membrane. So the larger and more numerous the pores, the more mannitol passes through.
- Lactulose, a larger disaccharide molecule, also lacks affinity for the carrier and is too large to pass through the pores. Lactulose molecules, which do reach the blood, do so by passing between the epithelial cells—that is, through the tight junctions. Therefore, if the tight junctions are weakened, lactulose molecules gain access to the blood in circulation.

Continues

BOX 46.1   A Closer Look: The Leaky Gut (*Continued*)

When these sugars gain access to blood, they are carried to the kidneys and excreted in urine. The ratio of mannitol to lactulose is measured in the patient's urine. The quantity of each sugar in the urine shows the degree of permeability of the intestinal membranes, and whether the tight junctions are weakened. Passage through weakened tight junctions is also presumed to be the way that peptides such as gliadin pass through a damaged intestinal membrane in celiac disease.

Method for Conducting the Lactulose/Mannitol Test[13]

The patient drinks a mixture of 5 g each of the sugars lactulose and mannitol (referred to as *compound* in the formula here) dissolved in water. Since these sugars are not metabolized, any absorbed sugar is fully excreted in the urine within 6 hours. The urine is collected, and concentrations of the two sugars are measured. Percent absorptions are calculated using the following formula:

$$\text{Percentage Absorption} = \frac{\text{Compound Concentration (mg/mL)} \times \text{Urine Volume (mL)} \times 100}{\text{Amount of Compound Administered (mL)}}$$

In the healthy intestine, the mean absorption of mannitol is 14% of the administered dose, whereas the mean absorption of lactulose is less than 1%. The normal ratio of lactulose to mannitol recovered in urine is less than 0.03. A ratio higher than 0.03 indicates that excessive lactulose was absorbed, indicating that it passed through a hyperpermeable barrier, and thus indicates a leaky gut.

There is a lack of evidence to suggest that casein, gluten, or their products cause the leaky gut. However, some researchers equate the process to celiac disease[15] in which immunological reactions to the gliadin fraction of gluten damage the intestinal villi that line the digestive tract epithelium and may result in hyperpermeability. Other studies[16] suggest that the improvement of autistic children on a gluten-free diet indicates that malabsorption of essential nutrients in celiac disease predisposes to symptoms of autism (see Chapter 41 for information on celiac disease).

Vitamin B-12 Deficiency and Nervous System Development

A deficiency in an essential nutrient has often been suggested as a possible contributor to some types of autism. Vitamin B-12 was thought to be a likely candidate because undetected and untreated vitamin B-12 deficiency in infants can result in permanent neurological damage. Furthermore, individuals with stomach and small intestine disorders may be unable to absorb enough vitamin B-12 from food to maintain healthy body stores.

According to the proponents of the theory that vitamin B-12 deficiency may play a role in certain types of autism, pathology in the lining of the ileal region of the small intestine in autistic children, which has been observed in a few studies, could interfere with vitamin B-12 being transported into circulation.[17] If absorption is severely inhibited, the resulting lower blood vitamin B-12 could interfere with the formation of *myelin*, the lipoprotein material surrounding the axon of certain nerve fibers. Myelin is necessary for normal conduction of the nerve impulse (action potential) in myelinated nerve fibers. Therefore, impairment in nerve conduction could result in the neurological deficits observed in autism. However, direct evidence of vitamin B-12 deficiency and impaired myelin formation in autism is lacking at this time.

A 2010 study[18] of 3- to 8-year-old autistic children indicated that vitamin B-12 supplementation improved autistic symptoms in 9 (30%) of their subjects, suggesting that a subset of children with autism disorder may benefit from B-12 supplementation. In general, authorities suggest regular monitoring of the B-12 levels in the blood of autistic children and supplementation, usually by injection, if the levels are found to be abnormally low. Ensuring that the diet includes adequate levels of vitamin B-12 is an obvious measure for ensuring optimal nutrition in any child, but especially autistic children whose diet may be rather unbalanced because of their own food preferences.

Magnesium, Vitamin B-6, and Autism

In the 1950s, megavitamin therapy became popular as a treatment of several chronic conditions. Autism was one of the conditions in which it was hoped that extremely large doses of vitamins might improve a child's mental processes. Vitamin B-6 (pyroxidine) was discovered to improve speech and language in some children with "autism syndrome." However, vitamin B-6 in high doses can be toxic, with several adverse effects, which were considerably reduced when magnesium was given at the same time.

Since 1980, numerous published studies have attempted to assess the effects of vitamin B-6 and magnesium on a variety of characteristics such as verbal communication, nonverbal communication, interpersonal skills, and physiological function in individuals with autism.[19] These studies were subject to scientific evaluation and review[20] in 2003. The authors concluded that due to insufficient evidence, they could provide no recommendations on the use of vitamin B-6 with magnesium as a treatment for autism.

Some clinicians have been investigating the possibility that magnesium alone as a supplement may improve symptoms in autism. This was based on the observation that children with autistic spectrum disorders had significantly lower plasma concentrations of magnesium than normal subjects.[21] Because magnesium is an essential element in several important physiological processes, it has been suggested that a deficiency might lead to impairment in certain brain functions that could contribute to the autistic disorder. However, studies on magnesium and its role in autism have not yet defined the deficiency or determined whether supplementation with the mineral is effective in treatment.

Dietary Preferences and the Restricted Diet

Children with autism tend to have strong preferences in their food selection. Many have intense dislikes for some foods, while they crave others and tend to select them repeatedly. They also tend to have very definite ideas about form and texture. For example, the author of this book had one client who would eat food only in the form of patties, but this was ideal because a wide range of chopped up foods could be incorporated into his patties, which in the uncut state he would reject outright. Consequently, the client was provided with a well-balanced diet, in spite of his limited food preferences, using fish-, meat-, or poultry-based patties containing a variety of chopped vegetables and fruit. However, in many cases, this selectivity means that an autistic child's diet is already limited, and parents and health care providers may be reluctant to restrict the child's food intake any further. Consequently, a gluten- and casein-restricted diet is not an attractive option for many.

Summary: Can Dietary Interventions Prevent or Treat Autism?

Many reports from parents and research studies have indicated that a variety of dietary interventions may have success in ameliorating symptoms in certain children with autism.[22] The most studied and successful have been discussed here.

Currently, experts do not agree on whether dietary manipulation can help prevent autism or aid in its treatment. Researchers in the field tend to agree that dietary manipulation is recommended if the child's behavior improves on the restrictions or supplements. However, many practitioners hold the opinion that "the link between autism and a gastrointestinal pathophysiology is not substantiated by research. The dietary approaches employed are cumbersome, not proven to be efficacious, and may further narrow the food choices of the child with autism."[23]

If any dietary manipulation provides some improvement, parents, caregivers, and clinicians are usually open to a trial on the suggested diet. If a parent feels there is a chance that their child might benefit from a gluten- and casein-restricted diet, it may be worthwhile to try the diet—for a limited time only. If the child's behavior does not noticeably improve after strictly adhering to the guidelines for a month, then the restrictions should be abandoned because it is unlikely that they are providing any benefit. As with any dietary manipulation, it is essential that any foods removed from the diet be replaced with those of equivalent nutritional value.

No evidence suggests that very high doses of any single nutrient are beneficial. In fact, the contrary is usually true. Excessive quantities of many vitamins and minerals can be toxic, and frequently, excess of one leads to deficiency in another, as they compete for absorption and metabolites. Each nutrient plays an essential role in keeping the body healthy; refer to the Dietary Reference Intakes (DRIs) published by the Institute of Medicine for recommendations about the levels of various nutrients that are ideal at each developmental stage.[24] The Tolerable Upper Limits set in the DRIs should not be exceeded except in specific medical conditions, which will be decided by a medical specialist in individual cases. Further studies are needed to establish the efficacy of any dietary intervention in the management of autism, to identify those individuals who would most benefit, and to determine the mechanism responsible for triggering any adverse responses.

References

1. Kaneshiro NK, Zieve D. Autism. PubMed Health. U.S. National Library of Medicine. National Institutes of Health. April 26, 2010. www.ncbi.nlm.nih.gov/pubmedhealth/ PMH0002494. Accessed May 4, 2012.
2. American Psychiatric Association. *Diagnostic and Statistical Manual of Mental Disorders (DSM-IV-TR)*. Washington, DC: American Psychiatric Association; 2000.
3. Tuchman RF, Rapin I. Regression in pervasive developmental disorders: seizures and epileptiform electroencephalogram correlates. *Pediatrics*. 1997;4:560-566.
4. White JF. Intestinal pathophysiology in autism. *Exp Biol Med*. 2003;228:639-649.
5. Lightdale JR, Siegel B, Heyman MB. Gastrointestinal symptoms in autistic children. *Clin Perspect Gastroenterol*. 2001;1:56-58.
6. Horvath K, Papadimitriou JC, Rabsztyn A, Drachenberg C, Tildon JT. Gastrointestinal abnormalities in children with autistic disorder. *J Pediatr*. 1999;135:559-563.
7. Black C, Kaye JA, Jick H. Relation of childhood gastrointestinal disorders to autism: nested case-control study using data from the UK General Practice Research Database. *BMJ*. 2002;325:419-421.
8. Lucarelli S, Frediani T, Zingoni AM, et al. Food allergy and infantile autism. *Panminerva Med*. 1995;37:137-141.
9. Knivsberg A, Reichelt KL, Nodland N, Hoien T. Autistic syndromes and diet: a follow-up study. *Scand J Educ Res*. 1995;39:223-236.
10. Whiteley P, Haracopos D, Knivsberg AM, et al. The ScanBrit randomized, single-blind study of a gluten- and casein-free dietary intervention for children with autism spectrum disorders. *Nutr Neurosci*. 2010;13(2):87-100.
11. Liu Z, Li N, Neu J. Tight junctions, leaky intestines, and pediatric diseases. *Acta Paediatr*. 2005;94(4):386-393.
12. Uil JJ, van Elburg RM, van Overbeek FM, Mulder CJ, VanBerge-Henegouwen GP, Heymans HS. Clinical implications of the sugar absorption test: intestinal permeability test to assess mucosal barrier function. *Scand J Gastroenterol Suppl*. 1997;223:70-78.
13. Paroni R, Fermo I, Molteni L, et al. Lactulose and mannitol intestinal permeability detected by capillary electrophoresis. *J Chromatogr B Analyt Technol Biomed Life Sci*. 2006;834(1-2):183-187.
14. de Magistris L, Familiari V, Pascotto A, et al. Alterations of the intestinal barrier in patients with autism spectrum disorders and in their first-degree relatives. *J Pediatr Gastroenterol Nutr*. 2010;51(4):418-424.
15. Barcia G, Posar A, Santucci M, Parmeggiani A. Autism and coeliac disease. *Autism Dev Disord*. 2008;38(2):407-408.

16. Genuis SJ, Bouchard TPJ. Celiac disease presenting as autism. *Child Neurol.* 2010; 25(1):114-119.

17. Wakefield AJ, Murch SH, Anthony A, et al. Ileal-lymphoid-nodular hyperplasia, non-specific colitis, and pervasive developmental disorder in children. *Lancet.* 1998;35:637-641.

18. Bertoglio K, Jill James S, Deprey L, Brule N, Hendren RL. Pilot study of the effect of methyl B12 treatment on behavioral and biomarker measures in children with autism. *J Altern Complement Med.* 2010;16(5):555-560.

19. Mousain-Bosc M, Roche M, Polge A, Pradal-Prat D, Rapin J, Bali JP. Improvement of neurobehavioral disorders in children supplemented with magnesium-vitamin B6. II. Pervasive developmental disorder-autism. *Magnes Res.* 2006;19(1):53-62.

20. Nye C, Brice A. Combined vitamin B6-magnesium treatment in autism spectrum disorder. *Cochrane Database Syst Rev.* 2002;(4):CD003497.

21. Strambi M, Longini M, Hayek J, et al. Magnesium profile in autism. *Biol Trace Elem Res.* 2006;109(2):97-104.

22. Srinivasan P. A review of dietary interventions in autism. *Ann Clin Psychiatry.* 2009;21(4):237-247.

23. Johnson TW. Dietary considerations in autism: identifying a reasonable approach. *Top Clin Nutr.* 2006;21(3):212-225.

24. Institute of Medicine. Dietary Reference Intake Tables and Application. http://iom.edu/Activities/Nutrition/SummaryDRIs/DRI-Tables.aspx. Accessed May 4, 2012.

CHAPTER **47**

Probiotics and Allergy

The gastrointestinal tract of the healthy human houses about 10^{12} to 10^{14} fairly harmless microorganisms per mL, mostly in the large bowel. More than 500 species have been identified, and together they form over 1 kg (2.2. pounds) of an individual's body weight. These microorganisms are essential for the health not only of the intestines, but also of the whole body. A complex symbiosis exists between the human host and the gut microflora that has developed to the advantage of each. Disruption of the balance between the two can lead to a variety of disease processes. Laboratory rats that are born and reared in a completely sterile environment, so that they never have microorganisms in their digestive tract, quickly sicken and die. Like rats and other mammals, humans are dependent on the digestive tract microorganisms for achieving and maintaining optimal health.

Microorganisms and Human Health

The microorganisms in the digestive tract aid human health in several ways:

- They break down undigested food that moves into the bowel from the small intestine (where most of the digestion of food and absorption of nutrients takes place). Micronutrients such as vitamin K, biotin, thiamin, vitamin B-12, and folate are produced as a result of their metabolic activities. These micro-nutrients are absorbed and form an essential part of the body's nutritional resources.
- Microorganisms in the large bowel defend the bowel from invasion by nonessential or pathogenic microorganisms by competing with them for space and nutrients.
- Microorganisms also perform a vital role in stimulating the immune system of the digestive tract—the gut-associated lymphoid tissue (GALT). This constant interaction between microorganisms and immune cells maintains a healthy

balance that aids in the GALT's defense against invasion by potential pathogens (the Th1 response). It is also the way in which a balance between the Th1
and Th2 response to microorganisms and foods may be maintained in oral
tolerance. (For a discussion about Th1 and Th2 responses in allergy and about
oral tolerance, see Chapter 1.)

■   Research in the past decade indicates that the risk of allergy in infants may be
reduced by using probiotic bacteria to maintain a good bacterial balance in
pregnant mothers and to modulate the intestinal flora of the infant. In addition, some strains of bacteria seem to have the potential to speed the recovery
from food allergy in babies and children.

What Determines Which Microorganisms Will Colonize the Bowel?

The environment of the large bowel determines precisely which microorganisms
survive therein. Factors such as the presence or absence of oxygen (eH); acidity or
alkalinity (pH); nutrients in a solid, liquid, or gaseous form; interaction with other
microorganisms and their metabolic products; and tolerance by the immune system
of the gut all play a part in determining which species survive and which do not.

Once the microbial flora is established, which usually occurs soon after weaning, it remains more or less unchanged throughout life unless significant modifying
events within the gut environment occur. People living in the same household, eating
more or less the same diet, can have quite different microorganisms in their bowel
(referred to as the *indigenous microflora*, or *microbiota*). Even if many species suc-
cumb to oral antibiotics used in treating an infection, over time the microorganisms
that were present prior to the antibiotic therapy tend to become reestablished in
more or less the same proportions.

Many studies have indicated the possible value of modifying the indigenous
microflora, especially in situations where the existing microbial activity appears
to be detrimental (see the later discussion, How Are Probiotics Used?). However,
this can be quite a challenge. Once the microflora is established, it can be likened to
a city in which all the houses are occupied by people of a specific race and culture.
Introducing a new group of residents, with different dietary and ethnic practices,
will require not only displacing the established populace, but also providing the
nutrients and environment required by the immigrants to allow them to survive
and flourish. This is where the science of probiotics aids in repopulating the large
bowel.

What Are Probiotics?

The term *probiotic* was coined in the early 1990s to describe a culture of living
microorganisms within a food that was designed to provide health benefits beyond
its inherent nutritional value.[1] Probiotics are live, nonpathogenic microorganisms

that improve the balance of microorganisms in the bowel. They are regulated as dietary supplements and foods.[2] The types of microorganisms used in such foods must have certain characteristics to be of any value: They must have a beneficial effect within the bowel, and they must be capable of living within the human bowel without causing any harm. To colonize the area, the microorganism must be able to survive passage through the hostile acidic environment of the stomach and upper small intestine; resist the effects of intestinal secretions, including evading the effects of digestive enzymes and bile salts; attach to intestinal cells on reaching the large bowel; and thrive within its physiological and nutritional milieu.[3] It is thought that probiotic microorganisms alter the gut microflora by competitively interacting with the existing flora through the production of chemicals that are toxic to other microorganisms (antimicrobial metabolites) or possibly by affecting the local immune response within the digestive tract so that it becomes hostile to the indigenous microorganisms.[2,4]

The microorganisms most frequently used in probiotics are human strains of lactobacilli, bifidobacterium, streptococci, saccharomyces, and a few enterococci. Given the enormous number of different species resident in the healthy human digestive tract, it is probable that many more types of bacteria will be identified as beneficial in the future. At the present time, however, research is being directed toward the saccharolytic strains, which use sugars for their nutrition and multiplication; these seem to promise the greatest benefit.

How Probiotics Work

The value of the probiotic microorganism lies in its ability to produce chemicals that are beneficial to the body. Microorganisms act on the substrate (nutrients) available to them and produce end-products which are determined by the enzymes that they are able to produce and the environment in which they are growing. The substrate and environment can be readily manipulated in the laboratory where most microbiological studies have been conducted. However, within the complex environment of the bowel, it is not so easy to achieve the desired end-products.

To ensure that the desirable microorganisms survive in the colon and that they produce the end-products that will be of greatest benefit, current research is focused on selecting the appropriate strains of microorganisms to incorporate into the probiotic food and the substrate that will yield the desired end-products.

Definition of Terms

The term *probiotic* refers to the strains of microorganisms selected to achieve a specific result when introduced into the digestive tract.

The term *prebiotic* has been coined for the nutritional substrate provided with the probiotic to achieve the optimal survival and establishment of the microorganisms in the digestive tract.

The term *synbiotic* refers to the combination of the specific microbial strain (probiotic) with its specifically selected prebiotic.

Prebiotics

Prebiotics are nondigestible food ingredients that move into the large bowel to act as a substrate for microbial fermentation. They provide the nutrients for multiplication of a desired probiotic and for other species of microorganisms in the gut that may be favorable for health.

Much of the research on prebiotics has centered on the oligosaccharides, which are carbohydrates consisting of chains of glucose molecules (from three to ten) that are indigestible by human enzymes. Their indigestibility means that they will pass unchanged into the large bowel, where they will provide a substrate for nutrition and multiplication of the bacteria that are being introduced. It is as if we are sending a population into an unknown region with food packages to ensure their survival.

In the United States and Europe, the fructo-oligosaccharides (FOS; also called *fructans*) and inulin-type fructans are the most common oligosaccharides in use as prebiotics because of their economy of manufacture and their proven value in human health.[5] Galacto-oligosaccharides (GOS) are also becoming available on the market in Europe and the United States but currently are not as widely used as the fructans. Many more oligosaccharides, such as isomalto-oligosaccharides, soybean oligosaccharides (raffinose and stachyose), xylo-oligosaccharides, and gentio-oligosaccharides, are available, especially in Japan. The precise metabolism of these substrates by specific strains of probiotic bacteria has only recently begun to be studied. Furthermore, if the substrate is not provided continuously, the newly introduced probiotic bacteria will not survive, and the original inhabitants of the area will quickly return and become reestablished.

Synbiotics

A synbiotic is a product containing both a selected strain (or strains) of probiotic microorganisms and the substrate (usually an oligosaccharide or a combination of oligosaccharides) that will provide nutrients to promote the growth and establishment of the probiotic bacteria.

Postbiotics

In 2009, a new term appeared in the research literature: *postbiotics*, defined as "the biologically active by-products of probiotic cultures (ie, short-chain fatty acids produced by bacterial fermentation such as butyrate), which can be added to health supplements."[6] Undoubtedly there will be more information on this topic available in the medical and scientific literature as the field develops in the future.

How Are Probiotics Used?

Probiotic microorganisms have been used in therapy for certain types of dysfunction within the colon in some quite specific ways. For example, it has been known for some time that yogurts containing live cultures of bacteria such as lactobacilli, bifidobacterium, and *Streptococcus thermophilus* assist in reducing the symptoms of lactose intolerance. The beneficial effects are due to the production of the enzyme beta-galactosidase (lactase) by the bacteria in the yogurt, which breaks down lactose. The thick, fermented milk itself delays gastrointestinal transit, thus allowing a longer period of time in which both the human and microbial lactase enzyme can act on the milk lactose. It has been suggested that lactose tolerance in people who are deficient in lactase (see Chapter 11) may be improved by continued ingestion of small quantities of milk. There is no evidence that this will improve or affect the production of lactase in the brush border cells of the small intestine in any way, but it seems that the continued presence of lactose in the colon contributes to the establishment and multiplication of bacteria capable of synthesizing the beta-galactosidase enzyme over time. Thus, when lactose reaches the colon undigested, large numbers of the resident microflora will break down the lactose, which will therefore not cause the osmotic imbalance within the colon that causes much of the discomfort of lactose intolerance.[7]

Another condition in which probiotics seem to be of benefit is in preventing diarrhea in infants and children who have been treated with oral antibiotics (antibiotic-associated diarrhea, AAD).[8] Antibiotics alter the microbial balance within the gastrointestinal tract, and the probiotics may prevent AAD by restoring the gut microflora. Antibiotics are prescribed frequently for children, and AAD is common in this population. The probiotic strains and doses with the most promising evidence for prevention of AAD were identified as *Lactobacillus GG*, *Lactobacillus sporogenes*, and *Saccharomyces boulardii* at 5 billion to 40 billion colony forming units/day.[6] However, the authors caution that, although the current data are promising, "it is premature to routinely recommend probiotics for the prevention of pediatric AAD."

Preliminary research also suggests that the *Lactobacillus* strain GG (LGG) may decrease the risk of upper respiratory tract infections, including rhinitis, pharyngitis, sinusitis, otitis, and the common cold in children. The researchers reported that the rate of absence from child-care centers due to infections was lower in children receiving LGG in comparison to those who were not.[9] However, the authors point out the limitation of their study in that diagnosis and treatment of the children was based on clinical judgment, and the rate of severe infections was very low; therefore, no clear effect of LGG could be proven.

Studies such as these indicate that it is likely that future research will determine a number of conditions in which manipulation of the bowel microbial flora may be beneficial. In this regard, there has been an increasing interest in using probiotics in allergy prevention and management.

How Probiotics Help in Allergy

Studies in the past decade have indicated that the intestinal microflora might be the major source of microbial stimulation that promotes maturation of the immune system in early childhood.[10] The appropriate microbial stimulus soon after birth may be important in balancing the Th1/Th2 response of the immune system, which is skewed to the Th2 (allergy) type at birth[11] (for details about the Th1 and Th2 response in the fetus and newborn, see Chapters 1, 41, and 42).

Research studies[11] suggest that harmless probiotic bacteria such as lactobacilli and bifidobacteria may stimulate a Th1 (protective) response in the digestive tract without causing disease. If these bacteria are introduced during the infant period, this might halt the atopic process.

Lactic acid bacteria and bifidobacteria are found more commonly in the intestinal flora of nonallergic children than in allergic children, and atopic children seem to have a different microflora composition than nonatopics, with higher levels of clostridia and lower levels of bifidobacteria.[12] These observations may pave the way for selection of probiotic strains that might promote the intestinal environment most beneficial in developing tolerance rather than sensitization to allergens in the immature infant. There are several studies suggesting that the appropriate selection of the bacterial strains used in probiotics may help in certain allergic conditions, but at the present time we have insufficient evidence to recommend probiotics as a therapy for allergy prevention in regular clinical practice.[13,14]

The use of probiotic therapy to prevent allergic disease has been demonstrated in a few studies using the probiotic strain *Lactobacillus rhamnosus GG* in neonates. This seemed to be particularly effective in reducing the incidence and severity of atopic eczema.[15] In a Finnish study, infants with milk allergy and atopic dermatitis had milder symptoms and fewer incidences of intestinal infections if their milk formula was fortified with lactobacilli.[16] However, a similar study from Singapore reported that administration of a cow's milk formula supplemented with probiotics (*Bifidobacterium longum* and *Lactobacillus rhamnosus*) for the first 6 months showed no effect on preventing eczema or allergen sensitization in the first year of life in Asian infants at risk of allergic disease.[17] Another study using the probiotics *Lactobacillus rhamnosus* or *Lactobacillus GG* in infant formula for 3 months in children younger than 5 months as prevention or management of atopic dermatitis (AD) concluded that the results "indicate that oral supplementation with these probiotic bacterial strains will not have a significant impact on the symptoms of infantile AD."[18]

A Swedish study in children between the ages of 4 and 13 months (89 in the study group; 90 in the control group) evaluated the positive effects of feeding *Lactobacillus F19* in cereals during weaning to help with symptoms of eczema. At 13 months of age, the incidence of eczema in the study group was reported as 11% and in the placebo group as 22%. The authors conclude that "feeding Lactobacillus

F19 during weaning could be an effective tool in the prevention of early manifestations of allergy, eg, eczema."[19]

Readers interested in recent studies on specific strains and the combination of strains that are being evaluated in prevention or management of atopic conditions in infants may wish to review the studies described in Tables 47.1 and 47.2. The strains investigated and the methodology and scope of these studies vary. Some of the strains are administered to the pregnant mother prior to delivery and are continued postnatally; some are given only to the neonate. In some studies, the subject group is limited to infants at high risk for allergy (at least one first-degree relative—parent or sibling—with diagnosed allergy), while in other studies the subjects are randomly selected. Generalizing from such studies is therefore difficult. Before any conclusions as to the effectiveness of probiotics, prebiotics, and synbiotics on childhood allergy can be made, many variables must be considered, including the following:

- The specific species and strains of the microorganisms
- The number of microorganisms required to be delivered orally (dosage) as colony forming units (CFU)
- The number of microorganisms surviving in their movement through the digestive tract
- The number colonizing (implantation and multiplication in) the bowel; usually measured as live organisms in the feces
- The age at which the probiotic is administered; whether prenatally or postnatally
- The duration of probiotic consumption
- The means of administering the probiotic (eg, in milk, formula, cereal, or other)
- The selection of an appropriate prebiotic (eg, milk, oligosaccharide such as fructo-oligosaccharide, or other)

Few studies on the long-term effects of probiotics in allergy prevention have been published, and even fewer are those on the use of probiotics in the management of established allergy in either children or adults. Most of the positive effects of prebiotics, probiotics, and synbiotics in adults are related to digestive tract disorders such as in acute diarrhea (most frequently due to pouchitis or rotavirus infection), ulcerative colitis, Crohn's disease, necrotizing enterocolitis, other inflammatory bowel diseases, and in modulation of the disordered digestive tract.[20] Many more large-scale studies need to be conducted, and we need to learn more about exactly how microorganisms interact with the immune system before we can state with any degree of confidence that probiotics are useful in allergy prevention and management.[21]

TABLE 47.1
Selected Studies of Effects of Individual Probiotic Strains on Allergy

Microorganism	Study Purpose	Design	Administration of Microorganism	Summary of Effects on Allergy
Lactobacillus rhamnosus GG	To determine potential role of L rhamnosus GG in allergy prevention.[a]	Follow-up to a randomized, placebo-controlled trial[b] of 132 infants at high risk for allergy (first-degree relative with allergic disease).	1×10^{10} CFU or placebo daily to (a) pregnant mothers 2–4 weeks before delivery; (b) mothers of breastfeeding infants for first 6 months of life; (c) nonbreastfed infants for first 6 months of life.	Compared with subjects taking placebo, those taking LGG had reduced risk of eczema at age 4 years.
Lactobacillus rhamnosus GG	To determine potential role of L rhamnosus GG as therapy for existing eczema.[c]	Randomized, placebo-controlled trial of 102 infants, ages 3–12 months, with mild to moderate atopic dermatitis.	5×10^9 CFU or placebo twice a day for 12 weeks administered as a food supplement.	No therapeutic effect of LGG against mild to moderate atopic dermatitis in infancy.
Lactobacillus rhamnosus GG	To study the preventive effect of the Lactobacillus GG on the development of atopic dermatitis in infants.[d]	Randomized, double-blind placebo-controlled trial of 98 subjects with a first-degree relative with allergic disease.	1×10^{10} CFU or placebo daily to (a) pregnant mothers of infants at high risk for allergy for 4–6 weeks before delivery; (b) mothers of breastfeeding infants for first 3 months of life then to the infants for 3 additional months; (c) nonbreastfed infants directly for first 6 months of life.	Supplementation with LGG did not reduce the incidence of atopic dermatitis at age 2 years or alter the severity of atopic dermatitis in affected children. LGG was associated with an increased rate of recurrent episodes of wheezing bronchitis.
Lactobacillus rhamnosus HN001 or Bifidobacterium animalis subsp lactis	To determine whether probiotic supplementation in early life could prevent development of eczema and atopy at age 2 years.[e]	Double-blind, randomized placebo-controlled trial of 474 infants with one or both parents with allergic disease.	Daily supplementation with (a) 1×10^{10} CFU Lactobacillus rhamnosus HN001; or (b) 1×10^{10} CFU Bifidobacterium animalis subsp lactis; or (c) placebo to (i) pregnant mothers from 35 weeks' gestation until 6 months postnatal if breastfeeding, and (ii) infants from birth to age 2 years.	Supplementation with L. rhamnosus, but not B. animalis subsp lactis, substantially reduced the cumulative prevalence of eczema, but not atopy, by age 2 years.
Escherichia coli serotype 083	To determine whether promoting after-birth oral colonization by a probiotic Escherichia coli strain to decrease colonization with pathogenic microorganisms reduces occurrence of allergy later in life in infants of allergic mothers.[f]	Randomized placebo-controlled clinical trial of 158 infants: (a) 56 infants of allergic mothers; (b) 57 control infants of allergic mothers; (c) 45 control infants of healthy mothers.	Infants of allergic mothers received (a) 1 mL of probiotic E. coli strain or (b) placebo within 48 hours after birth and subsequently 3 times a week for a period of 4 weeks. Infants of nonallergic mothers were also monitored.	Presence of the E. coli strain was monitored in stool samples throughout the study. At the conclusion, allergy symptoms were found in 14 infants of control allergic mothers, 7 infants of healthy mothers, and in 2 colonized infants of allergic mothers. Colonization affected levels of several cytokines and specific anti-E. coli antibodies.

Continues

TABLE 47.1

Selected Studies of Effects of Individual Probiotic Strains on Allergy (*Continued*)

Microorganism	Study Purpose	Design	Administration of Microorganism	Summary of Effects on Allergy
Lactobacillus acidophilus strain L10/ LAVRI-A1	To assess effects of *L10/LAVRI-A1* on allergic outcomes in children of women with allergy.[g]	Randomized placebo-controlled clinical trial of 153 children of atopic mothers.	Daily administration of (a) *L acidophilus (LAVRI-A1)* or (b) placebo for the first 6 months of life.	*L acidophilus* increased the risk of allergen sensitization at 1 year of age and did not have any significant effect on allergy at age 2.5 years.
Lactobacillus reuteri	To determine whether *L reuteri* prevents eczema and allergic sensitization in infants with a family history of allergic disease.[h]	Double-blind placebo-controlled trial of 188 families with any first-degree relative with allergic disease.	Daily oral administration of (a) 1×10^8 CFU *L reuteri* or (b) placebo to pregnant mothers from gestational week 36 until delivery, then directly to infants for 12 months.	The treated infants had less IgE-associated eczema compared to those in the placebo group (8% vs 20%) at 2 years of age. Wheeze and other potentially allergic diseases were not affected.
Lactobacillus paracasei strain F19	To evaluate the effects of feeding *L paracasei F19* to infants during weaning on the incidence of eczema and on Th1/Th2 balance.[i]	Double-blind, randomized placebo-controlled trial of 179 at-risk infants (infants with one first-degree relative [parent or sibling] with diagnosed allergy).	Cereals with or without probiotic administered to infants from ages 4 to 13 months during weaning.	The Th1/Th2 ratio in the treatment group at 13 months was higher than in the placebo group, indicating a possible reduced risk of allergy with treatment. At 13 months, the cumulative incidence of eczema was 11% in the probiotic group compared to 22% in the placebo group.

[a]Kalliomaki M, Salminen S, Poussa T, Arvilommi H, Isolauri E. Probiotics and prevention of atopic disease: 4-year follow-up of a randomised placebo-controlled trial. *Lancet*. 2003;361:1869-1871.

[b]Kalliomaki M, Salminen S, Arvilommi H, Kero P, Koskinen P, Isolauri E. Probiotics in primary prevention of atopic disease: a randomised placebo-controlled trial. *Lancet*. 2001;357:1076-1079.

[c]Grüber C, Wendt M, Sulser C, et al. Randomized, placebo-controlled trial of Lactobacillus rhamnosus GG as treatment of atopic dermatitis in infancy. *Allergy*. 2007;62(11):1270-1276.

[d]Kopp MV, Hennemuth I, Heinzmann A, Urbanek R. Randomized, double-blind, placebo-controlled trial of probiotics for primary prevention: no clinical effects of Lactobacillus GG supplementation. *Pediatrics*. 2008;121:850-856.

[e]Wickens K, Black PN, Stanley TV, et al; Probiotic Study Group. A differential effect of 2 probiotics in the prevention of eczema and atopy: a double-blind, randomized, placebo-controlled trial. *J Allergy Clin Immunol*. 2008;122(4):788-794.

[f]Lodinová-Žádníková R, Prokešová L, Kocourková I, Hrdý J, Zižka J. Prevention of allergy in infants of allergic mothers by probiotic *Escherichia coli*. *Int Arch Allergy Immunol*. 2010;153(2):201-206.

[g]Prescott SL, Wiltschut J, Taylor A, et al. Early markers of allergic disease in a primary prevention study using probiotics: 2.5-year follow-up phase. *Allergy*. 2008;63(11):1481-1490.

[h]Abrahamsson TR, Jakobsson T, Böttcher MF, et al. Probiotics in prevention of IgE-associated eczema: a double-blind, randomized, placebo-controlled trial. *J Allergy Clin Immunol*. 2007;119(5):1174-1180.

[i]West CE, Hammarström ML, Hernell O. Probiotics during weaning reduce the incidence of eczema. *Pediatr Allergy Immunol*. 2009;20(5):430-437.

TABLE 47.2
Selected Studies of Effects of Probiotic Combinations on Allergy

Microorganisms	Study Purpose	Design	Administration of Microorganisms	Summary of Effects on Allergy
Bifidobacterium longum (BL999) and *Lactobacillus rhamnosus (LPR)*	To assess whether probiotic supplementation administered in the first 6 months of life had an effect on eczema and allergic sensitization at 1 year of age in Asian infants at risk of allergic disease.[a]	Double-blind, placebo-controlled randomized trial involving 253 infants with a family history of allergic disease.	Cow's milk formula with or without 1×10^7 CFU *Bifidobacterium longum (BL999)* and 2×10^7 CFU *Lactobacillus rhamnosus (LPR)* administered daily for the first 6 months of life.	Probiotics in formula had no effect on prevention of eczema or allergen sensitization in the first year of life.
Lactobacillus rhamnosus GG and *Lactobacillus rhamnosus LC705* and *Bifidobacterium breve* and *Propionibacterium freundreichii* and prebiotics (galactooligosaccharides)	To evaluate use of pro- and prebiotics in prevention of allergic diseases.[b]	Randomized, double-blind placebo-controlled trial of 925 infants with one or both parents having allergic disease.	Pregnant mothers took (a) 5×10^9 CFU *L rhamnosus GG*, 5×10^9 CFU *L rhamnosus LC705*, 2×10^9 CFU *B breve*, and 2×10^9 CFU *P freundreichii* with prebiotics or (b) a placebo twice daily during the 2–4 weeks before delivery. Infants then took the same probiotics plus prebiotics or the placebo for first 6 months of life.	Compared with placebo, probiotic treatment showed no effect on the cumulative incidence of all allergic diseases (food allergy, eczema, asthma, and allergic rhinitis) by age 2 years but significantly prevented eczema and especially atopic eczema. A follow-up study[c] at 5 years concluded there was no difference in allergy (eczema, asthma, allergic rhinitis) between groups, except in a subgroup of caesarean-delivered children where less IgE-associated allergic disease was noted in the subjects that received probiotics.

Continues

TABLE 47.2
Selected Studies of Effects of Probiotic Combinations on Allergy (Continued)

Microorganisms	Study Purpose	Design	Administration of Microorganisms	Summary of Effects on Allergy
Lactobacillus lactis W58 and *Bifidobacterium lactis* W52 and *Bifidobacterium bifidum* W23	To study the primary prevention of allergic disease in high-risk children by pre- and postnatal supplementation with selected strains of probiotic bacteria.[d]	Double-blind, randomized placebo-controlled trial of 120 infants with atopic disease in either their mother or father and at least 1 sibling.	Administration of (a) 1 × 10⁹ CFU each daily of *L lactis* W58, *B lactis* W52, and *B bifidum* W23 or (b) placebo to pregnant mothers of high-risk for allergy infants from 6 weeks before delivery, then to infants for 12 months postnatally.	Parental-reported eczema during the first 3 months of life was significantly lower in the intervention group compared with placebo. Between ages 3 months and 2 years, the incidence of eczema was similar in both groups.
Lactobacillus rhamnosus GG and *Lactobacillus acidophiluis* LA5 and *Bifidobacterium animalis* subsp *lactis* Bb-12	To examine whether probiotics given to pregnant women in a nonselected population could prevent atopic sensitization or allergic diseases during the child's first 2 years.[e]	Randomized, placebo-controlled double-blind trial of 278 children from a nonselected population of pregnant women.	Pregnant women received probiotic milk or placebo from 36 weeks' gestation and while breastfeeding for 3 months postnatally.	At 2 years, cumulative incidence of eczema was reduced in the treatment group compared with the placebo group. There were no significant effects on asthma and allergic rhinoconjunctivitis.
Lactobacillus salivarius and *Lactobacillus paracasei* and *Bifidobacterium infantis* and *Bifidobacterium bifidum*	To identify any adverse effects of these probiotic microorganisms in potentially vulnerable populations.[f]	Randomized, double-blind placebo-controlled trial with 454 participants.	Placebo or a total of 1 × 10¹⁰ CFU of combined microorganisms administered daily to women during the last month of pregnancy and to their infants for the first 6 months of life.	Findings support the safe use of this grouping of organisms during pregnancy and early infancy. Compared with the placebo, the supplement did not demonstrate any effect on incidence of allergy.

[a]Soh SE, Aw M, Gerez I, et al. Probiotic supplementation in the first 6 months of life in at risk Asian infants: effects on eczema and atopic sensitization at the age of 1 year. *Clin Exp Allergy*. 2009;39(4):571-578.

[b]Kukkonen K, Savilahti E, Haahtela T, et al. Probiotics and prebiotic galacto-oligosaccharides in the prevention of allergic diseases: a randomized, double-blind, placebo-controlled trial. *J Allergy Clin Immunol*. 2007;119(1):192-198.

[c]Kuitunen M, Kukkonen K, Juntunen-Backman K, et al. Probiotics prevent IgE-associated allergy until age 5 years in cesarean-delivered children but not in the total cohort. *J Allergy Clin Immunol*. 2009;123(2):335-341.

[d]Niers L, Martín R, Rijkers G, et al. The effects of selected probiotic strains on the development of eczema (the PandA study). *Allergy*. 2009;64(9):1349-1358.

[e]Dotterud CK, Storrø O, Johnsen R, Oien T. Probiotics in pregnant women to prevent allergic disease: a randomized, double-blind trial. *Br J Dermatol*. 2010;163(3):616-623.

[f]Allen SJ, Jordan S, Storey M, et al. Dietary supplementation with lactobacilli and bifidobacteria is well tolerated and not associated with adverse events during late pregnancy and early infancy. *J Nutr*. 2010;140(3):483-488.

Which Organisms and Which Foods?

The current state of evidence suggests that probiotic effects are strain specific, meaning that each type of bacterium is likely to exert a specific influence as part of the intestinal flora once it has become established. Strain identity is important to link a bacterium to a specific health effect and to enable accurate surveillance of whether the microorganism is still in the colon.[2] When the strain can be demonstrated in fecal samples taken at intervals over a significant period of time, it can be assumed that the strain has colonized and is thriving in the bowel.

Because numerous studies have reported the ability of *Streptococcus thermophilus* and *Lactobacillus delbrueckii* subsp. *bulgaricus* in yogurts to enhance lactose digestion in individuals intolerant to lactose, the identity of the individual strains is not considered to be that critical. It is the final product—in this case yogurt—that is important (yogurt is discussed in greater detail below).

The World Health Organization has recommended that each probiotic strain considered for therapeutic use in humans should be investigated for its ability to do the following:[3]

- ▪ Resist destruction by gastric acid
- ▪ Resist destruction by bile acid
- ▪ Adhere to mucous and/or human epithelial cells and cell lines
- ▪ Exert antimicrobial activity against potentially pathogenic bacteria
- ▪ Reduce the adhesion of pathogenic microorganisms to cell surfaces so that they are prevented from becoming established in the digestive tract
- ▪ Cause no harm to the human who consumes it

A thriving industry has developed to manufacture products that contain live microorganisms within a food that will sustain their growth, in the expectation that they will be delivered to the bowel, where they will become established and thrive. At the present time, probiotic bacteria may be delivered to the bowel via the oral route in foods such as yogurts (bioyogurts), fermented milks, fortified fruit juice, infant formulas, cereals, and as supplements such as powders, capsules, tablets, and sprays. Each country tends to have its own regulations on probiotic foods and supplements.

Yogurt

Yogurt is a semisolid fermented milk product that originated centuries ago in Bulgaria. It is now consumed in most parts of the world. Although the consistency, flavor, and aroma may vary from one region to another, the basic ingredients and manufacturing are essentially consistent. Milk of various animals has been used for yogurt production in various countries, but cow's milk is used most frequently in large-scale manufacture. Whole milk, partially skimmed milk, skim milk, or cream may be used to make yogurt. In addition to milk, some manufactured yogurts may contain a variety of additional ingredients, including:

- Other dairy products that increase the nonfat solids content, such as concentrated fat-free milk, nonfat dry milk, whey, or lactose
- Sweeteners, such as glucose, sucrose, or aspartame
- Stabilizers, such as gelatin, carboxymethyl cellulose, locust bean guar gum, alginate, carrageenan, and whey protein concentrate
- Flavors, which may be natural or artificial
- Fruit preparations, including natural and artificial flavoring and color

Most yogurts produced in North America use a symbiotic blend of *Streptococcus salivarius* subsp. *thermophilus* (ST) and *Lactobacillus delbrueckii* subsp. *bulgaricus* (LB). The metabolic products of one strain stimulate the growth of the other. These microorganisms are ultimately responsible for the formation of typical yogurt flavor and texture. The yogurt mixture coagulates during fermentation due to the drop in pH. The streptococci are responsible for the initial pH drop of the yogurt mix to approximately 5. The lactobacilli are responsible for a further decrease to pH 4. The fermentation products that contribute to the flavor of yogurt are lactic acid, acetaldehyde, acetic acid, and diacetyl.

Probiotic yogurts will usually indicate the presence of live microorganisms on the label. The best is plain yogurt, which has only two ingredients: live cultures and milk (whole milk, low-fat, or nonfat). These products should contain at least 100 million (10^8) colony-forming units (CFU) per gram at the time of manufacture. In some highly sweetened yogurts, there are more calories in the sweetener than in the yogurt. The higher the protein and the lower the sugar content, the more actual yogurt in the container.

Those who seek probiotics should avoid yogurts with "heat treated after culturing" on the label. Such yogurt was pasteurized after the microorganisms were added, which defeats its purpose as a probiotic. In addition, pasteurization deactivates the lactase that the microorganisms produced during the manufacturing process. Therefore, two health benefits of yogurt have been completely eliminated by heating. Heat-treating yogurt trades economic gain for nutritional loss. It prolongs the shelf life, but spoils its nutrition and health value. Lactose-intolerant persons who can tolerate yogurt containing live bacteria will not be able to tolerate heat-treated yogurt.

Yogurt-covered products that do not contain live culture include such things as yogurt-covered candies, raisins, nuts, pretzels, and yogurt-containing salad dressings and dips. None of these are of any value as probiotics and should be eaten for their food (and additive) content alone.

Plain yogurt made with only milk and live cultures, with fresh fruit, raisins, nuts, and other tolerated natural foods, is far preferable to "fruit yogurts," which tend to contain several unwanted ingredients, including sugar and additives.

Yogurt can be frozen without destroying the bacteria, so frozen yogurt desserts and frozen yogurt popsicles are acceptable. Dips for vegetables can be made by adding herbs, garlic, and other appropriate natural additions to plain yogurt. For children younger than 2 years, whole milk yogurt rather than that made from fat-free or fat-reduced milk is recommended.

Probiotics for the Milk-Allergic Child

Most of the readily available probiotic products are bacterial cultures in milk, because this is the easiest way to grow probiotic microorganisms and keep them healthy and vigorous while they are delivered to the colon after consumption. However, for children who are allergic to milk, yogurts are not a suitable way of providing the live culture.

An alternative may be one of a variety of probiotics that are also sold in capsule or powdered form as supplements. There are several probiotic supplements on the market, which provide the probiotic and the prebiotic, which allow the organisms to get established in the bowel, together with the nutrients to get them started.

The parents or caregivers of children with milk allergies should be very careful of all probiotic products, because sometimes milk proteins may be included, particularly if the microorganisms have been cultured on a substrate that includes milk, especially casein. This should appear on the label and should be avoided: The casein in such a product may be sufficient to trigger a severe allergic reaction in a very sensitive child.[22]

A few vegetable- or cereal-based probiotic/prebiotic products are being developed that may prove useful in children with milk allergies, but like most of the probiotics, a great deal of research is needed to prove their efficacy in practice. One of these is a probiotic food product containing no milk constituents that was launched in Sweden in 1994. The product is a fermented oatmeal gruel that is mixed in a fruit drink.[23] It contains approximately 5×10^{10} colony-forming units of *L. plantarum* 299v/L. The strain *L. plantarum* 299v originates from the human intestinal mucosa and has been shown in rats to improve the immunological status of the digestive tract lining and reduce mucosal inflammation. The authors of the study claim that *L. plantarum* 299v not only improves the bacterial flora of the intestine but may also regulate the host's immunological defense. To make the fermented cereal gruel more acceptable to consumers, it is usually mixed into a fruit drink.

The Therapeutic Potential of Probiotics in Food Allergies and Intolerances: A Summary of the Current State of Research

In some research studies, several bacterial strains singly or in combination seemed to help prevent eczema in the high-risk infant.[17,19] The probiotic may be administered to pregnant women and to their newborns in an infant formula or to the breastfeeding mother and by spoon to her baby after birth, to continue its effects. Sometimes the probiotic is accompanied by a prebiotic, such as inulin or other fructo-oligosaccharide, which may provide further benefit in allergy management. Yogurt with live cultures of *Streptococcus salivarius* subsp. *thermophilus* and *Lactobacillus delbrueckii* subsp. *bulgaricus* may be of help in reducing the diarrhea and bloating in people with lactose intolerance.

However, there is a need for caution in recommending any of the probiotics outside the research setting at the present level of knowledge. The authors of a 2007 Cochrane review stated that, "There is insufficient evidence to recommend the addition of probiotics to infant feeds for prevention of allergic disease or food hypersensitivity. Although there was a reduction in clinical eczema in infants, this effect was not consistent between studies and caution is advised in view of methodological concerns regarding included studies. Further studies are required to determine whether the findings are reproducible."[14]

At the present time, there is no single food product or supplement that can be unconditionally recommended to the consumer specifically for allergy prevention or management. Furthermore, while some products may list the probiotic strains they contain, there are no laws requiring that labels identify specific strains or amounts of probiotics in a product, so selection of a food product for its specific probiotic is often not possible. Clearly, there is a need for additional large-scale, well-controlled trials to determine how, and if, probiotics are going to be of benefit in allergy prevention or for individuals with established food allergies.[24]

References

1. Thompson WG. Probiotics for irritable bowel syndrome: a light in the darkness? *Eur J Gastroenterol Hepatol.* 2001;13(10):1135-1136.
2. Williams NT. Probiotics. *Am J Health Syst Pharm.* 2010;67(6):449-458.
3. Food and Agriculture Organization of the United Nations, World Health Organization. *Guidelines for the Evaluation of Probiotics in Food.* London, ON: Food and Agriculture Organization of the United Nations and World Health Organization; 2002. www.who .int/foodsafety/fs_management/en/probiotic_guidelines.pdf. Accessed July 11, 2012.
4. Shanahan F. Therapeutic manipulation of gut flora. *Science.* 2000;289:1311-1312.
5. Rastall RA, Maitin V. Prebiotics and synbiotics: towards the next generation. *Curr Opin Biotechnol.* 2002;13(5):490-496.
6. Johannsen H, Prescott SL. Practical prebiotics, probiotics and synbiotics for allergists: how useful are they? *Clin Exper Allergy.* 2009;39(12):1801-1814.
7. de Vrese M, Stegelmann A, Richter B, Fenselau S, Laue C, Schrezenmeir J. Probiotics— compensation for lactase insufficiency. *Am J Clin Nutr.* 2001;73(suppl):421S-429S.
8. Johnston BC, Supina AL, Ospina M, Vohra S. Probiotics for the prevention of pediatric antibiotic-associated diarrhea. *Cochrane Database Syst Rev.* 2007;(2):CD004827.
9. Hojsak I, Snovak N, Abdović S, Szajewska H, Mišak Z, Kolače S. Lactobacillus GG in the prevention of gastrointestinal and respiratory tract infections in children who attend day care centres: a randomized, double-blind, placebo-controlled trial. *Clin Nutr.* 2010;29(3):312-316.
10. Bjorksten B, Sepp E, Judge K, et al. Allergy development and the intestinal microflora during the first year of life. *J Allergy Clin Immunol.* 2001;108:516-520.
11. Furrie E. Probiotics and allergy. *Proc Nutr Soc.* 2005;64(4):465-469.
12. Ozdemir O. Various effects of different probiotic strains in allergic disorders: an update from laboratory and clinical data. *Clin Exper Immunol.* 2010;160(3):295-304.
13. Murch SH. Probiotics as mainstream allergy therapy? *Arch Dis Child.* 2005;90:881-882.

14. Osborn DA, Sinn JKH. Probiotics in infants for prevention of allergic disease and food hypersensitivity. *Cochrane Database Syst Rev.* 2007;(4):CD006475.

15. Kalliomaki M, Salminen S, Poussa T, et al. Probiotics and prevention of atopic disease: 4-year follow-up of a randomized placebo-controlled trial. *Lancet.* 2003;361:1869-1871.

16. Majamaa H, Isolauri E. Probiotics: a novel approach in the management of food allergy. *J Allergy Clin Immunol.* 1997;99(2):179-185.

17. Soh SE, Aw M, Gerez I, et al. Probiotic supplementation in the first 6 months of life in at risk Asian infants—effects on eczema and atopic sensitization at the age of 1 year. *Clin Exper Allergy.* 2009;39(4):571-578.

18. Brouwer ML, Wolt-Plompen SA, Dubois AE, et al. No effects of probiotics on atopic dermatitis in infants: a randomized controlled trial. *Clin Exper Allergy.* 2006;36(7):899-906.

19. West CE, Hammarström ML, Hernell O. Probiotics during weaning reduce the incidence of eczema. *Pediatr Allergy Immunol.* 2009;20(5):430-437.

20. Williams NT. Probiotics. *Am J Health Syst Pharm.* 2010;67(6):449-458.

21. Johannsen H, Prescott SL. Practical prebiotics, probiotics and synbiotics for allergists: how useful are they? *Clin Exper Allergy.* 2009;39(12):1801-1814.

22. Moneret-Vautrin DA, Morisset M, Cordebar V, Codreanu F, Kanny G. Probiotics may be unsafe in infants allergic to cow's milk. *Allergy.* 2006;61(4):506-508.

23. Molin G. Probiotics in foods not containing milk or milk constituents, with special reference to *Lactobacillus plantarum* 299v. *Am J Clin Nutr.* 2001;73(2):380S-385S.

24. Gourbeyre P, Denery S, Bodinier M. Probiotics, prebiotics, and synbiotics: impact on the gut immune system and allergic reactions. *J Leukoc Biol.* 2011;89(5):685-695.

Glossary

acetylcholine: Neurotransmitter released at the synapses of the parasympathetic nerves and at neuromuscular junctions. It relays nerve impulses.

acidosis: Accumulation of acid or depletion of alkali (bicarbonate) in the blood and body tissues.

adrenaline: *See* epinephrine.

aerosol: Suspension of solid or liquid particle in a gas.

albumin: A type of protein classified on the basis of its solubility. Albumins are soluble in water at pH 6.6 (*see also* globulins; prolamins; glutenins). Albumins occur in different forms according to their function (eg, serum albumin in animals and humans, ovalbumin in eggs, parvalbumin in fish, α-lactalbumin in milk).

allergen: Antigen or hapten that causes a hypersensitivity reaction (allergy) in a sensitized individual.

allergen overload: A term used by allergists to indicate an excessive amount of antigen that in theory may result in a large volume of antigen entering circulation and triggering an immunological response when a lower quantity of antigen may be tolerated.

allergy: Hypersensitivity to an environmental, drug, or food antigen (allergen) caused by an altered or unusual immunological reaction to the antigen.

amino acid: Organic compound containing amino (nitrogen-hydrogen) and carboxyl (carbon-oxygen) groups. Amino acids are the building blocks of all proteins.

anamnestic response: Rapid production of antibody in response to an antigen subsequent to a first exposure, as in natural reinfection or a booster shot of vaccine. Requires the presence of memory B and T cells remaining from the first exposure.

anaphylactic reaction (anaphylaxis): Type 1 hypersensitivity reaction (allergy) due to the release of chemical mediators from cells caused to degranulate by complexing of antibody (usually IgE) with its homologous allergen.

anaphylactic shock: Acute generalized anaphylaxis in which edema; constriction of smooth muscles in the lungs, stomach, and blood vessels; a fall in blood pressure; circulatory collapse; and heart failure can lead to death.

anaphylactoid reaction: Reaction with anaphylactic symptoms not induced by an antigen-antibody complex.

anaphylatoxin: Substance produced during a complement cascade (specifically by complement components C3a and C5a) that causes the release of histamine and other vasoactive chemicals from mast cells and basophils.

anaphylaxis: *See* anaphylactic reactions.

angioedema: Localized swelling in tissues below the surface of the skin or mucous membrane caused by increased permeability of the capillaries from which fluid moves into the tissues to cause the swelling (edema).

antibiotic: Substance produced by microorganisms that can kill or inhibit the growth of other microorganisms by interfering with their metabolism.

antibody: Protein of the gamma-globulin type (immunoglobulin) produced by lymphocytes in the blood in response to a foreign antigen. Humans produce five types of antibodies, called IgA, IgD, IgE, IgG, and IgM.

antiendomysial antibody: IgA antibody detected in celiac disease. The presence of antiendomyssial antibody in a test is an indicator of active celiac disease. The antigen involved in eliciting the antibody has been identified as tissue transglutaminase (tTG).

antigen: Foreign substance that induces the production of specific (homologous) antibody by the immune system of the host it enters.

antigen determinant site: Part of an antigen's molecular structure that induces the production of antibody. Each cell has several different antigen determinant sites.

antigen processing: Display of antigens on the surface of a macrophage that has engulfed and partially degraded them, a preconditioning for recognition and a protective response by T cells.

antihistamine: Drug that inhibits the action of histamine (eg, chlorpheniramine, diphenhydramine, and mepyramine) and is widely used to treat hypersensitivity reactions in which histamine is the main cause of symptoms such as hay fever urticaria (hives) and pruritus (itching).

antiserum: Fluid portion (serum) of blood containing antibodies to specific known antigens. Used in diagnostic serology to identify unknown antigens and in passive immunization to transfer temporary immunity against a pathogenic microorganism.

antitoxin: Antiserum containing antibodies against a toxin or toxoid.

arachidonic acid: Polyunsaturated fatty acid component of membrane phospholipids. Tissue disruption by any cause, especially immunological mechanisms, allows enzymes to separate arachidonic acid from the phospholipid to be metabolized into a large number of chemicals (known as *eicosanoids*), such as prostaglandins and leukotrienes that contribute to an inflammatory response.

arthralgia: Pain in a joint.

atopic dermatitis: A chronic inflammatory skin disorder seen in individuals with allergy (atopy). Also called *allergic dermatitis, allergic eczema,* or *atopic eczema.*

atopy, atopic allergy: IgE-mediated hypersensitivity reaction with rapid onset of symptoms.

autoantigen: Antigen that is part of the body's own cells and induces the production of autoantibody, often leading to autoimmune disease.

autoimmunity: Production of antibodies against antigens of the body's own tissues. Often leads to autoimmune disease and tissue damage.

avirulent: Describes a strain of microorganism that cannot cause disease.

azo-: Prefix denoting a nitrogenous compound, as in the azo dye tartrazine.

basophil: White blood cell containing granules that stain with basic (alkaline) dyes. Degranulation in hypersensitivity reactions releases mediators of the allergic response.

B cell: Lymphocyte that produces antibodies in response to a specific antigen.

bifurcated: Having two branches; forked.

biogenic amines: Biologically active derivatives of amino acids that play a role in neural functioning. The most well known include histamine, tyramine, serotonin, dopamine, and acetylcholine.

biopsy: Removal of living tissue from a body site and examination, usually under a microscope, to establish a precise diagnosis.

bradykinin: Vasoactive peptide, released during a hypersensitivity reaction, that causes pain, dilation of blood vessels, edema, and smooth muscle contraction.

bronchitis: Inflammation of lung passages (bronchi) caused by infection with a microorganism or other agents that damage the bronchial lining.

bronchoconstriction: Narrowing of the bronchi by contraction of their smooth muscle sheath.

bronchodilation: Opening of the bronchi by relaxation of their smooth muscle coating.

bronchospasm: Narrowing of the bronchi due to spasmodic contraction of their smooth muscle sheath, caused by some stimulus. Usually allows air to be inhaled but requires great effort to expel it effectively. Occurs in such conditions as asthma and bronchitis.

bronchus (*pl.* bronchi): Air passages in the lungs that branch off from the trachea (windpipe), lined with mucus-secreting cells and sheathed with smooth muscle.

brush border cells: Cells in the epithelium lining the digestive tract. The name is derived from the appearance of the cells that results from the numerous appendages, called *villi* (sing. villus), projecting from their surfaces, giving the impression of a brush. The villi increase the surface area available for absorption of nutrients.

carbohydrates: Compounds containing carbon, hydrogen, and oxygen with the general formula $C_x(H_2O)_y$. They are one of the three main constituents of food (protein and fat are the others) and include the sugars and starches. They are an important source of energy in cellular metabolism. Carbohydrates constitute three-quarters of the biological world and about 80% of the caloric intake of humans. The most abundant carbohydrate is cellulose, the principal constituent of trees and other plants; the major food carbohydrate is starch.

catecholamine: A compound composed of catechol and an amine that conveys messages within the sympathetic nervous system. Types include dopamine, epinephrine (adrenaline), and norepinephrine (noradrenaline).

celiac disease: Gluten-sensitive enteropathy. A chronic intestinal disorder characterized by malabsorption of nutrients, caused by an immunologically mediated sensitivity to gluten.

chemotaxin: Chemical that promotes movement of a cell or microorganism toward a target in the process of chemotaxis.

chemotaxis: Movement of a cell or microorganism toward a target in response to a concentration gradient of a chemical known as a *chemotaxin.*

chitin: A white, insoluble, horny polysaccharide. Next to cellulose, it is the most abundant natural polysaccharide.

chitinase: An enzyme that hydrolyzes chitin to produce a linear homopolymer acetyl glucosamine.

cholinergic: Describes nerve fibers that release the neurotransmitter acetylcholine.

colostrum: First secretion from the breast after childbirth. Contains serum, protein nutrients, antibodies, lymphocytes, and macrophages.

complement: Group of over 20 enzymatic proteins in the blood that act together, in response to antigen and antibody, to destroy foreign cells by lysis.

complement cascade: Sequential activation of complement proteins resulting in lysis of a target cell. The cascade releases various chemical by-products that act as opsonins, chemotaxins, and anaphylatoxins to help destroy a threat to the body.

conjunctiva: Membrane covering the front of the eye and lining the eyelids.

conjunctivitis: Inflammation of the conjunctivae, causing redness, swelling, and a watery discharge.

cross-reacting allergens: A rather loose term that indicates that a person sensitized to one allergen will react to another allergen related to the first, either because it is from the same botanic family or is structurally very similar.

cyto-: Prefix denoting cell.

cytokines: Collective name for lymphokines and monokines (eg, the interleukins and interferons), peptides produced by immune system cells such as lymphocytes and macrophages and involved in sending signals between cells.

cytolysis: Destruction (lysis) of a cell, usually by disruption of its membrane and other outer structures.

cytotoxic; cytotoxicity: Mechanism that causes destruction of cells.

dalton: Atomic mass unit, equal to 1.6605×10^{-27} kg; $\frac{1}{12}$th the mass of an atom of carbon 12. The molecular weight of molecules is measured in daltons. A kilodalton (kDa) is 1,000 daltons.

DBPCFC: Double-blind placebo-controlled food challenge.

decarboxylase: An enzyme that catalyzes the removal of a molecule of carbon dioxide from a carboxylic group.

decarboxylation: Removal of a carboxyl group from a substrate chemical in the body by an enzyme called a *decarboxylase.*

degranulation: Release of chemicals from the intracellular granules of leukocytes in the process of inflammation.

dermatitis: Inflammation of the skin.

dermatographism: Skin reaction in response to moderately firm stroking or scratching with a dull instrument. The reaction appears as a pale raised welt or wheal, with a red flare on each side.

double-blind placebo-controlled food challenge: Provocation test in which the identity of the food to be challenged is unknown to both the patient and the supervisor of the test. A placebo is similarly concealed and the response to the food is compared to the response to the placebo. A positive test is the appearance of symptoms after consumption of the food, with no symptoms in response to the placebo.

eicosanoids: Collective name for chemicals derived from eicosanoic acid (a fatty acid with a 20-carbon chain), such as leukotrienes, prostaglandins, and thromboxanes.

ELISA: Enzyme-linked immunosorbent assay.

endo-: Prefix denoting *inside*. For example, *endogenous* means originating from inside an organism or body.

endocrine system: System of ductless glands and other structures, including the pituitary, thyroid, parathyroid, and adrenal glands; the ovaries, testes, and placenta; part of the pancreas; and the hormones they secrete internally and release into the bloodstream.

endorphins: Chemicals in the brain derived from beta-lipotropin, produced by the pituitary gland. Endorphins appear to influence the activities of the endocrine glands and have pain-relieving properties similar to those of the opiates.

endotoxin: Lipopolysaccharide that is part of the cell wall of Gram-negative bacteria, liberated only when the bacteria disintegrate. Endotoxins are responsible for the fever, gastrointestinal disorder, and shock of infections caused by pathogenic enterobacteria such as salmonella and shigella.

enteritis: Inflammation of the small intestine.

enterocolitis: Inflammation involving both the small intestine and the colon.

enteropathy: A general term that refers to any disease of the intestine.

enzyme: Protein produced by a living organism that catalyzes a biological reaction without itself being affected. Enzymes are essential for the normal functioning of the body.

enzyme-linked immunosorbent assay: Immunological test for identification of antigen-specific antibody in blood serum. Usually used to identify IgE or IgG antibodies to allergens. The "indicator system" for positive reactions is antibody linked to an enzyme, which acts on the enzyme substrate to form a product that is usually indicated by a change in color.

eosinophil: Granulocytic white blood cell whose granules stain with acidic dyes such as eosin. Eosinophils help defend the body against parasites and contribute to allergic reactions.

eosinophilic esophagitis: Esophagitis characterized by the presence of eosinophils in the esophagus, where normally none are found.

epinephrine (adrenaline): Hormone, secreted by the adrenal gland that prepares the body for "fight or flight." It has an important role in the control of blood circulation, muscle action, and sugar metabolism.

epitope: A single antigenic determinant. Functionally it is the portion of an antigen that combines with the antibody, at a site called the *paratope*.

erythema: Abnormal reddening of the skin caused by dilation of small blood vessels.

erythrocyte: Red blood cell. Its color comes from hemoglobin, which transports oxygen around the body.

esophagitis: Inflammation of the esophagus, the muscular tube that connects the mouth to the stomach.

estrogens: Steroid hormones, such as estrone, and estradiol that are produced mainly in the ovaries and control female sexual development.

etiology: Study of the cause of disease.

exo-: Prefix denoting *outside*. For example, exogenous means originating outside the organism or body.

exotoxins: Soluble toxic proteins, secreted by bacteria, that cause a variety of life-threatening diseases, including botulism, gas gangrene, tetanus, and diphtheria. Exotoxins are among the most poisonous substances known.

FAST: Fluorescence allergosorbent test. Immunoassay to identify allergens in which the indicator reagent is a derivative of fluorescein that emits polarized light.

fat: Chemical composed of one or more fatty acids and the principal form in which energy is stored in the body.

folic acid, folacin: Vitamin of the B complex that is an essential component in many major metabolic reactions in the body. Folate is a form of folic acid.

fructo-oligosaccharide (FOS): Sometimes called *oligofructose* or *oligofructan*. Oligosaccahride is a short chain of sugar molecules; in the case of FOS, fructose molecules (oligo = few; saccharide = sugar). FOS is not digestible by human enzymes and passes unchanged into the large bowel, where it acts as a substrate for microbial activities.

galactose: A hexose sugar consisting of a chain of 6 carbon atoms combined with oxygen and hydrogen in a structure indicated by the formula $CH_2OH(CHOH)_4CHO$. The major source of galactose is milk, where it is found combined with glucose in a 1-to-1 ratio to form lactose. Other food sources of galactose include sugar beet, several gums, seaweeds, and flax seed mucilage.

galactosemia: Refers to three types of genetic (inherited) disorders resulting from defective metabolism of galactose.

GALT: Gut-associated lymphoid tissue. Includes the tonsils, Peyer's patches, lamina propria of the intestine, and appendix.

gamma globulins: Blood proteins, rich in antibodies, that move in the "gamma" region in electrophoreses. Includes the five classes of immunoglobulin found in humans (IgA, IgG, IgM, IgD, IgE).

gliadin: An alcohol-soluble protein component of wheat and other gluten-containing grains. Several forms of gliadin occur in wheat; alpha-gliadin is the fraction most frequently associated with celiac disease.

globulin: Type of protein classified according to its solubility. Globulins (eg, β-lactoglobulin in milk) are soluble in dilute salt solutions at pH 7.

glucan: Polymer of glucose, often formed by the breakdown of sucrose by streptococci, especially *Streptococcus mutans*, in the mouth.

gluco-oligosaccharide (GOS): Also known as oligoglucan. A short chain of glucose molecules (gluco = glucose; saccharide = sugar). GOS is not broken down by human digestive enzymes and passes into the colon unchanged. There it acts as a substrate for microbial activities and growth.

gluten: A protein that is found in the endosperm of some cereal grains, especially wheat, rye, and barley, combined with starch. It is composed of gliadins and glutenins. Gluten makes up to 80% of the proteins in wheat. It is responsible for the elasticity of kneaded dough, which allows leavening (rising) with yeast and gives the "chewy" texture to baked products such as bagels.

glutenin: A protein classified on the basis of its solubility in acids (pH 2) or alkalis (pH 12); insoluble in water or ethanol. Glutenins are major proteins in wheat and other grains.

glyco-: Prefix denoting the combination of a sugar molecule (often glucose or galactose) with another type of chemical. For example, *glycoprotein* means sugar combined with a protein; *glycolipid* is a sugar combined with a lipid (fat) molecule.

glycogen: The main form of carbohydrate storage material in animals. It is a long chain of glucose molecules that is formed in and mainly stored in the liver and to a lesser extent in muscles.

granulocyte: White blood cell with a lobed nucleus, characterized by numerous granules within its cytoplasm (*see* polymorphonuclear granulocyte).

growth hormone (somatotropin): Hormone secreted by the pituitary gland that controls growth of the long bones and promotes protein synthesis.

hapten: Molecule too small to be an antigen by itself that induces the production of antibody when combined with an antigen or a body protein. The resulting complex is sometimes referred to as a *neoantigen*.

heme iron: A chelate of iron that forms part of the hemoglobin molecule. It is the form of iron that is found in animal tissues.

heparin: Anticoagulant chemical that inhibits the enzyme thrombin in the final stage of blood coagulation. Various cells, including white blood cells, produce it predominantly in the liver and lungs.

histamine: Chemical derivative of the amino acid histidine. It is produced in all body tissues, especially by mast cells. An important mediator of inflammation, it causes contraction of smooth muscle and increases the permeability of small blood vessels. It is the principal mediator of the wheal-and-flare skin reaction.

homologous: Means "the same." Describes the relationship between an antigen and the specific antibody whose production it induces.

hormone: Chemical produced by the body (eg, by the endocrine glands) that circulates in the bloodstream and has a specific regulatory effect on certain cells or organs.

human leukocyte antigens (HLAs): Antigens on the surface of body cells, coded for the major histocompatibility complex (MHC) and unique to the individual. They allow the immune system to recognize self and nonself.

hydrolase: Class of enzymes that catalyze the addition of the elements of water to a substance, thereby breaking it into two products.

hydrolysis: The process by which a molecule is broken apart with the addition of water. The process occurs under the influence of enzymes, known as *hydrolases*.

hyper-: Prefix indicating excessive, more, or above normal; for example, in hyperactivity, hypersensitivity, hyperresponsive, and hypertension (high blood pressure).

hypo-: Prefix indicating deficiency, less, or below normal; for example, in hyposensitive, hyporeactive, and hypotension (low blood pressure).

hypolipoproteinemia: Disease characterized by abnormally low levels of lipoproteins in blood serum.

IBS: Irritable bowel syndrome. A chronic noninflammatory disease characterized by abdominal pain, altered bowel habits consisting of diarrhea or constipation or both, with no detectable pathology. Also called *spastic bowel* or *spastic colon*.

idiopathic: Disease of unknown cause.

immunity: Resistance to a disease.

immunoglobulin (Ig): Glycoprotein that functions as antibody. The five classes (IgA, IgD, IgE, IgG, and IgM) differ in the structure of their polypeptide heavy chains. Immunoglobulins make up gamma globulin; all antibodies are immunoglobulins.

inflammatory mediators: Bioactive chemicals released in a defensive immunological response to an antigen that act on body tissues to produce symptoms of inflammation. In an allergic reaction, the inflammation results in symptoms typical of the allergy. Histamine, leukotrienes, prostaglandins, chemotaxins, and several enzymes are typical inflammatory mediators.

inter-: Prefix indicating *between*; for example, in intercellular (between cells).

interferons: Cytokines typically produced by cells infected with viruses. The known interferons (alpha, beta, and gamma) play a variety of roles in immunity, particularly the inhibition of viral multiplication. Usually written as *INF-* followed by the identifying Greek letter of the specific cytokine (eg, INF-α; INF-γ, etc.).

interleukins: Cytokines, produced principally by macrophages and T cells, act as signals in controlling various stages of the immune response. Usually written as *IL-* followed by the number that identifies the specific cytokine (eg, IL–1, IL–2, IL–4, and so on).

intra-: Prefix indicating *inside* or *within*; for example, in intracellular (inside a cell), intracytoplasmic (within the cytoplasm).

inulin: A group of oligosaccharides (a short chain of sugars) that are typically found in roots or rhizomes, where they are a means of storing energy (instead of the usual starch). They belong to the class of carbohydrates known as fructans, which are classified as soluble fiber.

in vitro: In glass. Describes biological activity made to occur outside a living body, usually under experimental conditions in a laboratory.

in vivo: In life. Describes biological activity within a living body.

kDa: Kilodalton: one thousand daltons.

ketone or ketone bodies: A class of organic compounds with a specific structure (the carbon atom of a carbonyl group [C=O] is attached to two other carbon atoms) that form as a result of unusual metabolic events in the body. Their presence is often indicative of a pathological condition.

lactoferrin: Iron-containing compound, present in secretions such as milk, that has a slight antimicrobial action due to its ability to bind the iron required by the microorganism.

lactose (milk sugar): A carbohydrate (disaccharide), present in milk that is metabolized by the body into glucose and galactose.

leaky gut: A descriptive term used to indicate a situation in which fluids and solids move more readily through the lining of the digestive tract. Usually results from inflammation caused by infection, allergy, or other insults to the epithelium. Synonymous with hyperpermeable digestive tract membrane.

leukemia: A progressive malignant disease characterized by distorted proliferation and development of leukocytes and their precursors in the blood and bone marrow.

leukocytes: White blood cells that defend the body against disease. Classified into three major types: granulocytes, monocytes, and lymphocytes.

leukotrienes: Hormonelike chemicals derived from precursor fatty acids, such as arachidonic acid, via the lipoxygenase pathway. Contribute to inflammatory and allergic reactions as powerful chemotaxins, and some cause constriction of smooth muscle.

lipids: Organic substances, including fats, steroids, phospholipids, and glycolipids, important as cell constituents and a source of energy and certain vitamins and essential fatty acids.

lipo-: Prefix denoting fat or lipid.

lipopolysaccharide: Molecule composed of a fatty acid (lipo-) and a sugar (-polysaccharide); for example, the endotoxin in the cell walls of Gram-negative bacteria that causes the symptoms of many intestinal infections.

lupus: Usual designation for lupus erythematosus: a group of connective tissue disorders usually resulting from an autoimmune process.

lymph: Transparent fluid in the lymphatic system that bathes body tissues. Similar in composition to blood plasma but with less protein and some lymphocytes.

lymphatic system: Network of vessels that convey lymph from body tissues to the bloodstream. Pathway for exchange of electrolytes, water, proteins, and other chemicals between the bloodstream and body tissues.

lymphocytes: White blood cells that mature within the lymphatic system. Classified as B and T cells, essential in immunity.

lymph nodes (glands): Small swellings, distributed in groups over the lymphatic system, that filter lymph and prevent foreign particles from entering the bloodstream. Most noticeable in the groin, armpit, and behind the ear.

lymphoid tissue: A lattice-work of reticular tissue in the interstices of which contain lymphocytes; lymphoid tissue may be diffuse or densely aggregated into lymph nodes and nodules.

lymphokines: Chemicals produced by lymphocytes that act as control signals between cells of the immune system. Commonly grouped under the general heading *cytokines.*

lymphoma: A progressive multiplication of cells that would interfere with the multiplication of normal cells of the lymphoid tissue.

lysis: Destruction of a cell by disruption of its membrane and outer structures, allowing cell contents to escape.

macrophages: Large phagocytes, closely related to monocytes, present in many organ systems such as connective tissue, bone marrow, spleen, lymph nodes, liver, and the central nervous system. Fixed macrophages (histiocytes) are stationary; wandering macrophages move freely and aggregate at the site of infection or trauma, where they remove foreign microorganisms and damaged tissue by phagocytosis.

major histocompatibility complex (MHC): Genes located on chromosome 6 and encoded for the human leukocyte antigens (HLAs), present on all body cells, that distinguish self from nonself. Their products are primarily responsible for the rapid rejection of grafts between individuals. The function of the products of the MHC is signaling between lymphocytes and cells expressing antigens.

MALT: Mucosa-associated lymphoid tissue. Term for lymphoid tissue associated with any mucous membrane–lined organs such as the bronchial tree, urogenital tract, etc.

mast cell: Large white blood cell, fixed within body tissue and characterized by numerous granules within its cytoplasm. The granules contain chemicals such as histamine, heparin, and enzymes released during an inflammatory or allergic reaction.

metabolic pathway: Series of reactions whereby enzymes transform organic molecules.

metabolism: Sum of the chemical and physical processes by which nutrients are converted into body tissue and energy. Includes catabolism (destruction) and anabolism (construction).

MHC: Major histocompatibility complex.

monocytes: Single-nucleus, granulocytic white blood cells that phagocytose foreign particle such as bacteria, viruses, and dead body cells.

mucus: Viscous fluid, composed largely of glycoproteins, secreted by mucous membranes lining many body organs, such as the respiratory, gastrointestinal, and urogenital tracts.

natural killer (NK) cell: Lymphocyte that destroys foreign cells, particularly aberrant cancer cells, apparently by releasing digestive enzymes that perforate the cells' membranes and cause cell contents to leak out.

neuropeptide: Peptide with significant effects on the nervous system, but not, strictly speaking, a neurotransmitter. Neuropeptides include the encephalins, endorphins, somatostatin, substance P, thyrotropin-releasing hormone (TRH), and luteinizing hormone–releasing hormone (LHRH).

neurotoxin: Nerve poison.

neurotransmitter: Complex chemical substance—for example, acetylcholine, norepinephrine, dopamine, and serotonin—that transmits signals across the synapses between nerve cells and across the minute gaps between nerves and the muscles or glands they control.

neutrophil: Granulocytic white blood cell containing a lobed nucleus and numerous granules within its cytoplasm that stain with neutral dyes. A powerful phagocyte that removes microorganisms and other foreign particles by phagocytosis.

norepinephrine: Hormone produced by the adrenal gland and also released as a neurotransmitter from nerve fibers of the sympathetic nervous system. Its actions include constriction and relaxation of smooth muscles (especially in blood vessels and intestinal walls), regulation of heart rate, and an influence on rate and depth of breathing.

OAS: Oral allergy syndrome.

oligo-: Prefix meaning *a few*, *little*, or *scanty*; deficient or less than normal.

oligoantigenic diet: A diet consisting of only a few antigenic foods; "few foods diet."

opsonins: Components of the immune system that facilitate attachment of antigen to the surface of phagocytes. Opsonins are antibodies and the C3b component of complement.

opsonization: Process by which opsonins aid attachment of antigen to the surface of a phagocyte.

oral allergy syndrome: A complex of clinical symptoms (eg, itching, swelling of lips and tongue, or blistering) in the mucosa of the mouth and throat that result from direct contact with food allergens in a sensitized individual who also exhibits respiratory allergy to inhaled allergens, usually tree, grass, or weed pollens (pollinosis).

ovalbumin: A major protein in eggs classified as an albumin on the basis of its solubility in water at pH 6.6.

panallergen: A term given to an antigenic protein that has an essential function or forms a structure in several different plants or animals. A person sensitized to a panallergen is likely to react to any of the foods containing the protein, regardless of their botanic or zoological relatedness. Parvalbumin in fish and certain lipid transfer proteins and pathogenesis-related proteins in plants are examples of panallergens.

parasite: Organism that lives in or on another living thing (the host), receiving food and shelter but contributing nothing to its host's welfare and potentially causing harm. Human parasites include bacteria, viruses, fungi, protozoa, and worms.

parvalbumin: A major protein in fish classified as an albumin on the basis of its solubility in water at pH 6.6.

pathogen: Microorganism that causes disease.

pathogenesis-related proteins (PRs): Proteins that are induced by pathogens, wounding, or certain environmental stresses in plants. PRs are presently classified into 14 distinct families of proteins, and include chitinases, antifungal proteins, lipid transfer proteins, inhibitors of alpha-amylases and trypsin, profilins, and proteases, among others.

peak flow meter: A measuring device, usually held in the hand, that measures the amount of air expelled from the lungs in a forced exhalation.

peptide: Chain of two or more amino acids linked together by peptide bonds between the end amino group of one amino acid and the beginning carboxyl group of the next. Peptides joined together form a protein.

phagocyte: White blood cell that is able to engulf and digest microorganisms, cells, cell debris, and other small particles.

phagocytosis: Process of engulfment and digestion of microorganisms and other small foreign particles by phagocytes.

phenylketonuria: A genetic (inherited) disease resulting from deficiency in the enzyme phenylalanine hydroxylase required to metabolize phenylalanine, an amino acid in many proteins. Management is a diet very low in phenylalanine. The diet prevents the neurological damage that can occur if the condition remains untreated.

plasma: Fluid portion of blood in which blood cells are suspended.

plasma cell: Cell, derived from a B cell that produces antibody.

platelet (thrombocyte): Disk-shaped blood cell principally involved in coagulation.

platelet activating factor (PAF): Phospholipid produced by leukocytes that causes aggregation of platelets and other effects such as an increase in vascular permeability and bronchoconstriction. Also acts on various other cells. Active form is known as *PAF-acether*.

polymorphonuclear granulocyte (polymorph, granulocyte): White blood cell distinguished by a lobed nucleus and fine granules within its cytoplasm. Classified according to the type of stain absorbed by the granules.

polysaccharide: Carbohydrate composed of monosaccharides (sugar molecules) joined together in chains.

prebiotic: The nutritional substrate on which probiotic microorganisms will grow and produce the by-products that give the food its health benefit. Usually consists of nondigestible fiber.

probiotic: A culture of living microorganisms within a food designed to provide health benefits beyond the food's inherent nutritional value.

profilins: Actin-regulatory proteins. Profilins are ubiquitous in plants and are usually associated with reproductive processes.

prolactin: Hormone secreted by the pituitary gland that stimulates milk production after childbirth and production of progesterone in the ovaries.

prolamins: Proteins usually found in plants, classified on the basis of their solubility in 70% ethanol. Zein and gliadin are examples of major plant proteins of the prolamin class.

prostacyclin: Hormonelike chemical related to the prostaglandins.

prostaglandins: Group of hormonelike chemicals derived from precursor fatty acids, such as arachidonic acid, by the cyclooxygenase pathway. They have many important controlling functions in the body, including smooth muscle contraction and relaxation.

proteins: Organic substances, composed of chains of amino acids linked by peptide bonds, essential as structural components of body cells and of regulators of function such as enzymes and hormones. One of the three main dietary constituents of food.

pruritus: Itching.

purpura: A small (less than 1 cm) hemorrhage in the skin or mucous membrane that may be caused by various factors such as blood disorders, abnormalities of blood vessels, and trauma.

pyogenic: Pus forming; for example, in pyogenic microorganism.

pyrogen: Substance that produces fever.

RAST: Radioallergosorbent test. Technique for measuring allergen-specific antibody in serum using radiolabeled reagents. Usually used to measure allergen-specific IgE or IgG.

receptor: Molecule on the surface of a cell that provides a selective attachment site for a particular substance, usually a protein.

reticulin: A protein derived from the fibers of reticular (netlike) connective tissue.

reticuloendothelial system (RES): Aggregates of phagocytes (monocytes and macrophages) spread throughout body tissues.

rhinitis: Inflammation of the mucous membrane lining the nose.

rhino-: Prefix meaning *nose*.

rhinorrhea: Runny nose with watery discharge characteristic of the common cold.

scarifier: An instrument with sharp points used to scratch or puncture the skin (hence, *scarify*, *scarification*), usually for introduction of a vaccine or skin test reagent.

secretory IgA (sIgA): A specific type of human antibody that is found in mucous secretions. It differs from serum IgA (written simply as IgA) in having an additional secretory piece that protects the antibody from acid and digestive enzymes, so it remains active, and protective, along the length of the alimentary canal.

sensitization: Alteration of a body's responsiveness to a foreign substance, usually an allergen. The immune system produces antibody to the allergen without symptoms on first exposure. Subsequent exposure releases more of the antibody and induces an allergic reaction.

serologically related: Applied to antigens; indicates that antigens have been demonstrated to be related because they react with the same antibody.

serological reactions: Serological tests.

serological tests: Immunological techniques to identify antigen-specific antibodies in serum.

serology: Study of serum, especially of constituents, such as antibodies and complement, involved in the body's defense against disease.

serum: Fluid portion of blood remaining after separation from clotted blood or clotted blood plasma. Similar to plasma but lacks fibrinogen and other coagulatory components.

somatostatin: Hormone that inhibits the secretion of growth hormone by the pituitary gland.

spirometer: An instrument used for measuring the amount of air taken into and expelled from the lungs.

synapse: Gap between nerve fibers across which neurotransmitters carry impulses from one nerve cell to the next.

synbiotic: The combination of probiotic microorganisms with their specifically designed prebiotic nutrient source.

synergism: Cooperative interaction between two systems that produces a greater effect than the sum of two systems acting alone.

T cells: Specialized lymphocytes that produce cytokines and participate in all functions of the immune system.

thrombocyte: *See* platelet.

thrombocytopenic purpura: A form of purpura in which the platelet count is decreased.

thymus: Organ at the base of the neck whose principal function appears to be the maturation of lymphocytes into T cells.

titer: Measure of the amount of antibodies in serum.

transglutaminase: One of a family of enzymes that catalyze the formation of a bond between proteins; the bond occurs between a free amino acid; for example, lysine on one molecule and a glutamine on the other. The enzyme is important in celiac disease because IgA antibodies formed against it are characteristic of the disease, and detection of these antibodies in a laboratory test (anti-transglutaminase test) is a sign of active disease.

urticaria (hives): Itchy rash with round red wheals ranging in size from small spots to large patches several inches in diameter.

urticarial vasculitis: Inflammation of a blood vessel associated with urticaria.

vascular: Relating to blood vessels.

vascular system: Network of blood vessels that circulates blood throughout the body.

vaso-: Prefix meaning *vessel*, especially relating to blood vessels.

vasoactive amine: Chemical (amine) that acts on smooth muscle, especially surrounding blood vessels, increasing or decreasing their diameter.

vasoconstriction: Decrease in the diameter of blood vessels, causing an increase in blood pressure, due to contraction of the muscles in their walls.

vasodilation: Increase in the diameter of blood vessels as a result of relaxation of the muscles surrounding the vessels, leading to an increase in blood flow and a decrease in blood pressure.

villus (*pl.* villi): A small projection from a cell that is part of a membrane. Intestinal villi are threadlike projections that cover the surface of the mucous membrane of the small intestine and absorb fluids and nutrients.

viral exanthem: Skin eruption or rash associated with a viral infection.

virulence: Measure of the disease-producing ability of a microorganism. Includes factors such as the organism's ability to invade the host, to evade the host's immune defenses, and to cause damage to the host's tissues.

wheal: Smooth, slightly elevated area on the skin, paler or redder than the surrounding area. Caused by the release of histamine and its action on the local tissues. The area is often itchy, and the wheal may change in size and shape. Usually disappears within a few hours.

wheal and flare: A positive response to a skin test. The wheal is a central "blister" that is surrounded by a flat reddened area (the flare). The reaction is caused by the release of histamine and other inflammatory mediators from mast cells in the skin in response to the application of the matching (homologous) antigen (allergen) applied in the test reagent.

Index

Page number followed by *b* indicates box; *f,* figure; *t,* table.